Praise for *Women, Ethics, and Inequality in U.S. Healthcare*

"Listening is an art. Hearing is an act of justice-making. Aana Marie Vigen does both as she opens up the world of Black women and Latinas fighting for their lives and their dignity when seeking treatment for breast cancer in a healthcare delivery system riddled with disparities from access to treatment. More than a study in medical ethics, this is a work of passionate concern that all of us count among the living."

—*Emilie M. Townes*, Andrew W. Mellon Professor of African American Religion and Theology, Yale University Divinity School

"Aana Marie Vigen has written an extraordinary book, bringing together the disciplines of medical sociology, ethnography, and theology. By careful analysis she displays the inequities in healthcare in the United States related to gender and class. By telling the stories of African American and Latina women living with cancer, she displays their courage and dignity. By attention to feminist and womanist theology—and to the theology of the women whose stories she tells—she displays the contributions of theology to the ethics of healthcare. I am humbled by this book, humbled by the strength of these women in the face of physical adversity and social injustice, humbled by their theological wisdom and virtue, and humbled by the author who grew both wise and passionate by attentively listening to them. All who hold privilege and power should listen as carefully to those who live at the margins of healthcare in this country. Anyone who is concerned about healthcare in this country should read this book, and anyone who is not concerned about healthcare in this country should have it assigned."

—*Allen Verhey*, Professor of Christian Ethics, Duke Divinity School, Duke University

"We have a consensus: healthcare is sick and broken. How to heal and fix it eludes us, however. A place to start is by listening to women of color who have cancer as if their voices really mattered. Aana Marie Vigen has. The results? Dispiriting, riveting, unsettling, inspiring. But most of all instructive: instructive for those giving healthcare, those receiving it, and those who worry over its indignities and injustice. How 'to count among the living' and how to begin to repair the breach is what Vigen rigorously engages—and offers."

—*Larry L. Rasmussen,* Reinhold Niebuhr Professor Emeritus of Social Ethics, Union Theological Seminary

"What really matters to Vigen is to understand health disparities not only as statistical differences in health outcomes, but as moral issues in the actual lives of poor women, especially poor Black and Latina women. And these vital issues turn on religious experience and understandings to such a degree that Vigen argues for a theological ethnography—a highly original method of studying the intersection of health and religion as lived experience. Vigen listens intensively to what her informants have to say about life, and through her we hear what poverty, illness, discrimination, and social injustice do to women, and how women respond through religious and moral practices.

Vigen practices an ethics of engaged advocacy and practical solidarity that itself is arresting and powerful."

—*Arthur Kleinman*, Esther and Sidney Rabb Professor of Anthropology, Chair, Department of Anthropology, Harvard University, Professor of Medical Anthropology, and Professor of Psychiatry, Harvard Medical School

"Beginning from the well-known realities of health-care discrimination against people 'of color,' Vigen shows how subtle and overt assumptions of white supremacy infect even the most well-intentioned care providers and theorists. This well-documented and innovative work creatively bridges 'mainstream' bioethics and womanist theology. Vigen provides a compelling and effective reeducation for white theologians who think we are already promoting healthcare justice."

—*Lisa Sowle Cahill*, Monan Professor of Theology, Boston College

"This book speaks to what we all know but seldom address: that healthcare in the United States is racially biased and that this bias works to our detriment both physically and spiritually. Vigen melds hard facts about racial inequalities in healthcare with easy to understand theological affirmations. She uses in-depth interviews to make the facts come alive. She does not shy away from strong critiques of both traditional and feminist views. Best of all, she offers solutions. It is heartening to know that even within an unjust system, individual actions can make a difference. It is helpful to hear from the stories of women with breast cancer what strengthened their resolve and what made them feel respected. This is a book for anyone who cares about justice in healthcare, about why spirituality matters, and about the future of race relations in America."

—*Karen Lebacqz*, Professor Emerita, Graduate Theological Union, Pacific School of Religion

"Aana Marie Vigen joins medical sociology, ethnography, and theology to provide not only a critical and incisive analysis of the political, economic, and societal forces that generate gross disparities in healthcare, but also opens a space for the voices of Latina and Black women who suffer from breast cancer. This work not only has implications for healthcare policy, it offers physicians, healthcare providers and healthcare system professionals an opportunity to rethink the quality of healthcare from the bottom up."

—*M. Shawn Copeland*, Associate Professor of Systematic Theology, Department of Theology, Boston College

"By adding the voices of Black and Latina women with breast cancer to ethics and policy discussions, Aana Vigen has enriched our understanding of the problem of health disparities in the U.S. The women's candid and revealing observations, as well as those of health care providers, provide often provocative, sometimes surprising, and always compelling insights into the way unfounded assumptions and past experiences enter the health care arena. The ethnographic narratives, framed by discussions of social ethics and theology, remind us of the value of listening attentively to the people who struggle not only with disease but also with inequities in health care."

—*Carol Levine*, Director of the Families and Health Care Project, United Hospital Fund

Women, Ethics, and Inequality in U.S. Healthcare

Black Religion / Womanist Thought / Social Justice
Series Editors Dwight N. Hopkins and Linda E. Thomas
Published by Palgrave Macmillan

"How Long this Road": Race, Religion, and the Legacy of C. Eric Lincoln
Edited by Alton B. Pollard, III and Love Henry Whelchel, Jr.

White Theology: Outing Supremacy in Modernity
By James W. Perkinson

The Myth of Ham in Nineteenth-Century American Christianity: Race, Heathens, and the People of God
By Sylvester Johnson

African American Humanist Principles: Living and Thinking Like the Children of Nimrod
By Anthony B. Pinn

Loving the Body: Black Religious Studies and the Erotic
Edited by Anthony B. Pinn and Dwight N. Hopkins

Transformative Pastoral Leadership in the Black Church
By Jeffery L. Tribble, Sr.

Shamanism, Racism, and Hip Hop Culture: Essays on White Supremacy and Black Subversion
By James W. Perkinson

Women, Ethics, and Inequality in U.S. Healthcare: "To Count Among the Living"
By Aana Marie Vigen

Black Theology in Transatlantic Dialogue: Inside Looking Out, Outside Looking In
By Anthony G. Reddie

African American Religious Life and the Story of Nimrod
Edited by Anthony B. Pinn and Allen Callahan
(forthcoming)

Womanist Ethics and the Cultural Production of Evil
Emilie M. Townes
(forthcoming)

Women, Ethics, and Inequality in U.S. Healthcare

"To Count Among the Living"

Aana Marie Vigen

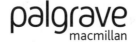
palgrave
macmillan

WOMEN, ETHICS, AND INEQUALITY IN U.S. HEALTHCARE
© Aana Marie Vigen, 2006.

First published in 2006 by
PALGRAVE MACMILLAN™
175 Fifth Avenue, New York, N.Y. 10010 and
Houndmills, Basingstoke, Hampshire, England RG21 6XS
Companies and representatives throughout the world.

PALGRAVE MACMILLAN is the global academic imprint of the Palgrave Macmillan division of St. Martin's Press, LLC and of Palgrave Macmillan Ltd. Macmillan® is a registered trademark in the United States, United Kingdom and other countries. Palgrave is a registered trademark in the European Union and other countries.

ISBN-13: 978–1–4039-7306–1
ISBN-10: 1–4039–7306–7

Library of Congress Cataloging-in-Publication Data

Vigen, Aana Marie.
    Women, ethics, and inequality in U.S. healthcare : "To count among the living"/Aana Marie Vigen.
        p. cm.—(Black religion, womanist thought, social justice)
        Rev. ed. of the author's Ph. D. thesis—Union Theological Seminary, New York, N.Y., 2004.
        Includes bibliographical references and index.
        ISBN 1–4039–7306–7
        1. African American women—Medical care. 2. Women's health services—United States. 3. Medical ethics. I. Title. II. Series.

RA564.86.V34 2006
362.1082—dc22   2006041561

A catalogue record for this book is available from the British Library.

Design by Newgen Imaging Systems (P) Ltd., Chennai, India.

First edition: September 2006

10 9 8 7 6 5 4 3 2 1

Printed in the United States of America.

With Gratitude and Love for
The Rev. Dr. Annie Ruth Powell
May 24, 1940–April 20, 2001

Contents

Series Editors' Preface   xi

Acknowledgments   xiv

Preface: A White Woman's Attempt to Listen   xvii

1. Introduction   1
   Statement of the Problem   1
   Method for Research   5
   Organization of the Chapters   10
   Health Status versus Healthcare Quality   11
   Conclusion   14

2. U.S. Healthcare 101: What Everyone
   Ought to Know about How U.S.
   Inhabitants are Treated (or Not)   17
   On the Outside Looking In: The Plight
     of the Uninsured   18
   The Overlapping Relationship between
     Access and Quality   28
   The Terrorizing Axis of (In)Access: A Story
     Three Headlines Tell When Told Together   29
   Beyond the Insurance Threshold: Additional Factors
     Contributing to Healthcare Inequalities   35
   The Bureaucracy of Healthcare Systems   50
   Implications of the Literature: Racial-Ethnic
     Disparities in Healthcare Quality Indict a Nation   57

3. A Call to the Particular: Contributions
   from Theology and Qualitative Research   63
   Introduction   63
   A Place and Role for Theological
     Anthropology   64

A Place and Role for Ethnography   84
Conclusion   109

4. Listening   111
    Eight Introductions   112
    Emergent Themes and Three Stories   126
    Additional Thematic Discussion   145
    Concluding Reflections: What I Did Not Hear   165

5. Resisting Death, Celebrating Life: Christian Social
    Ethics for Healthcare   171
    "God Has To Live in Each One of Us":
      Theo-Ethical Insights of Women with Cancer   172
    "I Didn't See [a] 'Doctor.' I Just Saw a Woman":
      Patient Expectations of Healthcare Providers   178
    "Keeping it Real" While Staying Out of the
      "Loony Bin": Social Ethics for
      Healthcare Systems   185
    Why These Stories Matter: Methodological
      Implications for the Doing of Ethics   200

Concluding Words for Beginning: (Re)Creating
the World through Scholarship   211

Appendices: The Recruitment Fliers   217

Notes   219

Index   259

Series Editors' Preface

Aana Marie Vigen deals with the thorny but everyday issues of dying, death, and dignity. Some U.S. Americans have privilege even amidst the human, vulnerable, and fragile state of serious illness while many, many of us have to battle not only the economics and pragmatics of survival and sickness, but our very existence as a human being comes under question. Yet Vigen's truth revealing and storytelling are a far cry from a postmortem on death. Rather, in this novel and well crafted book, she brings joy and insight on how to live ethically, even as we assert dignity while dying. She focuses on Black and Latina women with breast cancer as well as on the perspectives of healthcare providers. Through conversations with these women, we discover the spiritual resilience and upbeat viewpoint on life. Of course, these women do not naïvely succumb to a superficial innocence. The potential of answering death's knock on the door prevents such a sophomoric posture. In addition, their common sense wisdom gained from encounters with biased healthcare providers and a deleterious healthcare structure keeps these women sober. In a way, sobriety enhances the vibrancy of their outlooks and their hope in the face of morbidity.

Using ethnography, medical sociology, and theology to constitute the practice of Christian ethics, Vigen broadens the horizon of both (Christian) theology and (secular) healthcare discussions. She introduces the complexities of real people in the doing of theology. She offers healthcare talk metaphors of love of neighbor, child of God, and covenant. The hinge is Black and Brown women with breast cancer. These poor and working-class women have the right to human dignity in times of sickness and death. Professionals related to healthcare need to start their work by listening to and incorporating the voices and knowledge of marginalized communities. At root is the advancement of these women as human agents in their own lives and amidst the structural inequalities inherent in the U.S. health system.

Moreover, Vigen delves into cross-racial relations on several levels. How do those with privilege experience the revolutionary act of solidarity by listening to others without power and privilege? How does the socialization of being a white person in the United States work against the art of listening in solidarity? Undoing racialized existence requires a radical and loving change in ways of living. Vigen offers one powerful model from her research and personal experience with women of color in the healthcare system. One intriguing way out is Vigen's notion of double consciousness for white people. Playing on the poetics of W.E.B. DuBois' Black American double consciousness, Vigen calls on white citizens to do their own work, doubly so. They must remain present and listening in the conversations with people of color. And simultaneously they need to sincerely and critically step back to observe the larger racial factors present. The latter move ensures that whites can "check themselves."

Actually Vigen models a healthy way for us all to check ourselves. Her project fosters the craft of how the privileged can listen, leads to the practice of healthy interracial coalitions, and challenges public policy to redo the U.S. healthcare system. In this book, healthcare matters for all of us; for surely one leveling ground is the eventuality of death. Vigen presents to us again the role of women of color as they wed religion, Womanist thought, and social justice.

Aana Marie Vigen's book represents one definite dimension of the Black Religion/Womanist Thought/Social Justice Series—pioneering conceptual work and boundary-pushing effort. The series will publish both authored and edited manuscripts that have depth, breadth, and theoretical edge and will address both academic and nonspecialist audiences. It will produce works engaging any dimension of Black religion or Womanist thought as they pertain to social justice. Womanist thought is a new approach in the study of African American women's perspectives. The series will include a variety of African American religious expressions. By this we mean traditions such as Protestant and Catholic Christianity, Islam, Judaism, Humanism, African diasporic practices, religion and gender, religion and Black gays/lesbians, ecological justice issues, African American religiosity and its relation to African religions, new Black religious movements (e.g., Daddy Grace, Father Divine, or the Nation of Islam), or religious dimensions in African American "secular" experiences (such as the spiritual aspects of aesthetic efforts like the Harlem Renaissance and literary giants such as James Baldwin, or the religious fervor of the Black Consciousness movement, or the religion of compassion in the Black women's club movement).

Dwight N. Hopkins, University of Chicago Divinity School
Linda E. Thomas, Lutheran School of Theology at Chicago

Acknowledgments

No book is ever truly written alone, and in my case, seven distinct communities contributed various kinds of needed assistance. First, several organizations and individuals helped lay the groundwork needed in order to conduct ethnographic interviews. I am grateful to the Division of Medical Ethics of the Weill Medical College of Cornell University for our affiliation. Joseph J. Fins, MD, Cathleen Acres RN, MA, and the Reverend Curtis W. Hart helped me to bridge the worlds between healthcare and social/theological ethics. Dr. Linda Barnes offered helpful feedback, which facilitated the Institutional Review Board (IRB) approval process. In addition, the staff of New York area cancer support networks—Carmen Morales at Gilda's Club, Deborah Bristol at Kings County Hospital Center in Brooklyn, Ivis Febus-Sampayo at SHARE, and Yulinda Lewis-Kelly at The Witness Project of Harlem—were invaluable in helping me meet women with breast cancer.

A second community includes those who generously gave their time and practical expertise. Elaine Farris was an exceptional transcriber of the interview recordings. Kathryn Schifferdecker, Hella Von Unger, Robin Strickler, and Christine Sinnott all read portions of the manuscript with sharp eyes. My graduate assistant at Loyola University Chicago, David Creech, has been a blessing by taking on various (and often tedious) tasks that accompany publication. The text flows better and has far fewer typos because of these individuals. Any mistakes that remain are mine.

In addition, several colleagues have been faithful dialogue partners over the course of the evolution of this work. Kathryn Schifferdecker responded to my ruminations with both acuity and compassion. Christian Albert Batalden Scharen never fails to raise important questions, push edges, and offer constructive suggestions. A Qualitative Methods Writing group (Lourdes Hernandez, Hella Von Hunger,

Craig Fryer, and Kevin Robinson) helped me navigate the territories of qualitative fieldwork and the IRB process. Jennifer Harvey helped me to focus and to know what I needed to do (and what I did not) in order to bring the work to fruition. The insight of emilie m. townes contributed significantly to the scope and argument of several key sections. Mindy Fullilove not only welcomed this stranger to the aforementioned writing group, but also offered attentive feedback and counsel to myriad questions as they arose. Finally, for me, Larry L. Rasmussen will always set the standard of excellence for living out the vocations of teacher and colleague. There are no words to acknowledge fully all he has given to me in his years first as professor and advisor and now as colleague and friend.

Moreover, key individuals directly facilitated the publication of this work. It has been a pleasure to work with the Series Editors, Dwight Hopkins and Linda Thomas. They saw the value in this work from the beginning and urged it forward with prompt, constructive attention and grace. I am exceedingly grateful to them for their expert shepherding of this process. Amanda Johnson has been a responsive, highly competent, and friendly Editor at Palgrave Macmillan. She has consistently offered efficient and knowledgeable assistance at every juncture. My sincere thanks also go to Emily Leithauser and others at Palgrave for their able technical assistance.

The community of Loyola University Chicago also deserves a word of mention. I am deeply grateful to Loyola for both financial and moral support. I was granted a Summer Stipend in 2005 by the College of Arts and Sciences so that I could complete manuscript revisions and the Office of Research Services made funds available for a professional indexer. Moreover, I continually give thanks for tremendous colleagues at Loyola, especially (but not exclusively) those who inhabit the halls of the Department of Theology—staff, students, and educators. Because of their hard work, thought-provoking questions, able assistance, and genuine collegiality, I am reminded daily how fortunate I am to live out my vocation here on the western shores of Lake Michigan.

In a different vein, I owe much to my family and friends for many years of care and encouragement. In particular, Edward and Bertha Voss, Kathryn Voss Vigen and David Clifford Vigen, Amy and Michael Hemstad, Eric E. Vigen and Alison Anne Strickler have all been sources of constant love and faith. My niece and nephews, Sarah, Sean, and Christopher, bring much joy to my life and remind me why the hard work of ethics is worth the effort.

Finally, the most integral community to whom I am both profoundly grateful and accountable is comprised of the collaborators who were gracious and daring enough to speak with me. Without these 14 people, there would be no book. They gave me an incredible gift. None received compensation for their time or the sharing of their knowledge. The women who have faced or are facing breast cancer will not concretely benefit in their lives from this research. I owe a debt I cannot ever repay. Given this fact, I will try to make a difference in how discussions of adequate medical care, dignity, and respect are framed within the education of future generations of scientists, caregivers, theologians, and ethicists.

In a sense, I am an unusual scholar. I don't adore libraries; I would rather be out on the street or in a room with people. The gift of doing interdisciplinary scholarship in the work of ethics and of collaborating with a diverse body of people is this: The research has enabled me to understand that I am the kind of scholar who is as invested in people and in the transformation of society as much as in any publication. To these various communities who have not only helped bring this work to publication, but who have helped me identify this particular aim of scholarship, I owe a lot—including much of the mooring that anchors both my vocational identity and my hope for this broken but amazing world.

Preface: A White Woman's Attempt to Listen

There are many—ever multiplying and mutating—ways to discriminate against people. Environmental racism, unequal educational and unemployment opportunities, problematic stereotypes in mainstream media, and racial profiling are but a few. Embedded within all forms of discrimination is dehumanization. In order to justify to others (or rationalize to oneself) any kind of prejudicial treatment or aggression against a person or people, one always has to call into question (overtly or not) the humanity of the other. Only when a person or group can be perceived—even if on a subtle or unconscious level—as somehow less than fully human, is it possible to justify discriminatory practices.

While many troubling and systemic inequalities merit scholarly investigation, the topic explored in this book deserves close attention because it affects people when they are acutely vulnerable; namely, when they are seriously ill. Perhaps most critically ill persons seeking care in the United States experience some form of alienation during the course of their treatment.[1] Womanist[2] ethicist emilie m. townes observes, "As healthcare has become a big business, our lives have become far too much like commodities."[3] townes later observes that this objectification occurs not only because of profit motives, but also because of the predominant mindset of western[4] medicine that reduces human beings to individual body parts, divides the body from the mind, and narrowly defines health as the absence of disease.[5]

Yet, some persons seem to be more vulnerable to objectification than others due to the particularities of their socioeconomic, racial, and cultural backgrounds. Indeed, it is crucial that we lighter skinned people understand that darker skinned people are more susceptible to such commodification than we are due to structural inequalities within U.S. healthcare.[6] The prospect that significant populations of patients may not fully trust their healthcare providers, or that some providers may treat patients in moments of acute vulnerability (even if unintentionally) as somehow less than fully human, presents challenging theological and ethical issues for both religious and medical communities.

I am drawn to healthcare disparities because this issue touches upon one undeniable aspect of our common humanity: Mortality.[7] As human creatures, we must ask ourselves (as individuals and as a society), What kind of care do all human beings deserve in the moments we face the possibility or certainty of death? Some die in relative comfort; others are tortured before death, and still others are slowly brutalized over the course of their lives. Some are held by loved ones; others are alone or abandoned. Some die because their bodies have reached their limits; others have their lifeblood violently stolen from them well before their time. Those who die well—without pain, with love, support, and care, who are at peace with others, their lives, and the world—are intrinsically related to those who die in dehumanizing situations. And as a society, we are accountable to those who do not die well and to those who face the possibility of death without adequate support and care.

The specific route by which I came to this topic also deserves a brief word. The decision did not come about solely from intellectual reflection. Instead, three poignant experiences laid the groundwork for later intellectual thought. First, I accompanied my sister during the stillbirth of her first child. Apart from the tremendous grief and naïve surprise that a baby could be lost in an advanced U.S. hospital, I was deeply moved by the fact that my sister—an articulate, white, relatively privileged RN—felt a need for an advocate while a patient. Second, I participated in a nine-month chaplaincy internship at a hospital in northern California that served as the county's emergency trauma center. There I met many Latino patients and families who felt ignored and/or distrusted by the hospital. Moreover, many did not fully understand what was happening to or around them.[8] Finally, one of the most personally transformative experiences was witnessing the life and struggle of the Reverend Dr. Annie Ruth Powell as she faced her fourth diagnosis of cancer during the spring of 2001. She was an African American pastor and theologian who continually reasserted her agency and dignity in relating to healthcare providers and in making treatment decisions. Our friendship began when I started to work with her as her administrative assistant at Union Theological Seminary in New York. We became close over the course of her illness and I became an integral part of her support network.

At its most fundamental level, this book is about finding and giving voice. Specifically, it embodies both the effort to articulate my own voice and perspective regarding matters of healthcare quality and to listen intently to the wisdom and experiences of Black and Latina[9] women who have faced or are facing breast cancer. In one sense, it is simply an attempt at faithful storytelling for the sake of fostering moral imagination within U.S. healthcare provision.

And if I am going to tell others' stories and critique the care others provide, it seems appropriate to reveal one of my own in which my efforts to listen and to give care fell short of what was needed. This story represents one of the key moments in which the questions of this book started to brew within me.[10] And while I am not proud of it, I recognize that it is not unique to my individual experience or way of being. In a sense, it symbolizes a common failure of well-intentioned white people to see and hear fully communities of color. So I offer it up both as an effort at self-reflexivity and because it illustrates the some-times subtle—but nonetheless serious—missteps that hobble white attempts to listen.

My supervisor, who had become my friend, was having a difficult day. I did not realize how difficult. I called her to discuss when people would be coming to cook or to sit with her. Mine were among the few calls the Reverend Dr. Powell would take. She was gravely ill with cancer that had metastasized to her liver. The Reverend Dr. Powell was the Seminary Pastor and an Assistant Professor of Practical Theology; I was her administrative assistant. As her condition worsened, I served as a liaison for the seminary community she served and coordinated much of her home care and appointments.

On this particular March day, I wanted to talk about scheduling and the Reverend Dr. Powell wanted to breathe. I was frustrated by a number of schedule changes that I had not been made aware of and by not being able to tell how much assistance she wanted. I felt I had been getting mixed messages from her—alternating between not wanting to be alone and not wanting people around all the time. And, "I was try-ing to help her.". . . So, I kept asking questions, even as she kept trying to tell me that she could not focus on them at that moment.

Later that day, I went to see her and we sat on her bed. I apologized if my call had been an intrusion. In my mind, though, I still felt a bit defensive and indignant—telling myself that my intentions had been good, that I had her best interests at heart and that I was doing a "darn fine job" coordinating things. Somewhere deep inside me, I presumed to know best. The Reverend Dr. Powell looked me in the eye and spoke the truth in love: My priorities were not hers in that moment; I needed to listen to her; she needed to conserve her energy. When I asked her to turn her attention to the immediate things going on around her, that drained her. I learned that I needed to attune my ears so that I could make appropriate adjustments as best I could. Even more, I learned that although she counted on me, she was not asking me to figure it all out, to run the show or to take care of everything. She was asking me to listen and to be present.

This bit of my history illuminates a pernicious problem I have experienced in myself and in other white folk, even those seeking to work with darker skinned communities and to be informed by them: White people often do not listen—not fully—even when we think we are listening; yet, we can be so quick to speak. One might counter that this story has nothing to do with racial dynamics, but rather speaks more universally about how caregivers need to listen to those in their care. On one level, this retort is true. The critically ill and dying in the United States—across racial, socioeconomic, and cultural lines—often have difficulty getting their care providers to listen to them. On another level, however, presumptions and differing priorities have everything to do with differences in racial, socioeconomic, and cultural backgrounds. And these differences directly impinge upon dialogue and quality of care, even if they reside underneath the surface of what is being said.

I lament that my presumption to "know best" got in the way of hearing and responding to the Reverend Dr. Powell. While I cannot draw definitive conclusions regarding the origin of this presumption, it is important to note three possibilities. First, this presumption may stem from the fact that my personality (one, it is safe to say, often found among those in theology, ethics and/or ministry) is one inclined toward the care-taking of others. Thus, it may be true that regardless of the racial-ethnic background of the Reverend Dr. Powell, I may have done the very same thing—overstepped bounds in the desire to "fix, take care of, help." A second possibility is that my internal self-perception (even if not fully conscious) as "efficient, clear-headed, well organized, knowing best" has something to do with being socialized as a white person in this society.[11] Third, the combination of a general care-taking personality and white socialization having enculturated me with the sense that "I am right" may have been at work.

Regardless of its origin or my intentions, the flawed presumption that "I know best" deprived me both of awareness of the Reverend Dr. Powell's active decision-making skills *as well as* awareness of my

own emotions and inner chaos stemming from the reality that someone whom I loved deeply was very ill. I did not fully honor what was
going on within her *or* myself. Instead, focusing on "knowing best and
taking care of her" cost me my ability to be present to my own emotions as I identified only with the rational, problem-solving part of my
being.

Even more important to acknowledge, my personal presumption to
"know best" directly relates to a larger, collective history. For over
200 years in the United States, Black people were associated *only* with
their bodies—for the sake of white needs—for labor, for sex, to feel
psychologically superior to another, or for financial gain. To the white
mind and gaze, Black and Indigenous peoples were not ends in themselves nor considered fully human. They were tools employed in the
realization of white ends/desires. They were not presumed to have—
nor were they granted—the same human rights to dignity, respect, or
freedom. Furthermore, whites, especially men, claimed the domain of
rationality, civility, intellect, and even, humanity.[12]

This history continues to breathe in the present. Thus even if I do
not consciously hold such violent beliefs, I need to be aware of *how
the legacy of this history lives in contemporary relationships and contexts.* This legacy means white persons inherently bear responsibility
for making sure we do not replicate or participate in replicating a false
and destructive dichotomy that in any way (linguistically, symboli-
cally, relationally) denies or subverts the moral agency and intellect
intrinsic to people of color.

Ultimately, whether or not my care-taking and presumption
reflected my individual personality or are linked directly to white
socialization and identity (or both) matters very little. Regardless of
my intentions, my actions and attitude had certain effects due to the
knowable and concrete history that stands between lighter and darker
skinned peoples. This history continually infuses relational dynamics
with specific meanings in the present. I may be by nature a confident,
capable caretaker. But while paternalism is never helpful, it is imperative I understand that it can have particular ramifications across racial
lines. Part of responsible white listening and moral agency is being
attuned to this fact.[13]

The notion of a "double consciousness" is something people of
color live with in order to survive in a white supremacist society.[14] One
interpretation of this concept is that folks of color need to understand
the white way of seeing the world and the folks of color within it as
well as to cultivate ways of seeing themselves that are not dependent

upon or infected by white consciousness. In other words, communities of color need to understand—in order to survive—a white system that disparages "coloredness" as well as to understand themselves as inherently beautiful, precious, gifted persons and communities whose worth and identity are not at all what the white gaze sees.

White persons also need a double consciousness, but of a different kind and for different reasons. White people need to cultivate the skill to be fully present in interactions and work with people of color, while also being able to step back from the immediate dialogue and events in order to be cognizant of the larger picture and to check ourselves. Part of being responsible requires self-reflection both on how one may be perceived in a present context and on the actual effects of one's actions and decisions given the histories of the peoples involved and history's import for the current relationship, exchange or project.

Subtle but toxic presumptions that carry cultural and racial freight can be operative—even in a relationship where there is also genuine, mutual love and respect. Such presumptions may drive a wedge that obstructs communication and right relationship. The Reverend Dr. Powell and I worked hard to keep things honest between us because the relationship mattered a great deal to each of us. So rather than give up on me and distance herself, she held me accountable. Imagine for a moment how much racial and/or cultural stereotypes and presumptions might interfere between people who do not know or trust each other well.

Simply put, white people are accountable for the ways in which we fail to hear and understand the needs and claims that other communities make upon us. The tragedy is that in so many cases, as was true in mine, white learning comes at the expense of those already multiply harmed by white interpersonal and structural failures in perception, sensitivity, and justice. I regret that in the midst of contending with cancer, the Reverend Dr. Powell had to contend with my presumption as well. My learning came at a cost to her well-being during an acutely difficult time in her life.

Reflection on my own missed opportunities and mistakes has led me to want to do better. To paraphrase Nell Morton, if we cannot "hear one another into speech,"[15] our efforts at coalition-building will be continually and tragically undercut. Real differences must be intentionally respected in the midst of seeking solidarity.

Even as this book is finished, I continue to contemplate what has to be in place before coalition-building is possible (or even seen as worthwhile by people of color). One thing I know is that, fundamentally, racism is a white issue, just as homophobia is a heterosexual issue and poverty makes a claim upon the wealthy. White folk must "deal with our own stuff" and become more adept at recognizing racism than we usually are. This keen eyesight and insight will in turn make the quality of our hearing, cross-cultural discussions, and coalitions much richer and more productive than prior efforts.

Much of this book's argument could be summarized by one word: Humility. There may never have been a time when we (especially white scholars, but other white people as well) could less afford to separate our intellectual work from our daily practices and commitments. Engagement in messy dialogues, ethnography, or conversations in a second language will likely make white folk, especially "scholars," awkward and somewhat bumbling. But there is great learning to be had from such experiences. They may teach us what it is to be not the standard of humanity, but instead to be simply human.

1

Introduction

We must learn to count the living with that same particular attention with which we number the dead.

—Audre Lorde

Statement of the Problem

Black feminist essayist and poet, Audre Lorde, wrote the above words early in her battle with breast cancer.[1] She understood that honoring human life involves more than the tallying of statistics. Everyone counts, not simply in the sense of arriving at an accurate numerical total, but rather in the sense that everyone *matters*. Each of us, as a unique, precious human person, deserves to receive the particular attention that is owed to all human beings.

Healthcare access, commonly viewed through the lens of health insurance status, is a powerful and pervasive source of healthcare disparities. And it is not an insignificant fact that those without insurance are disproportionately people of color. However, access by itself is not an adequate lens through which to view disparities in the quality of care. Undeniably, healthcare access and quality issues are inextricably bound up with one another. Still, justice-oriented questions of race, gender, socioeconomics, and culture have not been adequately brought to bear upon U.S. healthcare systems in relation to healthcare quality.

Substantive research in medical sociology documents that even with comparable insurance and income, darker skinned communities receive a lower quality of care than their lighter skinned counterparts. In 2003, the Institute of Medicine (IOM) published a review of well over 100 such studies, covering a variety of medical issues—cardiac care, kidney transplants, mental health, pain management, and others—in various regions and care contexts, which showed clear evidence of such disparities. The IOM also cited research that indicates that racial bias and stereotypes are operative in healthcare providers that, along with a lack of culturally competent care and translation services, contribute to quality of care disparities.[2]

In 2003, the Henry J. Kaiser Family Foundation published a succinct summary of racial-ethnic health and healthcare disparities.[3] To illustrate some of its content, the report summarizes current data, which show the following:

1. Racial-ethnic minorities tend to report being in poorer health than non-Hispanic whites.
2. Racial-ethnic minorities tend to be more likely to have no usual source of healthcare and to go without healthcare visits than non-Hispanic whites. For example, Latinos, African American, and American Indian/Alaska Natives are at least "twice as likely than whites and Asian/Pacific Islanders to receive late or no prenatal care."
3. African Americans, across income brackets, have an infant mortality rate that is at least twice that of non-Hispanic whites.
4. There are significant disparities in various sectors of specialty care. For example, there are racial-ethnic disparities in procedures to diagnosis and treat heart disease,[4] in some forms of cancer screenings and treatments, and in the use of pain medication for pain management. Racial-ethnic disparities also exist in the treatment of asthma and HIV-AIDS.

In a related vein, the former U.S. Surgeon General, David Satcher, reviewed mortality rates between 1960 and 2000. In a special 2005 issue of *Health Affairs*, he concluded that "[m]ore than 80,000 black Americans die every year because of continuing disparities in health care. . . ."[5] Similarly, David Williams, a sociologist, also reported in this issue that "blacks had 30 percent higher death rates from cancer and heart disease than whites did in 2000. In 1950, blacks and whites were equally likely to die from heart disease and blacks had lower death rates from cancer."[6] Not everyone's health is improving (at least not to the same extent) despite the astounding technological advances in medicine in the twentieth century.

One additional area of healthcare merits a word: Mental health. This area definitely needs more research, but there are indications of significant racial-ethnic inequalities. For example, a survey published in 2005 of one of the largest psychiatric databases in the United States found that Blacks and Latinos are significantly more likely to be diagnosed with schizophrenia than non-Hispanic whites. The researchers analyzed 134,523 mentally ill patients in a Veterans' Administration registry. A *Washington Post* article reporting on the study explains, "Although schizophrenia has been shown to affect all ethnic groups at the same rate, [John Zeber] found that blacks in the United States were more than four times as likely to be diagnosed with the disorder than whites. Hispanics were more than three times as likely to be diagnosed as whites."[7] The article went on to explain that these results could not be accounted for by differences in wealth, drug addiction, or other variables.

Moreover, unlike other diseases (cancer, heart disease, AIDS) that are diagnosed with blood tests, brain scans, biopsies, et cetera, the subjective impressions of doctors largely influence whether a patient is deemed as mentally ill or not. One psychiatrist, Francis Lu, acknowledged the following: " 'Bias is a very real issue. . . . We don't talk about it—it's upsetting. We see ourselves as unbiased and rational and scientific.' "[8] Another psychiatrist, Michael Smith added, " 'Because we have no lab test, the only way we can test if someone is psychotic is, we use ourselves as the measure. . . . If it sounds unusual to us, we call it psychotic.' "[9] Indeed, racial assumptions and stereotypes can act as a powerful filter through which patients and their symptoms are interpreted. And in mental health cases, the opinion of the doctor carries a lot of weight in determining care plans, medications, whether someone is restrained or institutionalized and for how long, et cetera. The significance of provider bias and power dynamics will be explored in depth in subsequent chapters.

In 2005, the Applied Research Center and the Northwest Federation of Community Organizations jointly published a report that features a combination of a literature review and original research that documents the multilayered range of racial-ethnic health and healthcare disparities.[10] Specifically, the report explores two fundamental but distinct causes of racial-ethnic inequalities in current healthcare contexts: Structural/institutional racism and interpersonal racism. In addition, the report identifies the roots of these disparities and assesses the strengths of concrete programs and policies in place across the United States that were designed to ameliorate them.

This research should not surprise us. Healthcare environs and persons mirror the larger society in which they are situated. While significant advances have been made with regard to the legal prohibition of discrimination, in other arenas of U.S. society not as much has changed. For example, Lawrence Bobo recently reviewed sociological literature that shows that while white people voice positive attitudes toward integration in schools and neighborhoods, their comfort levels with actual integration diminishes the more integrated they become. "[M]ost Whites prefer to live in overwhelmingly White neighborhoods even though they are open to living with a small number of Blacks."[11] Similarly, white people are very divided regarding affirmative action policies even though they more strongly affirm equality in principle than in any other era of U.S. history. Bobo also notes that negative racial stereotyping pervades society, as seen for example in white fear of a Black stranger.[12] Surveying this conflicted reality, Bobo concludes,

> The death of Jim Crow racism has left us in . . . a state of laissez-faire racism. We have high ideals, but cannot agree on the depth of the remaining problem—we are open to integration, but in very limited terms and only in specific areas. There is political stagnation over some types of affirmative action, and persistent negative stereotyping of racial minorities; and a wide gulf in perceptions regarding the importance of racial discrimination remains.[13]

There is much difference of opinion in U.S. society regarding what integration, equality, and respect mean in actual relations and structures. These differences mean that not all U.S. inhabitants see current manifestations of racism and inequality in the same way, if at all.

With respect to healthcare disparities, for example, one recent study found a "growing proportion of Americans—from 43% in 1993 to 57% in 1999—who believe that [the] uninsured . . . are able to get the care they need from physicians and hospitals."[14] This belief may be common, but it is not accurate. Moreover, it illustrates the fact that when some communities (e.g., white, affluent, presently insured) distance themselves from confronting the struggles with which others routinely contend, the acuity of their moral vision suffers dramatically.

Given the breadth of existing documentation regarding racial-ethnic and socioeconomic healthcare quality disparities, this book does not have to prove they exist. Instead, it is able to make a different, but related case and to ask three distinct questions. Its focal argument is two-pronged: First, there is a theologically grounded claim to human dignity that patients, especially patients of color and of the lower socioeconomic classes, often do not have honored due to structural elements within U.S. healthcare. Second, ethicists, sociologists, chaplains, healthcare providers, and theologians only arrive at an adequate sense of respect and quality healthcare when we take seriously the experiences and voices of those most marginalized by structural inequalities.

Three questions guide this exploration: (1) At times of serious illness, what contributes to a sense of being well cared for and respected as a full human being? (2) Conversely, what dynamics and structural elements frustrate such care and respect? (3) What might the concept of human dignity, when bound up with a particular theological and social ethic, add to the care-giving imagination within U.S. society? With these convictions and questions in place, I prepared to listen to a few Black and Latina women with breast cancer.

Method for Research

This book brings together work from three distinct disciplines—medical sociology, ethnography, and theology—in the doing of Christian social ethics. While it articulates implications for healthcare policy, it is not grounded in this discipline. Instead, it stands a bit off to the side, looking in with the particular lens of social and theological ethics committed to liberationist endeavors.

It is also an attempt to begin a conversation among several distinct dialogue partners: Medical sociology, biomedical ethics, ethnography, theology, and feminist social ethics. Each makes a particular contribution to discussions of healthcare quality. This effort to bring these disciplines and perspectives into conversation with one another proposes a different method for how U.S. healthcare ought to be explored. Trying to start such a conversation is a significant endeavor in and of itself. For example, the use of ethnography is fairly novel to theology and the incorporation of social and theo-ethical claims is foreign to some streams within bioethics.

However, this book takes an additional step beyond interdisciplinary dialogue and description. It represents an attempt at normative social science and theology, meaning that both are done with the aim of positive social change.[15] Specifically, I hope this work will offer constructive possibilities and imagination for how U.S. healthcare might be (re)formed and (re)structured so that just and right relationships may flourish more widely than they do now.

A Word about Qualitative Research Methodology

By some standards, this research is already on the wrong foot. According to some understandings of the role of objectivity and neutrality in research, this project is woefully biased—riddled with subjective assumptions and aims. Substantive attention is given to such methodological questions in the second half of chapter 3. Here I will only respond briefly to this concern.

Unlike quantitative studies, qualitative investigations tend to focus upon the stories and perspectives of relatively small numbers of people. I intentionally limited the scope of this study as a way to illumine larger, structural patterns and issues present in a few concrete lives and that also extend beyond them. The purpose of the ethnographic fieldwork has been to learn from the experiences of a few particular people who have direct knowledge of healthcare systems, and especially from those who may have likely experienced healthcare inequalities. My hope is that by offering ethnography as a needed starting point for medical sociology, social ethics, and theology, the epistemological methods of each discipline will be reshaped in compelling and helpful ways.

The two primary learning objectives for the ethnographic fieldwork were as follows: (1) To learn what it means for members of vulnerable communities[16] to be treated as full human beings when critically ill; and (2) To hear why such respect is frustrated, according to patient and provider perceptions. To these ends, I conducted open-ended interviews with eight Black and Latina women with breast cancer and with six healthcare providers. In most cases, the Latina and Black women were members of local cancer support networks.[17] I paid attention to differences in socioeconomic class, ethnic/cultural backgrounds, and religious traditions among participants. I interviewed healthcare providers in order to understand how they feel fulfilled and/or frustrated by their work and by systemic healthcare realities.

The scope of the qualitative field research is relatively small. Future studies will be enriched by speaking with more people. For example, I am interested in dedicating one study to interviewing individuals from non-Christian faith backgrounds and another to interviewing healthcare providers in greater depth. However, even though the number of participants is limited, their stories are no less significant or valid. The point is that every story, every person, matters. And indeed, their insights have proven rather illuminative as is evident in chapters 4 and 5.

Throughout the fieldwork, I utilized a reflexive mode of study that emphasizes the dialogical relationship between the participants and myself. Such engagement means that I am critically aware of my own social location as well as my responses to the stories I hear from the research participants. It also means that I pay close attention to what participants say that either surprises me or disconfirms any assumptions that I have brought to the interviews. As part of holding myself accountable to all the participants, I followed up with them after the interviews and made transcripts and chapters available to them.

A Word about Theology within Healthcare Ethics

How might healthcare quality discussions benefit from the presence of theology? This explanation may take longer to give. Some may find that given our pluralistic and religiously diverse society, it is unwise to draw upon Christian theology as a source for ethical norms. Many ethicists address various topics within biomedicine and healthcare[18] without incorporating theological concerns or language. For example, John Evans traces the way in which explicit theological claims have become increasingly removed from genetic engineering debates.[19]

Theological values are often translated into the secular, virtue-oriented language of principlism, which focuses upon the principles of autonomy, nonmaleficence, beneficence, and justice.[20] White theological and medical ethicist Allen Verhey has also observed this secularization of bioethics. He explains that this move has "insisted that moral principles not be dependent upon any particular community or history. Moral principles had to be universal, compelling quite apart from any specific loyalty or identity, and that they had to be impartial, unbiased by any particular narrative that a community remembers or by any vision for human flourishing for which a particular community hopes."[21] I concur with Verhey that these four concepts in principlism along with dignity and respect may be enriched if they are understood as intrinsically social and theo-ethical matters. Undeniably, appeals to generic, secular principles across religions or cultures serve definite purposes in a pluralistic, democratic society. Yet something rich may be lost when the wisdom of particular peoples and traditions is rendered categorically obsolete or inappropriate.

Verhey also notes that as technological and scientific advances have moved forward in rapid succession (e.g., organ transplants and other lifesaving technologies), they have led to new questions that have been taken up more and more by scientists. However, he highlights the fact that while these questions are novel in one way, they also lead to very old "questions about life and its sanctity, questions about death and its dignity (or indignity), questions about human suffering and the appropriate response to it. . . ."[22] In other words, even as science advances, we as a society do not ever advance beyond the basic questions of what it means to live fully and in right relation with others. Such questions need ongoing exploration and reevaluation. And theology offers a language that is uniquely helpful to pondering these kinds of questions.

On a fundamental level, theology expands the conceptual framework for healthcare ethics and discussions. White Roman Catholic feminist ethicist Lisa Cahill argues that

> [t]he relevance of religion to bioethics does not lie primarily in any distinct or specific contribution to the process of moral argumentation, nor in lifting up "religious" behaviors, defensible only on faith, revelation, or church authority. Rather, it depends on the formation of socially radical communities that challenge dominant values and patterns of social relationship, not by withdrawing from the larger society, or by speaking to it from outside, but by participating in it in challenging and even subversive ways.[23]

Cahill and white feminist ethicists (e.g., Karen Lebacqz and Margaret Farley) along with Womanist ethicist emilie townes all understand that at their best, theology and theological ethics may help to critique the aspects of western biomedicine that objectify, commodify, and medicalize health and human persons.[24] townes sees that

> [h]ealth is not simply the absence of disease—it comprises a wide range of activities that foster healing and wholeness. . . . [It] is a cultural production in that health and illness alike are social constructs and dependent on social networks, biology, and environment. As it is embedded in our social realities, health also includes the integration of the spiritual (how we relate to God), the mental (who we are as thinking and feeling people), and the physical (who we are biologically) aspects of our lives.[25]

What might shift in our social structures, public policy, and medical arenas, I wonder, if we were to take more seriously than we often do as a society this understanding that an adequate account of health takes into consideration individual and collective social, psychological, and spiritual contexts?

With respect to healthcare quality issues and discussions, theology may very well add distinctive and useful metaphors. For example, I would like to see healthcare forums ponder together what notions such as covenant, child of God, and love of neighbor might add. We may enrich our collective understandings of dignity, dying well, respect, and justice if we incorporate, or at least entertain, such theological and moral visions. Perhaps secular philosophical language is not the only one needed. Clearly, such discussions and language would need to include various and diverse religious traditions both within and outside Christianity. Theology is not understood here to be the sole property of Christians.

In short, I am not content with a minimalist notion of justice that emphasizes giving each individual her or his due. Instead, as a white Christian social ethicist, I contend that justice means loving rightly—seeing and regarding one another rightly. For me (standing within a wide tradition of various liberation theologies and ethics), love necessarily involves justice. Love as an expression of justice means actively working for the care and healing of all God's creation—every bit of it. Nothing and no one is expendable; no person can be spared or discarded. In the language of the New Testament, each lost coin, each meandering sheep, each child—must be found and brought home.

This is just one example of the kind of language and imagination theology might bring to healthcare. Is it everyone's language? Surely not. Yet if it offers its provocative imagination without attempting to dominate the discourse, it might enlarge and enliven discussions focused upon giving all patients—of every race, culture, creed, socio-economic status, and ethnicity—the highest quality of care humanly possible. Without "baptizing" any sector of the public square, theological insights may nonetheless have an appropriate and constructive place in public policy discussions and deliberations. Specifically, this may happen when explicit theo-ethical voices—who engage their own traditions, scriptures, and communities of religious and moral memory—advocate for the equal care and regard of all persons, regardless of socioeconomic class, race, gender, or religious affiliation.

At their best, theology and ethics (like good public policy) are collaborative ventures. We need the wisdom of everyone—healthcare policy analysts, doctors, nurses, the sick, those who know poverty, those who have stared down the ugly face of racism, immigrants, the religious, and the secular. All are invited to come together in order to carve out an understanding of what it means to be human and to treat one another humanely. And it is together—by drawing upon various sacred scriptures, faith traditions, secular laws and virtues, emotional and embodied knowledge, articulations of principles and values, the natural and social sciences, the range of human experience and stories, and human intellectual capacities—that we can imagine and create at least a degree of love and right relationship. Such labor is an expression of God's incarnation and reign—embodied presence in and among us, even if imperfect and fleeting.

Finally, there is one connection that people of different faiths share with each other and with those who do not profess any faith at all: All persons and communities must discern their values, priorities, what they will love, and for what they will strive. In German theologian

Paul Tillich's language, a person or community's "ultimate concern" will shape in important ways concrete choices for living.[26] What ultimately matters to us, as persons or a people, what we see as worth dying for—*living for*—fundamentally shapes our societies and moral choices. Do we love something finite (e.g., wealth, power, status, health, material possessions, youth) as the ultimate goal for which we strive? People do not have to be Christian, or even religious, to benefit from exploring such conceptual terrain already well mapped by theology. Indeed, theology offers a unique gift that can help human beings to search and question our hearts and conscience—as persons and as a society—as we attempt to craft policies and legislation that will profoundly affect the lives of significant numbers and groupings of people.

Organization of the Chapters

The heart of this book is found in the ethnographic research. It seeks to explore the epistemological shift that occurs when dialogue with actual persons becomes a fundamental starting place for theological and ethical reflection. However, the ethnography does not stand by itself. Instead, it is triangulated by quantitative medical sociological literature and by feminist social and theological ethics. I invite readers to peruse the endnotes because they contain a lot of interesting details and illustrations on related topics. For example, the endnotes for chapters 4 and 5 include many additional comments from the interviews that flesh out even more facets of the participants' perspectives and experiences.

Chapter 2 situates the central argument and focal questions within present U.S. healthcare realities. Before listening to women of color with breast cancer and healthcare providers, attention to the larger socioeconomic context is needed. This literature review synthesizes relevant findings from empirical studies in medical sociology and U.S. Census data to demonstrate that healthcare disparities for communities of color stem from numerous sources and involve interrelated issues of quality and access.

Chapter 3 attends both to theology and to qualitative research methodology. The theological portion focuses upon Christian theological anthropology and summarizes certain contributions made by Lutheran, white feminist, and Womanist sources. Specifically, a particular theological commitment calls attention to the particular and serves as a rationale for attempting qualitative research into how healthcare disparities affect people. It is this: The basis for understanding what it is to be human has to be in relation to the most vulnerable of society.

The second half of this chapter then articulates the specific methodological approach that shaped how the ethnographic fieldwork was conducted. It begins with a general description of the value of qualitative research and then introduces the specific method for the ethnographic fieldwork. Finally, it reflects upon the unexpected learning that occurred during the Institutional Review Board (IRB) approval process.

Chapter 4 offers original ethnographic research borne out of conversations with eight Black and Latina women with breast cancer and with six healthcare providers. It attempts to (re)present faithfully what these women and care providers understand and experience with respect to quality healthcare. As I listened to these individuals, I tried to gain insight into what good (or poor) quality care looks and feels like and how quality of care disparities affect people. In keeping with the theo-ethical commitment articulated in chapter 3, this chapter foregrounds the experiences of Black and Latina women with breast cancer and draws on healthcare providers for additional insight. While not all of the interviews appear in detail, three stories are told in-depth which illustrate four recurring themes pertinent to healthcare ethics and policy.

Chapter 5 concludes the study by integrating ethnography, theology, and social ethics. Specifically, it begins with sharing how some of the women with cancer understand the divine-human relationship and what human beings owe to one another. It then focuses on their specific definitions of high quality patient-doctor relationships. Taking their insights seriously, the chapter then considers implications both for healthcare ethics and practice and for the actual doing of ethics and theology themselves. Thus, it reflects both on constructive suggestions for change in healthcare practices and structures as well as on methodological suggestions for the way in which scholars of various disciplines conceive of and carry out our respective vocations.

Health Status versus Healthcare Quality

Before pursuing the primary analysis of healthcare quality issues, a caveat is needed: I am aware that a discussion of healthcare quality disparities could potentially distract attention away from disparities in U.S. health status.[27] This is not a diversion I wish to enable. Disparities in health status are not synonymous with disparities in healthcare quality. The statement of the problem above highlights disparities in both health status and healthcare. To clarify, health status refers to a person or group's overall wellness or health—how well she or they function emotionally, socially, and physically. It is measured by people's self-reports of their own health along with quantitative indicators such as infant mortality rates, life expectancy, death rates, the prevalence of major diseases among specific populations, et cetera. In contrast, healthcare quality and access refer to the ability of a person or community to receive adequate healthcare—both in terms of quantity and quality of care provided.

This book's analysis focuses on disparities in access to, and quality of, healthcare. Yet, by discussing healthcare quality disparities with an emphasis on provider bias and stereotypes, for example, I do not want to ignore the fact that there are also pressing racial-ethnic and socioeconomic disparities in health status among the U.S. population. Here are a couple of the health status disparity statistics that most alarm me. In 2005, the U.S. Department of Health and Human Services (DHHS) together with the Centers for Disease Control and Prevention (CDC), and the National Center for Health Statistics reported the following:

1. In 2003 the life expectancy for blacks was 5.2 years shorter than it was for whites.
2. "The 5-year survival rate for black females diagnosed in 1992–2000 with breast cancer was 14 percentage points lower than the 5-year survival rate for white females."
3. "In 2003 breast cancer mortality rates for black females was 37 percent higher than for white females. . . . "[28]

Also in terms of cancer mortality statistics, the CDC has an Office of Minority Health and Health Disparities, which reported in 2005 that "African Americans are more likely to die of cancer than people of any other racial or ethnic group."[29]

Information on the health status of women with color is pointedly germane to this work. According to the Kaiser Foundation, "Among women 45 and older, African American women (37%) and Latinas (41%) are more likely to report being in fair or poor health than white women (23%)."[30] In terms of breast cancer, the CDC reported in 2005 that "[a]lthough deaths caused by breast cancer have decreased among white and black women, black women continue to have higher rates of mortality from breast cancer."[31] Indeed, understanding health status disparities, particularly as they relate to cancer mortality rates, is a crucial context to bear in mind as this analysis progresses. It will be especially important to recall as Latina and Black women with breast cancer describe their healthcare and experiences in the ethnographic sections of chapters 4 and 5.

Moreover, endemic to the health of certain U.S. communities are the festering ills of un and underemployment, racially and socioeconomically segregated neighborhoods, inadequate public education, the proximity to pollution, and a preponderance of fast-food chains combined with a lacuna of affordable grocery stores. These socioeconomic realities correlate strongly with national socioeconomic class and ethnic-racial differences in health status, as seen in such indicators as infant mortality; rates in asthma, diabetes, and heart disease; obesity; and life expectancy. These harsh realities must not be overlooked or ignored by those who focus on healthcare quality and access issues.

As an aside, sometimes healthcare professionals can be quick to point out that they cannot resolve these social problems that affect health when treating a person in a clinical setting. Such comments are often reflective of how overwhelming their responsibilities to provide medical care are given current realities. While this attitude is understandable and certainly not unique to healthcare providers, it nonetheless compartmentalizes what is "on the agenda" or within the boundaries of an individual's or professional group's responsibility and can be used as a rationale to abdicate responsibility to enjoin socioeconomic discussions. In other words, some healthcare professional sectors reason that they are charged to give equal, appropriate, effective medical care, but not to solve these larger problems. And in one sense, they are right. However, the problem with this view is that while symptoms indicative of these menacing social ills are addressed—even ameliorated—root causes of social, economic, and health problems are many times left untouched. Consequently, the results of their medical interventions are not as fruitful as they might be.

Yet, it is critical to not lay blame at any one provider's or community's doorstep. To do so would be simplistic and terribly unfair. Furthermore, such a convenient conclusion would miss the larger picture of structural social inequities. Physician and attorney Gregg Bloche issues an appropriate warning to those who focus more on healthcare provider bias or skill in healthcare delivery than on racial and socioeconomic disparities in health status:

> Why has racial bias in the clinical judgments physicians make on behalf of equivalently insured and socio-economically situated Americans generated a greater political response than has the racially unequal impact of allowing more than forty million Americans to go without medical

coverage? And, why have racial disparities in health status—a thing distinct from health care provision and not much influenced by it—received less political attention than has racial bias in physician judgment? The answers to both questions, I suspect, implicate our national tolerance for socio-economic inequality as a factor in disparities we deem unacceptable when they result purely and simply from racial bias. As a matter of law—and of politics—we tend to treat racial disparities in Americans' enjoyment of myriad goods, services, and benefits as less troublesome when they are mediated through socio-economic differences than when they arise from the overt bigotry of identifiable actors. Thus, racial disparities in access to health care (and in physicians' clinical recommendations) due to differences in insurance coverage are more "acceptable" than up-front racial bias at the bedside, despite the known correlation between coverage status and race (and despite the causal role of prior racial subordination in present socio-economic disadvantage).[32]

Bloche questions the predominant tolerance of structural socioeconomic inequalities that continue to divide U.S. society even when/if obvious (and oftentimes individual or personalized) racial bias is denounced. Simply put, it is more palatable to blame one person or sector of care provision for racial prejudice than to confront the fact that a social, economic, and political history along with the present structures of public life are to blame for the most profound health inequalities. The economic, political, and societal forces that make it possible for massive disparities in health status to continue with little public outcry must also be challenged. While I cannot take up myriad questions related to health status disparities here, I am grateful for those who do[33] and will continue to integrate this critical issue into my own research. What I have done is to address the crisis of the uninsured in chapter 2.

Conclusion

This book will not add to healthcare policy statistics, nor will it iterate a new classification of principles by which ethical decisions in healthcare ought to be made. Instead, it hopes to demonstrate two things: (1) Healthcare systems, providers, and ethics will learn much if they listen more fully to Latina and Black women with breast cancer; and (2) There is a place for explicit theo-ethical language and social analysis within the fields of medical ethics, bioethics, and healthcare discussions.

Three methodological claims about how scholarship is done undergird this work. It is important to identify them at the outset: First, qualitative research methods such as those found in ethnography are needed and ought to be more widely incorporated into research. Not only are they important for those in the social sciences, but they may also prove integral to theological and ethical inquiry as well. They also ought to be more widely valued by those in the natural sciences and in healthcare quality research. As it pays close attention to the particular, qualitative research may be a vehicle for honoring the sacred that is within each human being.

Second, bioethics as a discipline predominately focuses on biotechnologies (e.g., genetic research, artificial reproductive technologies, cloning) and on topics such as the principles of healthcare, informed consent, physician-assisted suicide, abortion, and euthanasia. While these technologies and topics merit sustained ethical reflection, the lens through which they are viewed matters a great deal. Simply put, analysis ought not be divorced from the social, economic, and political contexts in which they arise. Furthermore, bioethics needs to address the socioeconomics of healthcare provision (e.g., healthcare quality disparities, racism in healthcare, the crisis of the uninsured). Even more, it also ought to give more attention to the deleterious effects that poverty, malnutrition, poor education, and violence have upon the health and well-being of millions. In short, biomedical ethics needs to turn to the social in order to understand and elucidate how race, class, and the political economy pertain to all facets of healthcare, biomedicine, biotechnologies, and health in this country.

Third, as already noted, there is a place for theological language within healthcare and bioethics. Indeed, the complexity and magnitude of disparities in healthcare quality call for theological imagination. The voice of theology may help healthcare practitioners and ethicists turn more fully toward the particular—toward understanding what it means to be a person not only in the language of individual rights or autonomy but also in the language of various faith traditions—practiced by both providers and patients/families. There are important differences in meaning between contract and covenant, for example. As Verhey explains,

> [W]here the law is the major source for bioethics, morality is too easily confused with legality and moral questions too quickly reduced to legal questions. Moreover, the law is better at telling us what not to do than at providing ends and goals worthy of our humanity. The law is better at enforcing contracts than at nurturing covenants. The law is deliberately minimal, and it can be expected to give only a minimal account of what is morally at stake.[34]

Indeed, while one can post patient rights and the institutional mission on every hospital or clinic wall, it is not as easy to legislate the kinds of interactions and relationships that will make such dignity and respect real. Vibrant and concrete connections need to be made and remade between our stated principles, virtues and values and the actual practices, sensibilities, cultures, and policies of healthcare providers and systems.

Both health and illness are inevitable parts of human living, just like dying. The questions, then, become: How do we hope to be treated in times of illness? What do we hope for when it comes our time to face a health crisis—in our lives or the lives of those we love? These are important questions for us to ask not only individually, but as a nation. How people experience care in times of sickness fundamentally matters to the quality of life, both personally and collectively.[35] It is critical that we, as a society, learn and fully appreciate the fact that if the health of some communities is not promoted and cared for, the health of all is negatively affected.

Statistics sometimes move public policy, but they do not always move hearts out of complacency. At worst, they can obscure the persons who stand behind the numbers. When this happens, people become percentages. Not enough U.S. inhabitants are outraged that well over 45 million people in this country have no health insurance. Those who are insured and/or who are satisfied with the quality of their healthcare often disassociate themselves from those who are not. Statistics can act like smelling salts or they can numb people. One thing is for sure: Percentages alone never tell the whole story. The hope is that this work will help to narrow the conceptual gap between numbers and lives.

2

U.S. Healthcare 101: What Everyone
Ought to Know about How U.S.
Inhabitants are Treated (or Not)

Let's be frank: News stories about healthcare can be tedious. This may sound like a strange statement to make near the beginning of a book dedicated to exploring healthcare quality disparities. Yet it is the truth. The endless parade of numbers, factoids, and opinions—the mind-boggling figures spent on U.S. healthcare, the continual debates about prescription drugs, accusations and denials of medical malpractice, dizzying proposals about how to reform Medicare or Medicaid, the rapidly rising numbers of uninsured persons—can dull a person's interest rather quickly. And it is all too easy to skip to the next story, change channels, or surf a more scintillating website.

Ambivalence about healthcare reporting may have something to do with the way statistics are repeated in news and public debate. The use of the numbers—akin to the nature of many healthcare discussions themselves—is often highly decontextualized. Relevant social and economic conditions are often not addressed or even seen as pertinent to the discussion at hand. Instead, the specific features and costs of a new medical technology, healthcare organizational plan, or drug are discussed within a narrow frame. The technology or plan is divorced from its socioeconomic context.

Said differently, too many healthcare presentations and journalistic reports revolve around numbers or technologies not people, averages not particulars. I often find myself asking, "Where are all the people in this news story? Who are they? What do they look like? What do they think? How might they be affected by this new therapy or financial plan? Who is left out of the picture altogether?" In some healthcare circles, there seems to be a reluctance to move beyond statistics in order to pause long enough to see and consider actual persons—how they are affected on both personal and social levels by healthcare realities or by a disease and/or treatment regimen.

However, despite the fact that it can be divorced from context by reporters and analysts, current information from healthcare and sociological sources regarding racial-ethnic and socioeconomic disparities in the quality of healthcare is exceedingly important to understand. Statistics and studies testify to looming inequalities that gnaw at the well-being of our society. Indeed, healthcare quality disparities present a moral problem that threatens and implicates all U.S. inhabitants in some way or another. Consequently, one significant task of a theologian and/or social ethicist is to translate this information into meaningful terms for laypersons who live and work outside the walls of the healthcare industry, lobbyist camps, politicians' offices, and academia.

Thus, before attending to the wisdom of Black and Latina women with breast cancer or to any theological and ethical insights regarding these healthcare disparities, it is necessary to first lay some pertinent groundwork. Specifically, a review of relevant healthcare statistics and literature in medical sociology will situate the stories and ethical analysis of subsequent chapters. This chapter first highlights U.S. Census data that reveal the magnitude of the insurance crisis and show who disproportionately bears the brunt of it. Insurance status weighs too heavily within the context of U.S. healthcare disparities to ignore. Second, it illustrates the interrelationship between healthcare access and quality issues. Analyzing three recent headlines will make these connections especially visible. The third main section considers three factors eroding healthcare quality that cannot be accounted for simply by access-related disparities: Language barriers and a lack of cultural competency, healthcare provider bias and stereotypes, and the bureaucracy of healthcare systems. The conclusion then summarizes the implications of these healthcare quality disparities and why they matter to us as a society.

On the Outside Looking In: The Plight of the Uninsured

In August 2005, the U.S. Census Bureau estimated that 15.7 percent of the total U.S. population was uninsured for the entire year of 2004.[1] If you are poor by official standards, this percentage nearly doubles.[2]

In 2004, 24.3 percent of households with an annual income of less than $25,000 were uninsured.[3] The overall national percentage of 15.7 percent translates into 45.8 million uninsured individuals and represents an increase of 800,000 persons since 2003. This rise is part of a larger trend. While there was not a percentage increase between 2004 and 2003, 2003 was the third consecutive year of increases in the percentage of the uninsured.[4]

Among the 50 states, the numbers of uninsured vary significantly. Of all the states, Minnesota has the lowest percentage of uninsured (8.5 percent) and Texas has the highest (three year average of 25.1 percent).[5] This latter figure means that more than one in four residents of Texas is uninsured.[6] (New Mexico has the second highest percentage of uninsured—21.4 percent. All of the other 48 states are below 20 percent.)[7] Without a doubt, in the grand scheme of financial and institutional structures of U.S. healthcare, insurance status contributes more to overall disparities in the amount—and successful outcomes— of medical treatment than do racial dynamics by themselves.

Some healthcare analysts point out that often people are only without insurance for a couple of months; for example, when they are in between jobs. However, according to the Census guidelines, "People were considered 'insured' if they were covered by any type of health insurance for part or all of the previous year, and everyone else was considered uninsured."[8] The simple, but harsh fact is that the ranks of the uninsured are increasing significantly. The number of uninsured has increased from 41.2 million persons in 2001 to 45.8 million in 2004. Given recent changes to Medicaid programs, we can expect this number to surpass 46 million in the very near future. Kathleen Stoll, the Health Policy Director of Families USA, put these national numbers in startling perspective when she explained that the current number of the U.S.-uninsured population "now exceeds the cumulative population of 24 states plus the District of Columbia."[9]

Insurance is the most basic healthcare commodity. Depending on one's ability to purchase it or not, it opens up or seals off the pipeline to healthcare for millions of Americans. Undeniably, the most pervasive source of healthcare disparities is the inequality of access to healthcare provision. And it is not an insignificant fact that those without insurance are disproportionately people of color. In light of this reality, the first questions that a social ethicist needs to ask Black and Latina women may not be: How did the medical staff treat you? Did you feel respected in the interaction? Instead, they may very well be the following: How were you able to access medical care? Where do you go for the majority of your healthcare needs—a doctor's office? The emergency room? The neighborhood *botánica*?[10] Indeed, according to a 2004 Kaiser Women's Health Survey "Latinas (38%) have the highest rate of uninsurance of all groups of women examined by this survey— three times the uninsured rate of white (13%) women."[11] The report adds that Black women have an uninsured rate of 17 percent.

Undeniably, many uninsured individuals do receive medical care, often through public clinics and emergency rooms. However, the number and kinds of clinics and services often fail to meet the degree of need. One recent study found that both long-term and short-term uninsured adults, especially those in poor or only fair health, were "more likely than insured adults to report that they could not see a physician when needed due to cost."[12] The authors cite unmet needs to include routine checkups, cancer screenings, access to preventative services for a host of illnesses, and lack of assistance with the maintenance or prevention of chronic conditions such as diabetes, hypertension, and high cholesterol levels.[13]

As already mentioned in the introduction, "These findings challenge the views of a growing proportion of Americans—from 43% in 1993 to 57% in 1999—who believe that uninsured are able to get the care they need from physicians and hospitals."[14] Indeed, such flaws in our collective comprehension of the insurance crisis play into public complacency regarding healthcare reform. Unless they themselves have direct experience, people with insurance often fail to perceive adequately the realities that the uninsured encounter regularly. One of the fundamental claims of this book is that faulty assumptions such as this one both distance white and/or affluent people from the lives of others *and* obscure our moral vision.

For example, those of us who count among the ranks of the insured often miss the fact that many uninsured people delay seeking care. They do so both out of fear of what they might have *and* of the potential financial costs. Lamentably, they then often enter the healthcare system with advanced stages of disease and complications, which are usually more costly to treat than the options available at earlier diagnostic points. In addition, some complications and diseases are readily avoidable altogether if appropriate preventative and educative steps are taken.

Take cancer screening as an example. While rates of breast and cervical cancer screening have increased among uninsured women, the "absolute differences in cancer screening rates between uninsured and insured women have remained remarkably consistent when the findings are compared with earlier studies. . . . Lower rates of cancer screening among uninsured adults may be the principle reason why they are diagnosed at later, less curable stages of breast and colorectal cancer than insured adults."[15] In other words, even as more uninsured women are receiving breast and cervical cancer screenings, the gap between the proportion of insured and uninsured women who are screened has not diminished overall.

All U.S. inhabitants, especially the insured, ought to know the answer to these basic questions: Who are the uninsured? Is the burden of being uninsured shared equally across racial-ethnic communities? These questions are important because their answers begin to render the faces behind the statistics more visible. In keeping with the focus of this book, I will highlight the findings for three general racial-ethnic groupings. As of late 2005, the total U.S. population is estimated to be over 297.7 million people. (This number changes quickly. You can find the most up-to-date estimate by going to the www.census.gov webpage and looking at the prominent population clock.) According to 2003 Census estimates 197.3 million people identify as non-Hispanic whites;[16] 39.9 million as Hispanic (of any race); 38.7 million as Black; 13.5 million people identify as Asian; 960,000 identify as Hawaiian or Pacific Islander; and 4.4 million identify as Native Americans and Alaska Natives.[17]

The significance of racial-ethnic breakdowns regarding insurance status quickly becomes prominent in context of these overall U.S. population tallies. Table 2.1 summarizes U.S. Census Bureau statistics for 2004. To keep the human beings squarely in view, the numbers of people in each category are presented in bold-type.

Table 2.1 2004 Total U.S. Population Figures Compared with Uninsured Figures for Blacks, Latinos, Asians, and Non-Hispanic Whites:

Race-Ethnicity	Total Population* (Per 2002 and 2003 Data) (%)	The Racial-Ethnic Category Who Are Uninsured** (Per 2004 Data) (%)	Number of People Uninsured** (in Million)
Hispanics (of any race)	14	32.7	13.7
Blacks	13	19.7	7.2
Asians	4.4	16.8	2.1
Non-Hispanic whites	69.0	11.3	22.0

Note: According to these two Census documents, there are 4.4 million American Indians and Native Alaskans among the total U.S. population while 29% of all American Indians and Native Alaskans are uninsured (based on a three-year average).

Sources: * Total population estimates: U.S. Census Bureau, "The Face of Our Population," online: http://factfinder.census.gov/jsp/saff/SAFFInfo.jsp?_pageId = tp9_race_ethnicity. This information was last revised by the U.S. Census on October 13, 2004.
** Percentages and numbers of the uninsured by race-ethnicity: Carmen DeNavas-Walt, Bernadette D. Proctor, and Cheryl Hill Lee, U.S. Census Bureau, Current Population Reports, P60–229, *Income, Poverty, and Health Insurance Coverage in the United States: 2004* (Washington, DC: U.S. Government Printing Office, 2005); 16–18 and 61–66. This report is available online: www.census.gov/prod/2005pubs/p60–229.pdf.

Comparing the total population of the United States with the proportions of the uninsured reveals the depth of racial-ethnic disparities in insurance status. For example, by 2004 Latinos (of any race) represent 14 percent of the total U.S. are population while 32.7 percent of all Latinos in the U.S. are uninsured. Blacks represent 13 percent of the total population while 19.7 percent of all Blacks are uninsured. In contrast, non-Hispanic whites comprise 69 percent of the U.S. population, yet only 11.3 percent of all non-Hispanic whites are uninsured.

By doing some quick calculations, it is possible to see what percentage each racial-ethnic group makes up of the total uninsured population. For example, if we divide the figure of 22 million non-Hispanic whites who are uninsured by the total number of uninsured (45.8 million), we find that non-Hispanics whites comprise 48 percent of the total uninsured population. Similarly, Latinos represent 30 percent of the total uninsured population; Blacks represent 16 percent; and Asians account for 4.6 percent of the U.S. uninsured.

Let's look at the flip side of these statistics for a moment to see the implications of these numbers in even different light. In 2004, 67.3 percent of Hispanics were insured. In contrast, 88.7 percent of non-Hispanic whites, 80.3 percent of Blacks, and 83.2 percent of Asians had health insurance.[18] Latinos in particular suffer disproportionately from a lack of health insurance. In short, not everyone is served the same sized slice of the uninsured pie.

Similarly, the impoverished in this country—37 million people whose ranks continue to rise—are especially expected to swallow a big bite of an unsavory helping.[19] In 2004, the official poverty rate rose to 12.7 percent. This means that 1.1 million more individuals were considered poor in 2004 than in 2003. Again, this is not the first year of such an increase. In 2003, the "national poverty rate rose to 12.5 percent, up from 12.1 percent in 2002."[20] Akin to the uninsured statistics, a disproportionate number of people of color live in poverty as compared to their white counterparts. The U.S. Census Bureau reported that as of 2004, 8.6 percent of all non-Hispanic whites live in poverty. In comparison, 24.7 percent of Blacks, 21.9 percent of Hispanics (of any race), and 9.8 percent of Asians live in poverty.[21]

Another way of understanding the significance of these figures is to note that non-Hispanic whites "accounted for 45.6 percent of the people in poverty, compared with 67.1 percent of the total population."[22] Thus, non-Hispanic whites comprise a significantly larger proportion of the general population than they do of the impoverished population. If one were a utilitarian when it comes to conceptualizing justice, one would expect the benefits and burdens of society, in this case wealth and poverty, to be distributed fairly and perhaps proportionally. In this logic, one might conclude that if some poverty in society is unavoidable and that if a racial-ethnic group makes up 67.1 percent of the total population, then they ought to also make up 67.1 percent of the impoverished population as well (no matter how small the total percentage of impoverished is within the general population).

Philosophical musings aside, a tangible and pertinent question must be addressed: Who counts as poor in U.S. society? In order to be considered "officially poor" by the federal government, a family of two adults and two children under the age of 18 could earn no more than $19,157 in 2004. A single person under the age of 65 could earn no more than $9,827.[23] The stringent nature of these dollar limits causes me to wonder about those whose income hovers just above them. How well off and well insured are families who earn $25,000–30,000 a year or single adults who earn $15,000–20,000? The official line is set incredibly low. Many exist just above it and so do not officially "count" among the ranks of the impoverished and yet have serious difficulty accessing or affording healthcare.[24]

In fact, while many people technically have insurance, the coverage is often not adequate to meet their needs. Similar to the reality that the requirements for "offical poverty" masks who live in impoverished conditions, focusing on the "officially uninsured" obscures the plight of those who are underinsured. Cathy Schoen et al., found that in 2003 there were as many as 16 million underinsured adults. Being underinsured means for these individuals that "their insurance did not adequately protect them against catastrophic health care expenses. . . . An estimated total of 61 million adults, or 35 percent of individuals, ages 19–64, had either no insurance, sporadic coverage, or insurance coverage that exposed them to high health costs during 2003."[25] Indeed, the insurance crisis is significantly deep and wide, hurting both those who have absolutely no insurance as well as those who have a degree of coverage.

It is true that many impoverished people are insured by Medicaid programs. In 2004, Medicaid insured 37.5 million people or 12.9 percent of the U.S. population.[26] For its part, Medicare, the federal insurance program for seniors over 65 and others with permanent disabilities, insured 39.7 million persons (13.7 percent of the U.S. population). However, while Medicaid insures millions in poverty, an additional 15.1 million relatively poor people lacked health insurance—24.3 percent of people with household incomes less than $25,000 had no insurance in 2004. In addition, 14.9 million people with household incomes of $25,000–$49,999 had no insurance (20 percent of the total number of people in this income range).[27] In contrast, only 8.4 percent of people with household incomes of $75,000 or more had no health insurance in 2004. (Thus, 91.6 percent were insured). Indeed, there is a strong correlation between being uninsured and being among the poor and/or lower socioeconomic classes. Table 2.2 compares the current percentages of non-Hispanic whites, Hispanics, Asians, and Blacks in the general population with their respective proportions living in poverty and/or who are uninsured.

Table 2.2   A Comparison of Poverty and Uninsurance Rates by Race-Ethnicity for 2004

Race-Ethnicity	Total U.S. Population* (Per 2002 and 2003 Data) (%)	The Racial-Ethnic Category Living in Poverty** (Per 2004 Data) (%)	The Racial-Ethnic Category Who Are Uninsured** (Per 2004 Data) (%)
Hispanics (of any race)	14	21.9	32.7
Blacks	13	24.7	19.7
Asians	4.4	9.8	16.8
Non-Hispanic whites	69.0	8.6	11.3

Note: According to these two Census documents, there are 4.4 million American Indians and Native Alaskans among the total U.S. population while 29% of all American Indians and Native Alaskans are uninsured (based on a three-year average) and 24.3% live in poverty (also based on a three-year average).

Sources: * Total population estimates: U.S. Census Bureau, "The Face of Our Population," online: http://factfinder.census.gov/jsp/saff/SAFFInfo.jsp?_pageId = tp9_race_ethnicity. This information was last revised by the U.S. Census on October 13, 2004.
**Percentages of the uninsured and those in poverty by race-ethnicity: Carmen DeNavas-Walt, Bernadette D. Proctor, and Cheryl Hill Lee, U.S. Census Bureau, Current Population Reports, P60–229, *Income, Poverty, and Health Insurance Coverage in the United States: 2004* (Washington, DC: U.S. Government Printing Office, 2005); 9–10, 16–18 and 61–66. This report is available online: www.census.gov/prod/2005pubs/p60–229.pdf.

It is likely that more people who struggle financially may not find coverage from Medicaid and/or Medicare in the near future; obstacles to eligibility may only intensify. Given their rising costs, the U.S. Congress and the Bush administration want to slow the growth of both Medicaid and Medicare. For example, congressional budget proposals may significantly cut Medicaid benefits.[28] For its part, the Bush administration recently made a decision to give the state government of Florida tremendous flexibility in designing its Medicaid program and limits of coverage.[29] It is possible that Florida may well be a model for other states wanting to curb their own Medicaid programs.

Moreover, finding or being able to afford health insurance poses a serious challenge for a growing number of the middle classes as well. *The New York Times* recently reminded the nation, "The majority of the uninsured are neither poor by official standards nor unemployed."[30] The numbers of people who are working full-time but whose employers do not provide health insurance coverage are increasing. Furthermore, there are signs of a growing trend in which, whether to cut costs, survive as a business, or increase profits, employers hire more and more part-time or contract employees without offering insurance. It is a misconception to view the insurance crisis as only affecting low-income and officially impoverished persons.[31]

Furthermore, even those with insurance can still be hit by high costs that they cannot absorb (co-payments, deductibles, services not covered by the plan, etc.) Some are even strained to the point of filing for bankruptcy. Harvard researchers reported in 2005 that in their study of 1,771 individuals who filed for bankruptcy, 28 percent identified the cause as illness or injury. The researchers found that "most were middle class, educated and had health insurance at the start of the treatment."[32]

Another disconcerting trend in insurance status in the United States is that more people are shifting from having employer-based or private insurance to depending upon public insurance, mainly Medicaid and/ or Medicare. Of those who *were* insured in 2004:

- 59.8 percent had employment-based insurance (fourth annual decrease)
- 09.3 percent directly purchased their own insurance independently
- 12.9 percent were insured by Medicaid (fourth annual increase)
- 13.7 percent were insured by Medicare
- 03.7 percent were insured by military healthcare[33]

Therefore, not only are the numbers of the uninsured increasing, but the distribution among those who have insurance is also changing, and it is not for the better. People are moving from private insurance sources to the ranks of public insurance, which was created to meet the healthcare needs of those with low or nonexistent income levels.[34]

It is interesting to note here as well the racial-ethnic breakdowns with respect to employer-based versus Medicaid insurance levels. It is certainly true that a solid majority in each of these Census groupings has employer-based insurance. Yet it is also important to see that insured Blacks and Latinos are significantly more likely than whites to have Medicaid instead of employer-based insurance. Table 2.3 shows the contrast.

Table 2.3   Comparison of Type of Insurance by Race-Ethnicity for 2004

Race-Ethnicity	Total U.S. Population* (Per 2002 and 2003 Data) (%)	The Racial-Ethnic Category with Employment-Based Insurance** (Per 2004 Data) (%)	The Racial-Ethnic Category with Medicaid Insurance** (Per 2004 Data) (%)
Hispanics (of any race)	14	41.1	21.8
Blacks	13	49.6	24.5
Asians	4.4	61.8	10.3
Non-Hispanic whites	69.0	65.7	8.8

Note: According to the latter Census report, in 2004 61.8 percent of Asians had employer-based insurance and 10.3 percent had Medicaid. The charts did not give separate data for Native Americans or Alaska natives here.

Sources: * Total population estimates: U.S. Census Bureau, "The Face of Our Population," online: http://factfinder.census.gov/jsp/saff/SAFFInfo.jsp?_pageId = tp9_race_ethnicity. This information was last revised by the U.S. Census on October 13, 2004.
** Percentages of the uninsured and those in poverty by race-ethnicity: Carmen DeNavas-Walt, Bernadette D. Proctor and Cheryl Hill Lee, U.S. Census Bureau, Current Population Reports, P60–229, Income, Poverty, and Health Insurance Coverage in the United States: 2004 (U.S. Government Printing Office, Washington, DC, 2005), 62–66. This report is available online: www.census.gov/prod/2005pubs/p60–229.pdf.

In summary, Blacks and Latinos disproportionately bear three heavy burdens with respect to their non-Latino white counterparts: Being uninsured, being impoverished, and being more likely to have public insurance in a context where the most comprehensive and generous insurance plans are most often employer-based or privately purchased. While the insurance crisis hurts all U.S. inhabitants in some way or another, it is critical to see who is affected most directly and to understand that their portion of the burden is unfair. Given these facts, one might conclude that Blacks and Latinos—rather than being the ones "draining" U.S. healthcare of its resources—are, in actuality, the ones being asked to suffer the greatest costs to their individual and communal well-being.

Simply put, Blacks and Latinos have insufficient (and often unequal) choice in choosing, or gaining access to, any insurance. Indeed, not all insurance is the same in this country. And certainly not all plans are perceived as offering equal quality and benefits. Savvy consumers shop around for the best plans and providers if they have the luxury of choice or the ability to negotiate for certain benefits from a potential employer. Ask yourself this question: Would you be content with the current form of Medicaid insurance for your coverage if you could somehow afford or gain access to an HMO (Health Maintenance Organization) or PPO (Preferred Provider Organization) plan? Which would you choose?

It is interesting to note that for many who have always had it or who take it for granted, private, employer-based insurance is the only source that really counts as insurance at all. A personal anecdote illustrates the point: During our interview in Spanish, María spoke about the clinic she went to for her initial cancer care. I said, "So, you didn't have insurance." I was assuming that she had Medicaid as I made this comment. She replied, "Oh, yes, I had insurance. I had *public* insurance—and now I have both Medicare and Medicaid because I am over 65." For years, I had never realized that I equated having Medicaid with having no insurance—meaning no "real" insurance. I am grateful to María, a Puerto Rican grandmother for pointing out this flawed equation to me.[35]

Upon reviewing the Census statistics, I contend that the enormous numbers of uninsured living in the United States present not only a policy, but a moral crisis for all those who live in this nation. The unmet needs of the uninsured fester like infected wounds that assail the public body. If this foundational inequality is not corrected, the inequalities discussed below will never be eradicated either.

However, having acknowledged the significant role that insurance status plays in accessing adequate healthcare, focusing solely on this topic will not reveal every pertinent aspect related to healthcare quality and access concerns. Even after communities of color succeed in gaining entry to a hospital room or clinic office—with or without insurance—they often face additional barriers to quality care and full access. Racial-ethnic stereotypes, communication barriers, cross-cultural incompetence, and the dizzying maze of bureaucratic health-care all intertwine with insurance matters. For example, healthcare providers sometimes assume patients of color are uninsured, which speaks both to the ongoing prevalence of bias in healthcare *and* to the systemic insurance crisis. Said differently, the fact that some populations in particular have to scramble to acquire or retain a degree of healthcare coverage (whether private or public) influences provider perceptions. Simply put, issues of bias and linguistic barriers cannot be neatly divorced from the economics of healthcare.

The Overlapping Relationship between Access and Quality

When I initially conceived of this book, I emphasized that its focus would not be about healthcare access per se but rather healthcare quality. I had been alarmed both by recent experience and by recent findings that even when darker skinned peoples have comparable insurance and income, they often receive a lower quality of care than lighter skinned peoples. I was eager to seize upon evidence that racism, distinct from economic factors, is alive and operative in U.S. society. And I still believe that it is.

I now understand, however, that there were flaws in my definition of access and in my assumption that it is a wholly separate and distinct category set apart from quality. Initially, I set out to look at the quality of care for people of color with insurance—people "like me"—who, *unlike me*, might be more vulnerable to pernicious bias and discrimination due to racial and/or cultural factors. I mistakenly assumed that access to healthcare pertained only to the matter of obtaining insurance.

In the course of this research, I came to understand two things about access: First, "access to healthcare" involves more than simply being insured in some fashion. We cannot assume someone has no access to care if she is uninsured, and we cannot assume that another who is insured has decent access to the actual care they need. Second, comparable insurance and/or income levels *do not necessarily* equal comparable access to care.

My guess is that many in our society, especially white people with employer-based insurance, do not perceive the other factors at work that inhibit insured communities of color from getting a foot in the door. For example, if a person of color has public insurance, such as Medicaid, she/he technically has health coverage and should be able to access medical care. However, it is very possible that this same person will have difficulty finding a provider—especially a regular, ongoing physician—who will accept Medicaid as the sole payment source and thus, the patient. Some physicians complain that the reimbursement rates for doctors' services are simply too low to justify treating persons with Medicaid. Other factors that impede access include the distance of hospitals and clinics to communities of color as well as a lack of availability of certain drugs in pharmacies located in neighborhoods of color.[36] In addition, being of a particular racial, ethnic, cultural, or linguistic community different from that of the provider can complicate access. Simply having some form of insurance does not guarantee full or equal access to care.

In short, racism and prejudice cannot be neatly divorced from socioeconomic class when considering healthcare. Both sustain healthcare quality disparities. Indeed, to understand fully the kinds of social inequalities and obstacles darker skinned communities face in the United States, one needs to appreciate how enmeshed race and class are. For example, does the fact that children in the South Bronx have among the highest rates of asthma in the nation speak to economic or racial issues? The answer is both. Environmental racism was a factor in Robert Moses' creation of this section of the Bronx and still is a reason why city officials permit the continuance of such poor air quality.[37] Moreover, both racism and poverty are reasons why families have difficulty lobbying the government to do something about this chronic asthma problem and why many cannot simply pick up and move to more breathable environs.[38]

To summarize, healthcare access is a more multilayered concept than I had initially thought. Even if a person of color has insurance, especially if she is not affluent, she may still need to find affordable transportation and childcare in order to go to the doctor. Once at the clinic, she may not fully understand all of the directions and information given. Even murkier and harder to pin down is the fact that, even when communication seems clear on the surface, failures in cross-cultural competence or the presence of stereotypes and bias may obstruct trust in the relationship between the provider and patient. All of these issues affect *both* access to *and* quality of care. Yet unfortunately, such issues are often absent from the radar screen of healthcare policy.

The Terrorizing Axis of (In)Access: A Story Three Headlines Tell When Told Together

Scanning recent news stories can bring into sharp focus the relationship between healthcare access and quality. Sometimes, the mere juxtaposition of newspaper headlines tells an important story. Consider the picture these stories present when they are read in conjunction with one another rather than as isolated news items. All three appeared on the front page of *The New York Times* on September 3, 2003.

Emergency Rooms Get Eased Rules on Patient Care
Number in Poverty Grows
Africans Outdo U.S. Patients in Following AIDS Therapy

A bit of exegesis may flesh out details of the picture. Robert Pear succinctly condenses the news of the first headline to this kernel: "The Bush administration is relaxing rules that say hospitals have to examine and treat people who require emergency medical care, regardless of their ability to pay."[39] This decree eases the rules of a 1986 law, the Emergency Medical Treatment and Labor Act (EMTALA). The new rules limit the scope of what hospitals are obligated to provide in terms of emergency care by narrowing the definition of "hospital property" where persons are entitled to such care and by giving hospitals greater discretion in scheduling on-call coverage by doctors and staff. For example, hospitals will no longer have to have specialists available at all hours. Also, they may exempt senior physicians and other medical staff from on-call duties, as well as allow doctors to be on call simultaneously at two or more hospitals.[40] The administration hopes these changes will discourage people from seeking out free care in the emergency room (ER) and that hospital and physician costs in complying with the EMTALA will decrease.

It is hard for me to concur with the Bush administration's view that patient care will not be harmed by these changes. I am skeptical that patient care will not be compromised if fewer specialists are on call. Moreover, even those doctors who are on call will be able to schedule elective surgeries during their on call shifts and may be less available. The new restrictions may especially hurt those lacking insurance and financial resources. As noted earlier, those who are poor and without health insurance often delay seeking care, in part, for financial reasons. When they cannot avoid seeking care, they often turn to the emergency room, a place under EMTALA where they cannot easily be denied medical attention. Thus, the limiting of EMTALA is disturbing because the ER, whether the best place or not, has been for many impoverished and uninsured people a primary place to turn for care.

Also on September 3, 2003, a small boldface headline previewed an article found on page A16: "Number in Poverty Grows."[41] Lynette

Clemetson reports that the number of Americans living below the poverty line grew by over 1.3 million in 2002. However, this number turned out to be slightly off. On September 26, 2003, the U.S. Census Bureau reported that the number of those living in poverty grew by 1.7 million individuals in 2002, bringing the total then to 34.6 million people.[42] And, as noted earlier, the Census confirms that communities of color are disproportionately impoverished. (Recall that as of 2004, 37 million U.S. inhabitants live in poverty.) In 2001, a family of two adults and two children under the age of 18 could earn no more than $17,960 to be counted as "poor"; a single person under the age of 65 could earn no more than $9,200 for the year.[43]

One could counter that this increase in the number of poor might not be such a bad thing, at least in terms of healthcare access. For example, one might contend that it is an advantage to fall below the poverty level because doing so makes it easier to qualify for Medicaid benefits. However, another headline from September 2003 deflates such optimism. On September 23, Robert Pear was again the bearer of bad news: "Struggling through a third consecutive year of fiscal distress, states have again squeezed Medicaid, the nation's largest health insurance program, by scaling back eligibility, cutting benefits, increasing co-payments and freezing or reducing payments to doctors and hospitals." More specifically in 2003: "25 states restricted eligibility for Medicaid, 18 reduced benefits, and 17 increased co-payments. Moreover, . . . 21 states cut payment rates for one or more groups of health care providers."[44]

This trend continues in 2005. Numerous states are looking for ways to control Medicaid costs and many of the plans include restricting benefits and coverage. For example, Tennessee Governor Phil Bredsen decided in 2005 to cut 200,000 (or perhaps even as many as 323,000 according to a later account) of his state's residents from TennCare, the state's Medicaid program, in an effort to control costs.[45] Similarly, Florida received approval in 2005 from the Bush administration to reform dramatically its Medicaid program. This reform limits "spending for many of the 2.2 million beneficiaries there and gives private health plans new freedom in limiting benefits."[46] In this plan, the state will set a ceiling on spending for each Medicaid recipient and will increase the use of managed care. South Carolina has already developed a similar proposal and Georgia and Kentucky are watching the Florida plan closely.[47] Consequently, it is not a given that increased numbers of the officially poor will mean a proportionate increase in the numbers insured by Medicaid. Even as Medicaid insures many impoverished, millions of others at or near poverty levels are not, or may not be, covered.

Despite the fact that states share the cost of Medicaid with the federal government, many states need to slow the growth in enrollment because their revenues are growing more slowly than the national economy. This slow growth in revenue is due, in part, to recent tax cuts. "Economists and state officials said the cutbacks indicated the intense pressure on the states as a result of declining tax receipts. . . . 'The fiscal crisis facing states is far worse than the condition of the nation's economy,' said Donald J. Boyd, director of fiscal studies at the Rockefeller Institute of Government. . . . State tax revenue dropped sharply even as the nation's economic output grew at a slow pace in the past year. . . ."[48] Another main reason states and the federal government want to slow the growth is that the costs of giving care keep going up significantly—the price tags of medical procedures, equipment and tests, prescription drugs, provider fees, et cetera all continue to rise. According to this same article, the federal government spent $147.5 billion on Medicaid in 2002.

Before considering the third headline for September 3, 2003, another related story from September 8, 2003 deserves a brief mention: "Bush Seeks $87 Billion and U.N. Aid for War Effort."[49] Just four days after these two stories on changes to EMTALA and the increase in the number of U.S. poor, President Bush asked the U.S. Congress and the American people for an additional $87 billion in emergency spending for military operations in Iraq and Afghanistan. This amount is in addition to the $79 billion the United States had already spent up to September 2003 in these ventures. The phrasing and juxtaposition are ironic. U.S. inhabitants seeking emergency care in ERs may find it harder to come by even as emergency military operations subsequently received a rather generous increase in access to their desired technologies, specialists, equipment, and services.

My point is *not* that military troops should not be properly supported with the infrastructure they need to do their jobs. Instead, I only wish to suggest that there may very well a common thread that runs between militarism and the inadequate funding of healthcare, insurance, affordable housing, public education, et cetera. The link I see is this: To justify both military aggression in other countries *and* the refusal to fund basic public services in one's own society, the internal logic must distance itself on a significant level from the lives of the people being most directly affected by both decisions. Do enough U.S. citizens reflect on the very real and unsettling consequences of our military decisions for Iraqi and U.S. citizens civilians caught in the cross fire of invasion, occupation, and insurrection? Do enough consider the consequences for the American troops who are serving lengthy tours in Iraq and for their loved ones at home? Do enough U.S. citizens reflect on the very real and unsettling consequences that a lack of a healthcare safety net has for millions in the United States?

Interestingly, Carol Johnson made somewhat of a similar connection. Ms. Johnson is a single mother in Texas whose income is too high for Medicaid and who lost her insurance when she lost her job. She could not afford the Consolidated Omnibus Budget Reconciliation Act (COBRA)[50] payments to continue her insurance on her own; it would have cost over one-fifth of her unemployment check. She has two cysts in one breast and three in another but cannot afford to have them checked. She rhetorically asked a *New York Times* reporter in 2003: " 'Do I have to move to Iraq to get help? They have $87 billion for folks over there.' "[51]

The third *New York Times* headline for September 3 is as follows: "Africans Outdo U.S. Patients in Following AIDS Therapy." Donald McNeil reports that, much to the chagrin of some western physicians, drug companies, and politicians, recent studies indicate that Africans are more diligent than Americans in taking AIDS medications: "[S]urveys done in Botswana, Uganda, Senegal and South Africa have found that on average, AIDS patients take about 90 percent of their medicine. The average figure in the United States is 70 percent. . . ."[52] This evidence will be welcomed by Africans who have long argued that pharmaceutical and political rationalizations for resisting calls to bring drug therapies to Africa have been based, in part, on racism and racial-ethnic stereotypes. In 2002, "there was an outcry when the director of the United States Agency for Internal Development (USAID) said that AIDS drugs 'wouldn't work' in Africa because many Africans don't use clocks and 'don't know what Western time is.' "[53]

In contrast to such embarrassing assumptions, a Ugandan study of 29 patients—all poor and the majority of whom were women—revealed that they were taking 91 percent of their pills. One medical school professor who works in Uganda explained that "the whole extended family, possibly with several infected members, will chip in so that one member will be saved to care for the children."[54] When an entire family both counts on one person *and* makes sacrifices to their own health so that one might survive, the person receiving treatment has powerful incentives to take the medication.

Yet rather than understanding the concrete realities and choices HIV positive Africans face, many western politicians, pharmaceutical executives, and doctors (the majority of whom are likely white) have spoken about African "unreliability," which, they report, manifests as selling, sharing, or forgetting to take the drugs. They have then used this rationale to resist treating HIV infected Africans, resulting in the deaths of thousands upon thousands in the last decade.[55] Moreover, they criticize the choices and actions of Africans without looking at the social and systemic pressures within which these communities live. What would make an impoverished African person with AIDS sell or steal a drug? Poverty and desperation are just as (if not more) likely reasons as greed or financial gain. What motivates an African woman to share her drugs with her family members? Ignorance? A lack of education? Or might the reason stem from the wisdom of deep love and a generous heart? This kind of decision may very well be borne out of love that is willing to risk and sacrifice, even if the odds of saving her or her loved one's life are against her.

Why did I include this last story in this chapter? It does not pertain to U.S. healthcare realities. Or does it? The sometimes subtle but potent biases on the parts of administrators, politicians, and insurance companies have discernable effects upon the lives of vulnerable populations, whether they live in South Africa or the South Bronx. In both contexts, the common questions are these: Do those in institutional powers value all persons and communities equally? Do stereotypes around race, socioeconomic class, ethnicity, culture and education come into play in ways that affect a person or community's access to or quality of care? These questions pertain not only to nations within the Two-Thirds World, but they are also highly relevant for U.S. healthcare settings, even as we pride ourselves on democratic principles and some of the best (and most expensive) healthcare in the world.

The "axis of (in)access," then, refers to the formidable obstacles posed by the interlocking realities of racial inequalities/stereotypes, poverty, and a lack of adequate insurance. In various combinations, these three components frustrate the attempts by numerous members of U.S. society to access equal, decent, and affordable healthcare. Indeed, one could ask these questions: Do enough professionals—hospital CEOs, physicians, insurance company and Medicaid administrators, pharmaceutical executives, politicians—see vulnerable persons and honor their full personhood? Do they adequately perceive the multiple obstacles and stressors that they confront on a regular basis? How do their policies and programs respond to these issues and barriers? Do their responses place an inordinate burden on the individual to make up the difference? In other words, do they ask vulnerable persons and communities to prove they are worthy of care or drug therapies—to find ways to work out all of the complications of their lives that are not directly related to a medical condition (childcare, racial assumptions or prejudice, transportation, rent, food money, neighborhood violence)— so that they can get to the doctor appointment on time, wait for hours if needed, and follow the prescribed treatment plan to the letter? Such questions merit sustained and self-critical reflection. Whether or not a given healthcare provider or policy expert adequately perceives the heavy demands and terrible choices with which such communities wrestle can make an enormous difference in both the present quality and future prospects of these lives.

In brief, there are many levels and nuances of access-related issues that bleed into quality of care issues. Quality and access concerns flow back and forth, continually complicating one another. Understanding the ways in which insurance affects both quality and access, it is then possible to consider in more depth forms of inequalities that cannot be fully accounted for by insurance status alone.

Beyond the Insurance Threshold: Additional Factors Contributing to Healthcare Inequalities

Vast amounts of literature document numerous kinds of disparities in healthcare that insured communities of color regularly confront. In its landmark review of more than 100 studies investigating these health-care inequalities, the Institute of Medicine (IOM) found ample evidence of widespread disparities—across medical conditions, regions, and healthcare contexts. The IOM summarizes its findings in unambiguous terms:

> Racial and ethnic minorities tend to receive a lower quality of health-care than non-minorities, even when access-related factors, such as patients' insurance status and income, are controlled. The sources of these disparities are complex, are rooted in historic and contemporary inequities, and involve many participants at several levels, including health systems, their administrative and bureaucratic processes, utilization managers, healthcare professionals, and patients. Consistent with the charge, the study committee focused part of its analysis on the clinical encounter itself, and found evidence that stereotyping, biases, and uncertainty on the part of healthcare providers can all contribute to unequal treatment. The conditions in which many clinical encounters

take place—characterized by high time pressure, cognitive complexity, and pressures for cost-containment—may enhance the likelihood that these processes will result in care poorly matched to minority patients' needs. Minorities may experience a range of other barriers in accessing care, even when insured at the same level as whites, including barriers of language, geography, and cultural familiarity. Further financial and institutional arrangements of health systems, as well as the legal, regulatory, and policy environment in which they operate, may have disparate and negative effects on minorities' ability to attain quality care.[56]

Most often, the literature reveals the evidence of racial-ethnic disparities in the amount and type of medical care received along with the outcomes of such care. For example, studies document that people of color experience disparities in terms of follow-up, aggressive treatment, and access to referrals. Common areas of research have included the differences in renal transplantation referrals, mental health, cancer screenings, and cardiac care.[57]

For example, one recent study found that Black Medicare patients enrolled in managed care health plans were significantly less likely than others to receive breast cancer screenings, eye exams if they had diabetes, beta-block use after a myocardial infarction, and follow-up after hospitalization for mental illness.[58] All of these disparities diminished once socioeconomic factors (income, education, Medicaid, rural versus urban) were controlled, but they were still statistically significant even after this adjustment. The researchers conclude the following:

> Our descriptive analysis of the interaction of race with health plan characteristics suggests that a subset of health plans (for-profit, decentralized model types, and health plans in some regions of the United States) may need to make special efforts to improve rates of breast cancer screening. For the other 3 clinical services we studied, the similarity of disparities across all categories of health plans suggests that all health plans should attend to racial disparities in care.[59]

As this study indicates, racial disparities in the amount and quality of care are not localized anomalies found in only a few regions or care settings. While not experienced to the same degree or in the same ways everywhere, disparities are nonetheless widespread, entrenched in one form or another within the U.S. healthcare system.

The IOM study committee underscores the fact that racial-ethnic disparities occur at two fundamental levels: Systemic and individual. Their analysis distinguishes between these two, identifying in turn kinds of disparities that have to do with how systems function and those that relate to interpersonal dynamics between patients and caregivers. While this distinction is helpful in organizing such voluminous data, it is important to note that systemic and interpersonal dynamics mutually shape and reshape one another. Individual care providers work, and have been trained in, particular systems that have their own cultures and significantly affect how care providers both view and carry out their responsibilities. For their part, individuals bring their values and perspectives to these care systems and can contribute to, and/or alter, the vision and procedures of these institutions.

The following discussion identifies three sources of healthcare disparities that cannot be accounted for solely by using the lens of insurance status: Language and cultural competency barriers, the existence of bias and stereotypes, and healthcare system bureaucracies. In naming these three, it is important to note that both systems and individuals are implicated in each. Language barriers and bias, for example, are not problems that can be solved merely by individual initiative. On the other hand, lamenting the tedious and complicated ways that healthcare systems function ought not be a way to excuse healthcare practitioners from their obligation to think critically and independently regarding decisions and interactions with patients. Both individuals and systems are responsible for the ways in which they perpetuate disparities.

Language Barriers and Poor Cultural Competency Skills

This discussion on language and cultural competency barriers focuses on Latino populations. However, they are certainly not the only ones who suffer due to shortcomings in this area. Various languages and cultures can clash in healthcare settings in sometimes tragic ways. For example, Anne Fadiman masterfully documents the extended collision between a Hmong family and their white, western doctors in California.[60] Indeed, many linguistic/cultural communities would benefit from the presence of increased professional translation services and culturally competent practices. Moreover, research specifically focusing on the numerous Asian, Asian American, Pacific Islander, and Indigenous communities living in the United States is very much needed in order to know how they are impacted by quality of care disparities.[61]

The rationale for a focus on Latinos stems from the dual facts that they have been largely underrepresented in healthcare policy research and that they represent significant proportions of the U.S. general population, of the impoverished, and of the uninsured.[62] In addition, more data in the area of language translation is available for them than any other linguistic group. Moreover, Latinos often do not get the same amount or quality of care even when insured.[63] Finally, Latinos do much of the grunt work that keeps this nation running. In large numbers, Latinos work in areas of hard physical labor: Assembly lines, textile and fabric industries, construction sites, fields, home and business custodial care, and meat-packing plants.[64] Overall, they work hard and long at physically demanding tasks, are not paid well, and far too many do not receive health benefits from their employers.[65]

There are many levels of linguistic and cultural understanding. Adequate communication across two languages is the most basic. Even when rudimentary understanding across languages is present, however, other degrees of mutual understanding may not be. In what follows, I will discuss a couple of these levels, beginning with the most fundamental, in order to develop a sense of what is needed to achieve comprehensive understanding.

Presently, approximately 14 million U.S. inhabitants do not speak or understand English fluently. Professional translators can make an important difference in the quality of communication. "Physicians who have access to trained interpreters report a significantly higher quality of patient-physician communication than do physicians who used other methods."[66] A 1998 study compared the degree of understanding and satisfaction among Spanish-speaking patients proficient in English with Spanish-speaking patients who were not. The patients who did not need a translator were more likely to report that the side effects of medications were explained and also greater satisfaction with their care.[67] In fact, limited English proficiency is often cited as a pivotal reason for the underutilization of medical services by Latinos.[68] For example, a 2002 study compared the results of Latinos who speak English fluently with those who do not and found the following: "After adjustment for predisposing factors, English-speaking Hispanic patients displayed a use pattern similar to non-Hispanic white patients. In contrast, Spanish-speaking Hispanic patients had a significantly lower likelihood than non-Hispanic white patients of having had a physician visit, visit with a mental health provider, influenza vaccination, or mammogram."[69] All 31,003 participants (18–64 years old) of this study were insured, either by private insurance or Medicaid. Thus, another possible explanation for underuse, namely being undocumented, is not as likely here.

Upon assessing the findings of recent studies on language barriers, one group of healthcare policy analysts summarizes the scope of the problematic consequences for Latino patients:

> Research in this area has shown that Spanish-speaking patients discharged from emergency rooms are less likely than their English-speaking counterparts to understand their diagnosis, prescribed mediations, special instructions, and plans for follow-up care; less likely to be satisfied or willing to return if they had a problem; more likely to report problems with their care; and less satisfied with the patient-provider relationship.[70]

Language barriers clearly compromise healthcare quality in several ways and have various effects even when Spanish-speaking Latino patients have comparable insurance to English-speaking patients. Yet adequate language translation services are often not made a priority in every care setting where they are needed.

Indeed, professional translators are often not utilized as often as they are needed. In one 1996 study, 467 Spanish-speaking patients and 63 English-speaking patients who came to a hospital emergency room with nonurgent medical problems were surveyed. The researchers found that translation was provided to just 26 percent of the Spanish-speaking patients. They report,

> 52% of the Spanish-speaking patients who were seen without a translator felt that interpretation was not necessary, but an additional 22% of the patients who did not receive interpretation felt that it was necessary. Of the patients who received interpretation services, almost half (49%) received interpretation services by a physician or nurse. But when both the providers' Spanish and the patients' English were poor, interpretation was not called in over one third (34%) of encounters. In these instances, 87% of patients felt an interpreter should have been called.[71]

Reasons for this lack of use are both logistical and financial. The use of translators is largely up to the discretion of the care provider, not the patient. It can take time to find a trained translator, if one is even available, within the hospital. Many times, doctors cannot, or do not wish, to wait. The care provider may be satisfied with the degree of communication and understanding they perceive in the exchange unaided by an interpreter. In addition, professional translation services can be expensive and may not be provided for within hospital budgets. Indeed, to my knowledge, insurance companies, Medicaid, and Medicare cannot be billed for translation services provided. Thus, any costs related to them cannot be recouped by the healthcare provider or institution.

Given these facts, some hospitals have a volunteer team of trained translators; however, since they are just that, they are not always available or in adequate supply to meet the needs of everyone. Other hospitals rely on telephone translation services. This service is expensive, and, given logistics, its use may limit the time a patient and family has to get all of their questions answered. Once the telephone is hung up, the time for clarification is also up. Also, a disembodied voice interpreting may feel a bit impersonal to some patients.[72]

Many times, instead of using professional translators, doctors and other staff will use whatever knowledge they have of the patient's language to communicate important medical information. There is a wide range of skill level in doing so and even if providers are able to convey certain information, this ability does not ensure that they will correctly understand comments or questions on the part of the patient. The problem with such practices is that there may appear to be sufficient communication between a patient and caregiver, at least from the provider's perspective, when in actuality there are significant gaps in mutual understanding. Hurried doctors may settle for a rough medical and social history and use medical tests to fill in the blanks.[73] In these cases, they may adequately communicate that the patient is going to have tests and what they are, but the reasons for these tests may not be as clear to the patient and/or family.

Often, when patients and healthcare providers cannot communicate sufficiently in the same language, an ad hoc translator will translate. These persons can be a family member, another staff person (a nurse, member of the custodial staff, desk clerk), or another patient. While on the surface these strategies may seem to suffice, they also pose particular problems. It can be emotionally difficult for a family member to translate for their loved one. For example, they may be charged to convey "bad news," or they may be put in the awkward position of having to ask their parent or sibling about their sexual history. I have personally witnessed children (youth well under the age of 18) who have translated for their hospitalized parent and other family members in the room. For their part, while hospital staff may speak the patient's language well (it may even be their first language) they may lack formal translation training. One study analyzed actual ad hoc translator situations and found that "23%–52% of words and phrases were incorrectly interpreted."[74] In the absence of training, hospital staff, other patients and family members may not know the needed medical terminology even as they may be willing to help.

In short, for a number of reasons, ad hoc translators may fail to translate well everything that either the patient or doctor says. Instead, due to the emotional difficulty, other family dynamics, or a lack of knowledge of medical and physiological terms, such translators may condense or alter information. They may rephrase what the doctor is saying without retaining the same degree of specificity. They may also fail to convey the breadth and depth of patient concerns and questions. Furthermore, both patient privacy and confidentiality are concerns. Staff may share inappropriate information with others in the hospital or clinic. Family members may be given (and pass on) information that the patient does not want divulged.

As serious as these concerns are, an absence of qualified translators is just the tip of the iceberg in terms of barriers to adequate communication. Indeed, while many current studies emphasize a lack of patient understanding due to limited English skills and a lack of translators, it is also critical to stress that providers may be missing things as well. Beyond the possibility that they may not correctly or adequately understand a patient's language, they may very well miss other important but more subtle cultural clues. It is not sufficient to make sure that the patient understands the provider's words, instructions, and information. The provider needs to understand the patient just as well, if not more so.

Indeed, the significance of language and cultural understanding goes far beyond whether crucial facts of someone's health, medical history, or present ailment are conveyed between patient and provider; this is merely "triage"—what is minimally necessary. It is the *beginning* of understanding and effective communication, not its culmination. However, it is the level most regularly reached in healthcare contexts. Given time, workload, and cognitive demands (and perhaps a lack of interest on the part of some providers) more advanced levels of shared understanding and respect are not as often achieved.

In particular, a physician's ability to communicate across languages and cultures is imperative for the delivery of quality care. This competence must include an understanding and appreciation of sociocultural differences related to values, health beliefs, and behaviors. As one example, how patients report and experience pain often varies across cultures. Not all will experience or articulate the same symptoms.[75]

Communication barriers along with a lack of shared cultural understanding strain patient-provider relationships. Many healthcare providers themselves are aware of the weight of linguistic and cultural differences. A 2001 survey published of Los Angeles physicians

> who participate in the "Healthy Families" programs, L.A. Care (the
> local health authority of Los Angeles County) found 71% of providers
> believe that language and culture are important in the delivery of care to
> patients. Slightly over half (51%) believe that their patients did not
> adhere to medical treatments as a result of cultural or linguistic barriers.
> Yet over half of these providers (56%) report not having had any form
> of cultural competency training.[76]

Indeed, *both* cultural and linguistic barriers can lead to poor understanding, which then results in patient dissatisfaction and/or poor adherence to treatment plans as well as to disease prevention strategies.[77]
Moreover, these shortcomings can frustrate efforts at building trust
between patients and providers.

In sum, a sophisticated degree of linguistic and cultural understanding is important on a number of levels. In particular, providers
need to understand and appreciate the particular cultures, religions,
and socioeconomic contexts of their patients. Beyond the fact that
such understanding enhances the likelihood that patients will follow
through with treatment regimens, appointments, and prescriptions if
they fully understand why doing so is beneficial (and why not doing so
would be detrimental), it also creates empathy—a vital component in
provider-patient relationships.[78] Doctors who understand how their
patients conceive of health and quality of life issues are often better
able to come to decisions with the patient that correspond well with
patient values and priorities. They are able to collaborate effectively
with the patient because they are attuned to hearing and understanding
both the content of and the rationale behind patient preferences and
needs.[79]

For Latinos, these cross-cultural sensitivities and abilities are especially important because there are so few Latino physicians. The
Association of American Medical Colleges reports that as of 2000,
Latino graduates comprise 2.25 percent of the total population of
medical graduates.[80] This figure mirrors the percentage of Latino
physicians that is approximately 2 percent of the total number of doctors
nationally.[81] In September 2004, the Sullivan Commission on Diversity
in the Workforce reported that even though together they account for
over 25 percent of the national U.S. population, Blacks, Native
Americans, and Hispanics only comprise "nine percent of the nation's
nurses, six percent of doctors and five percent of dentists."[82] Given the

size of Latino communities within the general population (14 percent of the total), such small numbers of Latino physicians and graduates fall far below what is needed in order to care for an increasingly diverse and complex society. Some research supports the notion that care providers may often understand descriptions of symptoms better from members of groups who are racially, culturally, linguistically, and/or socioeconomically similar to them. For example, a white male doctor may pick up more on important clues when speaking with a white male patient than when he listens to a Latina woman who speaks limited English.[83]

Provider Bias and Stereotypes

Here is where things can get a bit dicey for some. Healthcare practitioners, perhaps most especially physicians and nurses, are enculturated by their professional training to hold tightly to egalitarian principles. The Hippocratic Oath, dearly known to every physician, insists that doctors be uncompromisingly committed to the well-being and alleviation of suffering of every patient she or he treats. "Physicians are generally expected and expect themselves to be unaffected by the patient's social or demographic characteristics in forming judgments of patients. . . . [They] are generally expected to view each patient objectively and impartially, using biomedical information obtained from physical examination and diagnostic test results to develop a diagnosis and effective treatment plan."[84] Doctors are trained to zero in on medical conditions and physiological clues, and to find the best course of treatment for each person—without taking into account race, class, insurance status, language, culture, or sexual orientation.[85] The idea that healthcare providers would favor the lives of some over others goes against every ethos ingrained within the healing professions. In fact, to suggest so would be deeply offensive to many.

So how could it be that of all people, healthcare professionals—those with an explicit mission to care, heal, help—might view or treat patients differently on the basis of race and/or socioeconomic class? Overall as a society, perhaps we expect a lot of our care providers, especially physicians. Many of us expect them to fix us "like new," to delay (or at least hide) our aging, to keep our libidos active, to help us beat our cancer, to prevent that next heart attack, to buy us more time. Perhaps, we tend to hold them to a higher ethical standard as well. And in so doing, perhaps we may forget that they are human—limited in knowledge and abilities by particular social contexts, and susceptible to all the other nagging imperfections that come with being mere mortals. Of course, to acknowledge their humanity does not excuse ignorance.

While numerous researchers have long documented the fact that insurance status and socioeconomic status (SES) (and more recently, language and cultural barriers) create serious disparities in the quality of care that communities of color receive, a few more recent studies make the case that provider perceptions harm these communities as well.[86] While the IOM and others are cautious in citing direct links, more and more healthcare researchers acknowledge that there are important indications of such a connection.[87] A. I. Balsa and T.G. McGuire have elaborated a theoretical framework that distinguishes three ways in which providers may (often unwittingly) discriminate against communities of color. Specifically, they cite provider prejudice, greater clinical uncertainty, and beliefs and stereotypes about such communities.[88] There is the least concrete evidence documenting overt prejudice or racism active in healthcare systems or provider practices.[89] However, significant empirical findings support the claim that both stereotypes and clinical uncertainty negatively affect patients of color.

In 2000, Michelle van Ryn and Jane Burke published results from a study of 842 patient encounters with cardiac physicians in New York State. In all, 193 physicians provided information on 618 of these encounters. Of these 618 encounters, 57 percent of the patients surveyed were white and 43 percent were African American; 53 percent were male and 47 percent female; and 84 percent of the encounters took place with white doctors.[90] The summary of their findings merits extended quotation:

> Black CAD patients were more likely to be seen as at risk for noncompliance with cardiac rehabilitation, substance abuse, and having inadequate social support. In addition, physicians rated Black patients as less intelligent than White patients, even when patient sex, age, income and education were controlled. Physicians also report less affiliative feelings toward Black patients.
>
> In general, physicians gave lower SES patients more negative ratings on personality characteristics (lack of self-control, irrationality) and level of intelligence. In addition, lower SES patients were rated as less likely to be compliant with cardiac rehabilitation, less likely to desire a physically active lifestyle, less likely to have significant career demands, less likely to have responsibility for care of a family member and more likely to be judged to be at risk for inadequate social support. Again, the effect of patient SES on physician perception remained when patient age, sex, race, frailty/sickness, depression, mastery and social assertiveness as well as physician characteristics were controlled.[91]

Thus, doctors' perceptions of their Black and lower socioeconomic class patients fell into common stereotypes of these populations. Strengths of this quantitative study are that it explores the dynamics of actual clinical encounters and samples a relatively significant number of patients and physicians.

One might counter that the physicians surveyed did not stereotype patients, but rather accurately assessed the patient's background, life situation, and preferences. The authors themselves note that there is a positive correlation between lower socioeconomic class and less exercise and that most of the Black patient participants did have fewer years of education than white patients. The doctors' perceptions of these differences remained, however, *even when the actual facts of a patient's case contradicted such views.* Even when Black patients had the same level of education as whites, they were more likely to be described by their doctor as less intelligent, less educated, and less rational. Similarly, in the cases of patients who reported that they were responsible for the care of others and that they worked several hours a week, these facts, too, were not reflected in physician perceptions.[92]

Doctors can make assumptions that limit what they see when looking at patients. The authors offer this explanation of their findings: "Physicians may fail to correctly incorporate individual diagnostic data, instead being swayed by their beliefs regarding the probabilities of individuals in a socio-economic category having a given characteristic."[93] Population-based generalities may be grafted onto certain individuals, even if there are specific facts that contradict such generalization. Simply put, doctors may not always see the actual person in front of them but instead see only a generic representative of a larger group. The question at the crux of this book surfaces here: What does it take for each and every person to be seen and treated *as* a person, in her or his own right, and not merely as an individual embodiment of a stereotype?

There are additional unsettling aspects to these findings. Specifically, van Ryn and Burke found that doctors had less affiliative feelings toward their Black and/or lower socioeconomic class patients—the same patients they tended to rate as less intelligent and rational. The doctors rated these patients as "less pleasant" than their white and higher socioeconomic class counterparts.[94] As mentioned above, the presence or absence of empathy and affinity can influence both the provider's behavior toward the patient and the patient's degree of trust, satisfaction, and adherence to a suggested treatment plan.[95] "When patients perceive that physicians like them, care about them and are interested in them as a person, they are likely to volunteer more information and be more active in the encounter, more satisfied, and more compliant with medical regimens."[96] Van Ryn and Burke cite numerous studies that demonstrate that doctors' attitudes, perceptions, and beliefs influence their behavior toward patients and that patients' satisfaction and behavior are affected by the attitudes of their doctors.[97]

Finally, it is important to highlight one other finding of van Ryn and Burke's study. The authors found that physicians spent less time in their encounters with Black and/or lower-socioeconomic-class patients. Given their findings and that of other related research, van Ryn and Burke note the disturbing possibility that it is conceivable that doctors "may be less likely to listen to or respect the contribution of patients who are perceived as less intelligent or rational."[98] In addition, they also cite other studies that document that doctors give less information to darker skinned patients and to those of lower socioeconomic classes than they do to lighter skinned and affluent patients. The authors hypothesize that physicians' differences in perceptions of intelligence, rationality, and education may, in part, account for these disconcerting facts.

While this data cannot be taken as evidence that such biases by doctors are the norm—across regions, healthcare settings, and medical specialty—still the findings cannot be dismissed lightly. Other studies support such data with related findings of their own. Moreover, even if such perceptions and tendencies are not equally evident everywhere, or not found in every physician, they are nonetheless potent wherever they do exist.

Yet, it may be likely that they are more common than not, given the predominance of similar biases in the larger society.[99] One recent study published in 2000 examined the assumptions of first- and second-year medical students. Saif Rathore et al. randomly asked 164 medical students (57 percent male, 86 percent white, 14 percent racial-ethnic minorities) to view either a video of a Black female or white male patient actor who used an identical script containing sufficient clinical symptoms for a definite diagnosis of angina.[100] The researchers found that overall the students assigned a lower value to the quality of life or health status of the Black woman than to the white man, even though they had identical symptoms. "The quality-of-life ratings for the black woman were lower, yet students considered the white male patient actor's condition to be more severe. . . ."[101] The students were also less likely to identify the Black female patient's symptoms as definitely angina. She was also viewed as "friendlier, a better communicator, and as having more positive affect than the white male patient actor. However, [she] was perceived to be less likely to obtain follow-up care."[102] Interestingly, however, the medical students of color *did not* differ in their assessments of the quality of life of the two patients (meaning they did not express a bias that determined the white patient's quality of life to be better than the Black patient's), but instead they rated the two similarly.[103]

These findings lead the authors to conclude the following:

> If patient race or sex influences physician recommendations about treatment, then our study indicates that these biases may be present at the earliest stages of medical training. Our subjects were first and second year medical students who had not been acculturated to clinical medicine. They lacked clinical experience that may have influenced perceptions about the effects of race and sex on coronary disease. Thus, differences in diagnosis and health state rating may derive from preformed ideas brought to medical training. These biases may not be conscious but may still influence clinical decisions. These findings are consistent with reports of race and sex bias in the general population.[104]

The researchers understand that biases around race and sex do not originate in medical school, but instead reflect biases and assumptions present within the larger society. Even more, some medical school programs may reinforce them in particular ways, especially if they tend to emphasize the doctor's expertise and superior knowledge over that of patients. Consequently, unless intentionally addressed in the curriculum, the experience of medical school will not necessarily interrogate or alter these stereotypes present within the mindsets of many students. Healthcare systems are a microcosm of society—not an escape from it. Indeed, they can constitute a concrete ground in which larger structural and social inequalities and biases are played out. Far from being immune to such social ills, healthcare—embedded in a particular sociopolitical context—can replicate them in their sites of care.

More studies investigating the relationship among provider beliefs, perceptions, and behaviors as they relate to race and SES, the experiences and degree of patient satisfaction and clinical outcomes for patients of color are needed. Yet to date, enough quantitative evidence exists to make the case that such beliefs and perceptions negatively affect both provider behavior and patient outcomes and that they thus contribute to quality of care disparities. For example, Michelle van Ryn followed up her 2000 study with a well-documented article in 2002 that reviews current literature and findings related to these issues.[105] She first summarizes the research related to four medical problems (kidney transplants, cardiac procedures, psychiatric treatment, and treatment of pain) and how racial-ethnic disparities have been shown to influence the amount and kind of information given to the patient, the amount and kind of referrals made, and the kind and degree of actual treatments administered.

To note just one illustration, I will highlight her findings with respect to mental health.[106] Van Ryn explains,

> [P]rovider bias has been most heavily studied in relation to mental health services, resulting in substantial evidence that patient race/ethnicity influences psychiatrists' clinical decision-making. Both United States and British psychiatrists are more likely to prescribe antipsychotic medications, hospitalize involuntarily, and place nonwhite patients in seclusion once hospitalized than their white counterparts, independent of appropriateness and clinical factors.[107]

Van Ryn goes on to cite research indicating that Black patients are more likely to be diagnosed as schizophrenic but less likely to have their depression diagnosed. Simply put, unchecked (sometimes subtle and hard to pin down) biases can have very tangible and deleterious consequences for patients.[108]

Thus, the presence and potency of stereotypes operative within healthcare seem hard to dispute. Yet a question remains, How exactly do they function? Similar to van Ryn's incorporation of social cognition literature, the IOM drew upon the sociological analyses of J.F. Dovidio and others to flesh out the ways in which stereotypes and biases function and to understand their effects.[109] They define stereotypes as a "process by which people use social categories (e.g., race, sex) in acquiring, processing, and recalling information about others. The beliefs (stereotypes) and general orientations (attitudes) . . . help organize and simplify complex or uncertain situations and give perceivers greater confidence in their ability to understand a situation and respond in efficient and effect ways."[110] This definition understands that stereotypes are a common means for helping to make sense of and organize a complex world.[111] However, I would add the caveat that while they may increase "efficiency" in navigating one's world, they ought not be understood as benign. Indeed, one of their most nefarious attributes is that they are not recognized for what they are but are taken to be accurate observations of reality.

Social psychologists emphasize that stereotypes often function at an unconscious level and may be present within persons and communities who hold overtly egalitarian principles. They also explain that stereo-types tend to be self-perpetuating, evidence of which was seen in van Ryn and Burke's 2000 study discussed above. As they extend them-selves, stereotypes may create self-fulfilling prophecies in which doctors' assumptions encourage the very responses they anticipate. To illustrate, if patients feel less respected and listened to, they are more likely not only to be dissatisfied with their care, but also to fail to follow through with treatments and appointments. This behavior then reinforces the physician's stereotype that initially assumed the patient would be "noncompliant" or "a problem." It is also important to add that if, in general, stereotypes shape how information is interpreted, then their power may be even greater in the case of interactions and relationships across cultural, racial-ethnic, linguistic, and socio-economic class lines.[112]

The implications of the ways that stereotypes function are many. First, since they are commonly used by human beings, physicians, nurses, social workers, healthcare administrators, and insurance repre-sentatives are not immune to them. Second, stereotypes often filter new information so that any information that might contradict the stereo-type is not emphasized or seen by the person holding the stereotype. Third, and perhaps most significant for healthcare contexts, stereotypes are often invoked automatically, almost as a reflex, in unconscious ways. They do not need to be consciously owned to be operative.

Indeed, physicians and healthcare professionals may be especially prone to stereotypes. They work within context of high cognitive and time-pressure demands, which may make the unconscious use of stereotypes all the more pernicious:

> There is evidence that time pressure, the need to make quick judgments, cognitive load, task complexity, and "busyness" increase the likelihood of stereotype usage. Physicians may be especially vulnerable to the use of stereotypes in forming impressions of patients since time pressure, brief encounters, and the need to manage very complex cognitive tasks are common characteristics of their work.[113]

Hectic, complex, high-pressure environs incubate stereotypes, which then serve as a "survival" strategy in managing large amounts of infor-mation and in making critical decisions. Doctors in particular are trained to take "cognitive shortcuts" so that they may arrive at treatment deci-sions with great efficiency. What is important to realize is that even if there are benefits to their use, there are also discernable costs to taking these shortcuts.

In addition to the pace and pressure inherent in most healthcare settings, Balsa and McGuire theorize that the inevitability of clinical uncertainty fuels healthcare quality disparities for vulnerable populations in particular.[114] Despite technological advances, many healthcare professionals and researchers alike emphasize that much discretion and ambiguity are still integral parts of medical treatment.[115] When care providers are less certain of the information they receive from patients, they may substitute tests or simply make an educated guess based on what they observe. Consequently, clinical uncertainty does not necessarily mean that patients of color and/or lower socioeconomic class patients receive *less* care than white and/or affluent patients. Instead, they may also be more at risk of receiving care that is *more poorly matched* to their specific needs. For example, they may have more tests ordered than a white, English-speaking patient might if the tests substitute for a substantive medical history created through mutually informative dialogue between patient and provider.

To summarize, it is critical to see that the levels of ideation, perception—and even unconscious beliefs and assumptions—have concrete, often devastatingly real, effects upon human lives. Healthcare providers cannot be expected to be exempt from what are human tendencies. The problem is not that doctors, nurses, and social workers work within subjective analyses and perspectives that limit their objectivity. Instead, the problem is a lack of awareness of, and accountability for, this fact. Under the guise of objectivity, caregivers may fail to account for the ways in which they filter information through subjective assumptions. In doing so, the accuracy and adequacy of their interpretation of the symptoms and the social conditions of patients, who are often noticeably different from them in terms of racial/ethnic/cultural and socioeconomic-class background, may unknowingly be warped. Furthermore, if they miss seeing the patient at this juncture, it is also possible they will miss finding, and communicating, the best and most appropriate course of treatment for the patient.[116] At worst, healthcare providers may even fail to present options or other important information out of an assumption that the patient will not follow through with the therapy prescribed or is not deserving of it.

The Bureaucracy of Healthcare Systems

The United States spends a lot of money on healthcare. How much? As of 2004, health spending accounted for close to 15 percent of the nation's economy. In 2002, healthcare spending equaled $1.55 trillion, which means that on average, the United States spends $5,440 per person on healthcare each year.[117] (In comparison, in 2001 the United States spent $4,887 while Canada spent $2,792.)[118] According to 2001 data, the United States spent 13.9 percent of the total gross domestic product (GDP) while the median expenditure for other industrialized (OECD [Organization for Economic Cooperation and Development]) nations was just 8.3 percent.[119] The question then becomes: Are we the best—is U.S. healthcare worth the high price tag? Canadians live on average two and one half years longer than U.S. citizens. Spaniards also live two years longer and the Japanese live almost four longer than those in the United States.[120] Emilio Carrillo et al. highlight an embarrassing irony: "The health care system in the United States is the most expensive and yet arguably among the least cost effective in the developed world. Despite the highest per person health care spending among the Organization for Economic Cooperation and Development (OECD) nations, the United States still ranks below many along a variety of health indicators."[121] Indeed, U.S. healthcare does not compare as favorably as many Americans assume it would to that of other countries.

For example, the World Health Organization (WHO) reported in 2000 that "[t]he U.S. health system spends a higher portion of its gross domestic product than any other country but ranks 37 out of 191 countries according to its performance. . . . The United Kingdom, which spends just six percent of its gross domestic product (GDP) on health services, ranks 18th."[122] Being ranked thirty-seventh puts the United States between Costa Rica and Slovenia. Specifically, the WHO looked at five indicators to determine the ranking:

> [O]verall level of population health; health inequalities (or disparities) within the population; overall level of health system responsiveness (a combination of patient satisfaction and how well the system acts); distribution of responsiveness within the population (how well people of varying economic status find that they are served by the health system); and distribution of health system's financial burden within the population (who pays the costs).[123]

Of these five criteria, the United States was ranked at the top only in terms of overall health system responsiveness. In terms of the fairness of distribution of the financial burden of healthcare, the United States ranks 54 among the nations. With respect to health indicators such as infant mortality, life expectancy, and immunizations, the United States consistently ranks in the range of 20–25. In addition, among the OECD nations, only six others had a slower growth rate of physician and nurse to population ratios than the United States. According to 2001 data, nationally, the United States has 2.7 physicians and 8.1 nurses per 1,000 persons in the population. From 1991 to 2001, the "supply of U.S. physicians per capita grew only 1 percent per year. . . ."[124]

To illustrate the significance of these statistics, let us look briefly at infant mortality rates. According to the CIA *World Factbook* and a recent report from the Centers for Disease Control (CDC) the U.S. infant mortality rate is 7 per 1,000 live births, meaning that seven babies die for each thousand live births. This rate is significantly higher than that of Singapore (2.3), Sweden (3.4), Japan (3.2), France (4.6), and Denmark (5.3). In all, 41 countries have a better infant mortality rate than the United States, including Cuba. Nicholas Kristof, reporting on these statistics, puts the numbers in context: "If we had a rate as good as Singapore's, we would save 18,900 babies each year. . . . [W]omen are 70% more likely to die in childbirth in America than in Europe. . . . For all their ruthlessness, China's dictators have managed to drive down the infant mortality rate in Beijing to 4.6 per thousand; in contrast, New York City's rate is 6.5."[125] It is startling that the United States spends the most on healthcare of any nation, yet we are not ranked even close to the top ten in terms of so many indicators of good health and performance.

In short, U.S. healthcare consumers pay among the highest bills for services that are not consistently excellent. Nationally, there is significant variation in healthcare quality, depending both on the comprehensiveness of one's insurance as well as on the site in which the care is given. While there are important differences among healthcare contexts (HMOs, teaching hospitals, public hospitals and clinics, urban versus rural healthcare), it is nonetheless true that in all contexts, there are significant pressures stemming from finite time and funds. All aspects of the healthcare industry are in the business of cost containment, whether for survival or profit maximization.

This insight does not mean that all public hospitals are inherently inferior to private ones, or that all teaching hospitals are better than HMOs. It *does* mean that holes and leaky patches in the overall quality of U.S. healthcare prevent this nation from boasting to others that "while we may be the most expensive, we're also the best." Nationally, U.S. inhabitants receive uneven care and may often suffer the anxiety and stress of hustling to make sure that they get into one of "good sites" instead of one of the "flunkies." When one takes into account the collective costs of healthcare services, prescription drugs, insurance premiums, and co-payments—all of which are ever increasing—it is possible to argue that U.S. consumers of healthcare are not getting the best value for their dollar. Some might even contend that they are getting taken to the cleaners.

While noting that line of argument, I will instead focus upon what Carrillo et al. observe next: "In a complicated health care system where the rules are many and economic forces drive both structure and function, the needs of vulnerable populations inevitably suffer."[126] To illustrate, while the long lines and waits, in addition to the laborious intakes and admission processes, can be aggravating for all, they can rise to the level of prohibitive hurdles for some. In short, the burdens and frustrations of current healthcare configurations do not have the same consequences for every person who confronts them.

For example, it is likely that all U.S. healthcare consumers have battled with seemingly endless piles of forms and bills/account statements, automated telephone trees, insurance representatives, and even harried desk clerks and receptionists at some point or other.[127] Yet not all are affected in the same way or degree. The IOM notes, "Maneuvering through the bureaucratic and administrative 'maze' commonly found in modern hospitals and clinics is essential in accessing clinical resources, yet some racial and ethnic groups, for a variety of reasons, may experience less success in navigating through such bureaucracies."[128] Simply put, the sticky red tape of healthcare policies and reimbursement procedures may entangle vulnerable persons and communities more than white persons and/or those of higher socioeconomic classes.

Indeed, what might amount to a frustrating annoyance and loss of a couple of hours to an educated, assertive, English-speaking, white, middle-class person (who can afford to take time off of work) can translate into daunting and prohibitive obstacles for someone who does not speak or read English fluently and/or who does not have the luxury of "sick days" or time off for medical appointments. I do not mean to infer that people of color are less assertive, less intelligent, or less educated, or less able to advocate for themselves than others. The point is that they may find that they have to work harder to get through the bureaucratic maze due to certain realities not faced by a white, middle-class counterpart. For example, they may have to contend with stereotypes in a different way and when they advocate for themselves, rather than being respected as assertive, they may be viewed as "emotional" or "irrational."

Beyond paper and organizational mazes, geographic and physical ones also affect vulnerable communities in particular ways. As noted earlier, in addition to the need for more interpreter services, there is often a lack of language-appropriate health education materials and signs within hospitals and clinics. Many offices and care centers are not conveniently located within communities of color, which makes it hard for members of these communities to reach them via public transportation. The limited operating hours of some clinics and services can also present serious obstacles.[129] One group of researchers recently concluded after exploring racial-ethnic disparities within Medicare managed care that "having a usual source of care may not suffice to overcome financial barriers such as co-payments, or non-financial barriers, such as the location of facilities in areas with limited transportation, inadequate interpreter services, or a lack of cultural sensitivity on the part of clinicians or staff."[130] My sense is that partial fixes offered by state and federal health initiatives in lieu of overhauling the Medicare and Medicaid systems themselves may not resolve all of these logistical and location issues.

Present healthcare configurations are cumbersome for all involved—patients, families, and providers. In the best scenarios, all collaborate together to "work" the system so that bureaucratic obstacles are diminished rather than intensified. Current research indicates that mutual respect and understanding can be essential ingredients for achieving such collaboration.

Indeed, empathy contributes more than warm feelings between patients and their caregivers. It can also provide the impetus needed for care providers to the make extra effort to help patients and families negotiate what can be a tedious and overwhelming system. The presence of empathy, respect, and affinity on the part of care providers can make it more likely that the doctor will do all in her or his power to refer the patient to needed therapeutic services. Patient advocacy on the part of doctors plays a big role in a system where physicians have a lot of discretion in terms of what course of treatment they recommend and pursue, as well as one in which insurance utilization managers make decisions about what the insurance will or will not cover. In order to dispute a decline of coverage, patients need a strong medical advocate to advance their case and/or dispute the initial rejection. My concern is that darker skinned patients and/or lower socioeconomic classes may receive less advocacy from care providers who do not have the same degree of understanding and empathy that they do for lighter skinned and more affluent patients.

As it turns out, even when doctors attempt such advocacy, the desired results can be difficult to achieve. For example, it is a labor-intensive and time-consuming process to appeal a denial of insurance coverage. In a related vein, there are indications that when physicians of color make referrals for their patients, they may have more difficulty doing so than their white counterparts. The IOM cited a recent study that explored the experiences of physicians of color in referring their patients to specialists and in admitting them to hospitals. They report these findings:

> Controlling for physician characteristics (e.g., years in practice, gender, specialty, group or private practice, revenue from managed care, Medicaid, and Medicare) and market characteristics (e.g., local physician participation in managed care, supply of hospital beds, and specialists per capita), minority physicians were found to have greater difficulty in gaining access to care for their patients. Hispanic physicians were more likely to report problems with obtaining referrals for specialty care than their white colleagues, and African-American physicians reported experiencing greater difficulty than white physicians in arranging hospital admissions for their patients.[131]

Thus, not only do patients of color push up against bureaucratic walls more often than whites, but providers of color may do so as well. One study is not sufficient to prove definitively that such problems are experienced everywhere and more research is needed. Yet these findings ought to awaken us to the degree and complexity of racial-ethnic barriers to quality care and equal access that need to be addressed.

One final kind of bureaucracy merits a brief word. It is more abstract than reimbursement forms, automated telephone trees, and language appropriate signs, but it is just as important. It speaks to the culture of medicine and the medical gaze.[132] Mary-Jo DelVecchio Good and Byron J. Good underscore that implicit in all healthcare contexts is a gaze and culture that tend to reduce human beings to medical conditions and body parts. Through several decades of research, they have come to conclude that " 'the medical gaze' soon becomes the dominant knowledge frame through medical school, that time and efficiency are highly prized, and that students and their attending [physicians] are most caring of patients who are willing to become part of the medical story they wish to tell and the therapeutic activities they hope to pursue."[133] In this culture, physicians regularly screen out information that they deem as medically insignificant as they are predominantly interested in very specific questions related to the physiological history and facts of the patient.[134]

Good and Good note that in the last two decades, increasingly U.S. medical programs have integrated cultural competency and social medicine into their curricula, drawing upon materials from anthropology and sociology. However, these curricular changes have not helped students critically assess their own training or the implicit assumptions on which it is based. They observe,

> [M]any schools have produced formal and informal curricula, which on paper appear to be promoting cultural competence. Rarely, however, does medical training focus on the culture of medicine itself; rarely do students have the time or the formal sanction to critically analyze the profession and the institutions of care to examine how treatment choices, quality of care and research practices are shaped; or how medical culture may produce processes that evolve into institutional racism or aversive racism in clinical practice.[135]

Given this deficit, Good and Good are not surprised that racial-ethnic and socioeconomic disparities have not abated in U.S. healthcare. Moreover, this lack of transformation has led them to ask several questions. I will highlight just this one: "Does the culture of medicine—as exemplified in the medical gaze and its underlying ideologies and political economy of what constitutes legitimate medical knowledge, bioscience, and appropriate medical decision-making—too readily exclude patients whom clinicians assess as likely to pose 'problems' and compromise the efficacy and efficiency prized by the medical world?"[136] In their present work, Good and Good have begun to explore this question and I encourage readers to seek out their subsequent publications.

To be viewed with a narrow biomedical lens can be frustrating to any patient who wants to be seen as a whole person with a larger social history, life, and relationships. However, in the context of racial, ethnic, linguistic, cultural, and socioeconomic barriers, it can leave a darker skinned patient feeling even more alienated than her or his lighter skinned and/or affluent counterpart. Indeed, it is not that communities of color encounter problems that never happen to white patients. Rather, the point is that racial-ethnic disparities in the quality of care mean that darker skinned communities often experience particular and intensified kinds of alienation and frustration, even as lighter skinned and affluent communities may also experience similar frustrations and isolation in medical care. What is unique and so important about this research is that, in contrast to the vast majority of cultural competence literature and curricula, Good and Good call for self-critical research into the culture of medicine itself. This research is imperative because a predominant medical gaze may very well create yet another layer of bureaucratic and systemic healthcare inequalities for communities of color. In fact, such a constricted lens may contribute to rendering certain persons nearly invisible.

Implications of the Literature: Racial-Ethnic Disparities in Healthcare Quality Indict a Nation

Reviewing current literature makes it impossible to dispute the breadth and depth of racial-ethnic disparities in U.S. healthcare, although some have tried. H. Jack Geiger blew the whistle when officials within the U.S. Department of Health and Human Services (HHS) significantly edited and rewrote a portion of the first annual national report on disparities in healthcare for the most vulnerable in the United States. This report was written by the Agency for Healthcare Research and Quality (AHRQ), which is part of the HHS. Geiger says that the AHRQ had done its work well:

> Its draft report was a clear and massive presentation of the data on disparities in care associated with race, ethnicity and socioeconomic status. Its summary was blunt, noting that such disparities are "national problems that affect the health care at all points in the process, at all sites of care, and for all medical conditions," affecting health outcomes and entailing "a personal and societal price."[137]

However, Geiger goes on to reveal this fact:

> After "review" by HHS, those truthful words are gone, as are most references to race and ethnicity, now described as problems that existed "in the past." Prejudice is "not implied in any way." Disparities are simply called "differences," and—incredibly—"there is no implication that these differences result in adverse health outcomes."[138]

Following public outcry from healthcare researchers such as Geiger, then Secretary of the HHS, Tommy G. Thompson, told Congress, "There was a mistake made. It is going to be rectified."[139]

As a nation, we dare not turn from facing this profound and complex healthcare quality and access crisis. These disparities mean many troubling things for darker skinned communities in particular. They range from the most obvious—receiving less medical care and/or care poorly matched to their needs resulting in poor outcomes—to those harder to quantify—a lack of trust, understanding, and respect between darker skinned patients and lighter skinned providers, which then can mean less advocacy and assistance in navigating bureaucratic webs. Provider stereotypes and behaviors can play off and reinforce one another, which then leave the patient feeling alienated. As discussed above, if care providers view a patient as passive, unintelligent, emotional/irrational, or not very likeable, they may very well interact less and advocate less for her than they do for those they like and respect more.

Van Ryn and Burke summarize the significance of such interplay:

> This dynamic is especially worrisome because information flow and physician affective and affiliative behavior has been found to influence patient satisfaction, trust in physician competence, and the level of stress or anxiety experienced during the encounter. These factors, in combination with physician information and affect, are associated with patient adherence.[140]

Patients of color and/or lower socioeconomic class are especially vulnerable to the force of negative assumptions that can have palpable effects on their care. They may receive less information, may be considered inappropriate or unworthy candidates for certain medical interventions, and may feel less secure and more afraid than white and affluent patients.

Certainly, patients and families may come into the interaction with biases and assumptions of their own. They may not trust the provider, given other experiences they may have had in the past with healthcare or in other societal arenas. Thus, they may be more likely to misconstrue what care providers are saying to them out of a misunderstanding of the provider's culture, communication style or out of mistrust of the system or the provider. However, I concur with the IOM that healthcare institutions and providers of care are the more powerful actors in exchanges with patients and families. To a large degree, they determine the policies and boundaries with which the patient and family must contend. So, when language or cultural barriers exist or when negative assumptions and bias sour a provider-patient relationship, even if both parties have contributed to the situation, the lion's share of the responsibility goes to the provider and institution. The healthcare provider and system, given their relative power and the historical legacy of racism and prejudice both in U.S. healthcare (e.g., The Tuskegee Syphilis Study) and in the society at large, are also the ones most responsible for building trust and for breaking through patient fears and mistrust.

There are a couple of brief conclusions I wish to draw from this literature review: First, U.S. inhabitants must learn as a society that if the health of some is not valued and protected, the health of all suffers. This observation may seem an obvious truism at first. However, it actually seems to run counter to many mindsets in U.S. society. For many, healthcare is a commodity that one purchases through insurance or individual resources. The main goal is to access the best care available for one's self and one's dependents, through good insurance and long-term relationships with providers. The logic I sometimes hear is that if others are not able to gain entrance to the same quality of care, it is an unfortunate reality, that fact does not directly affect their own care or health per se. If a connection is made at all, it is made in terms of taxes; namely, the government's taxation of citizens to cover the escalating costs of Medicare, Medicaid, and treatment of the uninsured. This connection often leads people to denounce the presence of the poor, the unemployed, welfare mothers, and undocumented immigrants. Sadly, stereotypes can substitute for a reasoned assessment of these complicated social issues.

Yet, it is possible to make a different connection: This nation depends upon human labor. Even in the context of a technologically advanced society, it still needs human beings to do the hard work that others find unattractive—digging ditches, building roads and buildings; manufacturing any number of goods and services; planting, tending, harvesting, processing, packaging, and shipping food; cleaning offices, hotels, homes, streets; picking up and processing garbage; providing childcare. The vast majority who occupy these positions are persons of color. Thus, it is tenable to argue that it is in the self-interest of the society that these laborers be healthy so that they will be productive. At first hearing, this argument may sound like an appeal to crass self-interest of the white and/or affluent sectors of society. On one level it is. Yet in spite of this fact, it also points to our inherent interdependence as a society—a truth that does not fit well with the myth of and devotion to individualism and independence so prevalent in the United States.

Second, the crisis of the uninsured presents a fundamental obstacle to the fulfillment of U.S. democratic principles. It is impossible to contend that all lives are valued equally or are regarded with the same respect when some are forced to plead for Medicaid coverage or for the charity of a hospital, drug company, or physician. If some more than others—by virtue of insurance—are able to access care or perhaps more care and more options, then already there is discrimination. This argument does not mean that everyone should get every single treatment, drug, or therapy that they want. The point, instead, is that a lack of universal coverage in this country mocks our claims to equality and to an end of structural discrimination.[141]

In sum, if structures inherent in healthcare systems—managed care, cost containment initiatives, insurance policies, the financing, and strictures of Medicaid—are not addressed, we as a society will never get to the root of the disparities. Diversity or cultural sensitivity trainings will not help much if these levels are not directly confronted as well. On the other hand, universal healthcare by itself will not equalize access and quality issues either. As long as biased assumptions and prejudice go unchecked in societal and institutional mindsets and practices, the quality of care for some will continue to be detrimentally affected.[142]

A third conclusion I draw from the above research was highlighted already in chapter 1: Ethical principles in medicine are not enough to ensure the equal care and respect of all. A person, professional community, or society can simultaneously hold egalitarian views and still have unconscious bias and prejudice at work. Disparities in care due to combinations of access and quality issues transgress the moral obligations of a democratic society that espouses a healthcare doctrine of a respect for autonomy, beneficence, nonmaleficence, justice, and equality.[143]

As I reflect upon the volumes of quantitative research on healthcare disparities, one thing is clear: Medical, sociological, and healthcare researchers are excellent collectors of data. Yet one question remains, How does the collection of this information transform the problematic realities it documents?[144] Gathering facts is just not enough.

For example, one ambitious endeavor that has been criticized for not accomplishing much in terms of actual transformation and reform is the HHS' "Healthy People 2010" initiative. This federal initiative, originally named "Health People 2000," has set as its goal to have 100 percent of the population insured by the year 2010.[145] In addition to this lofty goal, "Healthy People 2010" lists 467 specific objectives, grouped within 28 focus areas. However, some public health analysts are not overly optimistic with respect to the prospects for achievement. Marilyn Aguirre-Molina, Carlos Molina, and Ruth Enid Zambrana, all experts in Latino health policy, comment, "After several decades of the 'Healthy People' initiative, it is not clear what it has accomplished other than document and track the morbidity and mortality patterns of the American people and minority populations."[146] Indeed, it is one thing to document healthcare inequalities or the plight of vulnerable people; it is another matter altogether to enact change—grounded in a nuanced understanding of the sources of these social ills and relationships between the various problems and root causes. Adequate healthcare policy does not stop at verifying inequalities; it must do something constructive to ameliorate them.

This is an important insight for social and medical ethicists to bear in mind as we evaluate congressional reports and healthcare policy presentations. What are they recommending? Are the recommendations fitting, feasible, sufficient? How will improvements be identified and tracked? As members of this society, we must not let ourselves off the hook by simply denouncing inequality; we must hold ourselves accountable to offering concrete and creative means for change. The task of social ethics and healthcare policy is to help create viable and worthy alternatives to those conditions, structures, and practices that are woefully unacceptable.

As this chapter concludes, I am left with several questions encircling my brain: How does one break through predominant stereotypes and biases in a person or society? How might self-critical awareness be enculturated into both systems and human hearts so that, collectively and individually, people reflect ever more deeply on their behaviors, assumptions, and practices? How does a system or society facilitate moving beyond stereotypes and statistics so that harried and hurried healthcare providers are able to see the faces and to understand more fully the lives, needs, and values of the particular persons and families seeking their care? The research of this chapter cannot answer any such questions with much satisfaction.

Indeed, even as the mammoth body of statistical data is impressive, there are still more and different kinds of information that are needed to move beyond the mere documentation of disparities. This one broad lens of medical sociological literature will not suffice for getting at the depth of why disparities are so problematic nor will it suffice for envisioning alternatives. In order to take these next steps, different languages are needed—specifically, I argue, those found in theology, ethnography, and social ethics. In particular, a precise theological anthropology (an understanding of what it means to be human) may expand the moral imagination for healthcare provision in critical ways. For its part, qualitative, ethnographic methods might open human beings up to a kind of information that no amount of quantitative research or reporting can tell. Attention both to theology and qualitative research methods, then, will set us upon a path toward attentive and faithful listening to the stories of a few people who intimately know the dynamics of healthcare and the sometimes menacing consequences they can have for human lives.

3

A Call to the Particular: Contributions from Theology and Qualitative Research

Introduction

> *All women are white;*
> *All blacks are men;*
> *Some of us are brave*
> —Cherrie Moraga

To know and experience in one's own bones that one's worth is accurately seen and fully respected by others amounts to basic sustenance for human living. Akin to air, food, and water that expand the belly and breast, such embodied knowledge replenishes ephemeral storehouses that perpetually ache for meaning, joy, love, and hope. It is, in short, a requirement for human life—as integral as any physical need.

Yet this quality of human living evades precise measurement. Its presence or absence cannot be calculated on an index like the Gross National Product (GNP). To know deeply that one matters—that one's individual, fragile and temporary life matters in the larger context of a society, within the even larger sweep of human history and for those who are religious even to God—is both as essential to living as oxygen and as vaporous. This quality may be hard to capture or pin down, and yet most people know in their hearts when it is present in their lives or not.

While quantitative studies serve vital purposes in many forms of scientific research, they may not be the best methods to explore such amorphous qualities of human existence, especially if they are used as the sole, or even primary, method of inquiry. Consequently, in an effort to heed Audre Lorde's call to pay attention to the particular, I have turned to theology and ethnography. The expertise of ethnography is strong exactly in the area where positivistic science is weak: Thick descriptions of particular lives that may then spark moral imagination regarding larger dimensions of human living. For its part, a precise theological anthropology elaborated here, which incorporates nuanced reading of particular lives, can help vulnerable people to know and experience that they are loved and that their lives matter. In short, by drawing upon these two distinct tools, I am attempting to craft a theological and liberationist ethic for healthcare.

In this chapter, I describe a particular theological anthropology and explain why it is needed, as well as discuss the rationale and method for the ethnographic research I have undertaken. Chapter 4 will then share insights from the ethnography itself. First, however, I think it is important to share the methodological approach that has informed the way the ethnography has been done and how it relates to specific theo-ethical convictions. My hope is that theology and ethnography may help to expand social-, medical-, and bioethical understandings of what it concretely means to treat human beings with dignity and respect. Chapter 3 is divided into two main parts. First it considers what the language of theology might bring to healthcare ethics. To do so, it explores the respective theological anthropologies of Martin Luther, select twentieth-century white feminist theologians, and contemporary liberation theology as seen in the work of Roman Catholic Womanist theologian, M. Shawn Copeland. The second section describes the contribution ethnography might make. It begins by highlighting the distinctiveness of qualitative research and the specific methodological commitments that have informed how I have sought to do ethnography. It then turns to introducing the actual fieldwork and shares pertinent methodological learning from going through the Institutional Review Board (IRB) approval process.

A Place and Role for Theological Anthropology[1]

At the outset, it is important to clarify the meaning of a term that is central to this discussion: "Theological anthropology" refers to a faith tradition's or theologian's conceptualization of what it means to be a human being in light of the reality of divine being. Those who explore the notion of theological anthropology ask, How does a faith community's understanding of God (and/or creation, Jesus, redemption, sin, etc.) shape its understanding of what it means to be human? Any answer to such a question largely depends upon the particular theological perspective, interpretation of scripture, and embodied, historical memory operative within each community or theologian who asks the question. The particular theological anthropology I advocate will soon be apparent.

To say that theological anthropology has a place in healthcare forums will raise the eyebrows of some who believe that theology has no place in biomedical or healthcare ethics.[2] Many who currently engage in healthcare debates are more comfortable with the language of human rights than that of theological anthropology. Some, especially those who work in healthcare or the natural sciences, may greet a discussion of theological anthropology by a Christian social ethicist with suspicion—fearing a Christian overlay onto what is a complex and pluralistic humanity. These concerns are justified. Undeniably, religious sensibilities that identify what it means to be a human being or to be God's "chosen" always carry with them the danger of categorizing others as neither fully human nor chosen—by God, by the community, or by society.

Furthermore, attention to place matters. Even as exclusion and oppression have happened, within numerous religious, historical, and cultural contexts, Christians living in the United States must own Christianity's bloody legacy as it has uniquely materialized within the history of this nation. Christianity was intentionally wedded to the brutalizing pursuits of colonization, empire, and segregation in the Americas. And Christians, most notably white Christians, have fully participated in and profited from, these pursuits—as slave owners/traders, members of the military, politicians, entrepreneurs, judges, farmers and ranchers, industrialists, members of the clergy—in short, as citizens.[3] This history still breathes in the present. Whites, the majority of whom identify themselves as Christians, predominate in both numbers and spheres of economic and political influence in U.S. society. The current historical moment in the United States is no less complex or tenuous than earlier periods.

Hospitals, for their part, can be some of the most diverse gatherings of people found in the United States. They are often run not by particular denominations or religions anymore, but by Health Management Organizations (HMOs). Consequently, in most settings no common theological orientation can be assumed among the managers, boards of directors, practitioners, or patients. With a few notable exceptions, the names of hospitals that still bear adjectives such as "Lutheran" or "Presbyterian" constitute merely an archeological clue to their origins. Their survival on hospital walls and letterhead serve as left-behind residue that reveals something of the distance hospitals have traveled from being originally a ministry of faith communities to the sick and impoverished to their current existence as corporate centers of medical treatment, research, and technology whose efforts are continually aimed at maximizing cost-effectiveness, state of the art healthcare delivery, prestige, and productivity.[4]

To sum up, the legacy of (white) Christian activity and influence upon U.S. socioeconomic relations, especially with regard to race and empire, constitute an important cautionary context for anyone attempting Christian social ethics. Moreover, there exists today an amazing degree of plurality and diversity (including, but not limited to that of religion) found within U.S. healthcare settings. Finally, the ownership and orientation of most hospitals themselves has shifted away from being faith-based/operated.

Given these facts, one might ask, Why introduce theological anthropology into a discussion of healthcare quality disparities? Is not theological language misplaced in healthcare discussions—antiquated and misguided? My response to this concern is that if it is not careful, and done with a significant degree of humility and self-criticism, theology can very well be out of place. However, it is not necessarily so. Even in this complicated society, theological anthropology can make a distinct contribution. Here is why: To understand fully what it means to be human, it is not sufficient to think in individualistic terms often found in rights and entitlement language in the United States. It is also not sufficient to think in abstract, universalized terms. Instead, at its best, theological anthropology offers the insight that to understand what it means to be human, one has to think concretely, relationally, and contextually.

In various historical contexts, albeit with differing nuances and emphases, theologians have claimed that *human being* is inextricably bound up with *divine being*. The logic generally argues that to respect fully the dignity and worth of each person, one needs to appreciate that each person is intrinsically precious, without price, because she/he is both a child of the divine and also imbued with the divine within her/his very being. Furthermore, the crucial claim has often been made by theologians that human beings are not only inherently related to God but to *all* of creation.

The vision of humanity I wish to bring to healthcare discussions is grounded in particular theological and ethical norms: Human beings are both fragile and beloved children of God. We are relational beings at our core. As we are able to embody love and justice in our relationships, we image or participate in divine being. We cannot divorce ourselves from God, from other human beings, or from the rest of creation. When we attempt to do so, we place ourselves, others, and creation in dire peril. We need God and each other in many and varied ways for our individual and collective survival and well-being. Moreover, we profoundly depend upon all within creation that brings forth and sustains life.[5] These claims will be fleshed out in the following theological discussion, but because they so integrally inform the lens I bring to social and healthcare ethics, they need to be explicit at the beginning.

Beyond this general statement, an additional word about the operative theological anthropology in this book is needed. The present work not only seeks a place for theological language within healthcare ethics, but more specifically advocates for a fundamental shift in what is employed as the subject of theological anthropology. An adequate anthropological subject must be particular, not abstract in its conceptualization. Specifically, for theological anthropology to be both sufficient and of use to social ethics, the basis for understanding what it is to be human ought to take as its frame of reference the most vulnerable of a society. This argument is the theological and ethical axis upon which this book turns.

At the most basic level, what this theological anthropology may contribute to healthcare and social ethics (and to the moral formation of persons) is this: Humility. It may rekindle a vibrant awareness of both our shared sacredness and finitude. This embodied consciousness may then serve to engender mutual respect and caring among us. In the words of Brazilian feminist theologian, Ivone Gebara, "Because we are going away, it is necessary to have tender embraces; because we are going away, people who are hungry today must eat, and I must share my bread."[6] Each of us, and all of our children and children's children, will one day die. And because of this fact, we must attend to one another in times of illness with great care, especially those at most risk of being forgotten or invisible.

Human beings are fragile and temporary creatures. Across important differences, we all need some very basic elements to survive and thrive for the time we are alive. These include not only material resources such as food and water, but immaterial ones as well, namely, love and recognition. Human beings have a choice. We can either turn inward and hoard whatever we have acquired or we can heed the command, expressed in the language of Christianity, to "love one another as one's self"—to honor all precarious and fleeting lives as much as we cherish our own. My hope is that as we human beings tap into our ability to sense the sacred in others—other persons and other life forms—we may be more able to respect and care for them in real and concrete ways.[7]

To understand how I have arrived at these theological and ethical norms, it is important to lay a bit of theological groundwork. Specifically, I need to make two brief stops at the doors of Martin Luther and of twentieth-century white feminist theology.[8] While neither brought me all the way to the point of making the lives of the most vulnerable the subject of theological anthropology, each has played a crucial role in my theological and moral evolution. Again, the purpose of sharing this theological background is to show how I have arrived at a particular theological anthropology that then informs the ethical claims I make in subsequent chapters. Thus, I will limit my discussion here to a relatively fast-paced overview of Luther and twentieth-century feminist theology that make these connections most clear. For those interested in further reading, the endnotes are rich in examples from the primary sources.

In what follows, I both honor what I have gained from these particular roots with respect to anthropology and demonstrate the need to move beyond their strictures. While both Luther and contemporary white feminism have made important contributions to an understanding of humanity, neither has wrestled sufficiently with particularity. Consequently, I will conclude this discussion of theological anthropology by showing why a sustained turn to the particular is needed.

Martin Luther

In a nutshell, here is what Luther's theological anthropology offers to the moral life: By definition, to be a human being on this planet is to depend radically upon God's love and to be in intrinsic relation with God and with all creation.[9] Insofar as human beings are able to accept God's absolute gracious love and acceptance, we can then be vehicles of the same in the world. Not only can we become agents of love, healing, and justice, but *we are called to do so*. In Luther, theological anthropology is thoroughly *moral* anthropology. Because God has secured humanity's salvation, instead of anxiously brooding about and scheming to win our ultimate reward, human beings can be free to take up the responsibility of attending to the concrete, material communities and relations of which we are an inextricable part. In fact, we must attend to these realities *not* as a way to save ourselves but out of our moral obligation as human persons to contribute to the life and well-being of others. Our escape from death does not hinge on this activity, but the viability of our world does. The justifiable needs and demands of others make a claim upon each human being and community.

In Luther, I first glimpsed a vision of a God who does not hover above the earth, but who is embedded within it; who charts not only the courses of stars and planets, but who is invested in me—in each person, and in every conceivable community of life.[10] Luther's theology is richly incarnational. He delights in the human body and in the earthly realm as God's own good creation. He emphasizes that all finite creation bears God's true and infinite presence. In Luther's work, I found a God who is wholly committed to the flourishing of all life and to just relationships among all facets of creation.

In terms of anthropology, I found Luther's descriptions of human beings as intrinsically relational children of God to be compelling and fresh.[11] Luther was the first theologian to open up for me the mystery of God's connection to humanity in a way that revealed an intimate love affair in which God is present to the most mundane aspects of human existence. Luther's vivid, often provocative theological language is saturated with earthy metaphors taken from daily communal life. In doing theology and ethics, Luther drew upon visceral descriptions (e.g., of bowels, diapers, the pleasures of food, and companionship) to create images that related to people's immediate experience.[12]

In Luther's anthropological vision, to understand what it means to be human, one must first understand this about God: God loves all creation, including human beings—and all creation exists in utter dependence upon God. In our creatureliness, God comes to creation and pervades all of it. God closes the distance between the earthly and the divine and claims us as beloved. To be loved, human beings do not have to become perfect, leave our bodies behind, or attain enlightened reason. In fact, we cannot affect this love. It is God's action, God's choice and gift. Our identity as beloved of God is part of the deepest core of our being.

In agreement with the church's teaching of his time, Luther grounds this understanding of humanity in scripture, specifically in the claim in the book of Genesis that all human beings are created in the image of God (*imago dei*).[13] However, Luther soundly rejects what he calls the Augustinian tradition, which identifies *imago dei* in terms of memory, intellect, and will. Instead, Luther continually stresses the inability of natural human capacities, apart from the word of God, to know God and to act in accordance with God's will.[14] Human beings cannot move toward God by their own powers; instead it is God who comes to humanity through scripture, incarnation, and the presence of the Spirit.[15]

Ultimately, for Luther, what matters is not our (dis)similarity to God, but rather that we are *loved* by God—infinitely and intimately—in the midst of our finitude and imperfections. We do not ascend to God; instead God comes to dwell with *and* within us. Because of this relationship to God, human beings are set free to be *who we are* in the deepest sense and to live into *who we are called to be for others*, namely, servants, neighbors, and lovers of creation.[16]

While Luther consistently assails human attempts at self-salvation, an even stronger theme in his thought is the power of the Gospel to create a new creation within this state of separation.[17] We cannot move to any kind of perfection in this life; nonetheless, the Gospel and God's grace have real and visible effects upon the lives and hearts of human beings. Moreover, divine love and revelation are found not only in scripture, but also in our relationships with other human beings.

Thus, it is crucial to distinguish between what Luther says are limits in terms of knowledge of God and what we can hope to accomplish in the moral life with regard to love of neighbor. For Luther, human relationships are a real way in which human beings experience divine grace. In actual relationships and interactions, human beings may become expressions of divine grace and love for one another.[18] People image God in terms of how they relate to God and to one another. When we live in right relationship with God and others, we actively participate in this imaging of the divine. The image of God is perceived in the fruits of a person's life, in concrete relationships.

Dwelling upon one of Luther's key writings will show this distinctive theological vision in action. Specifically, Luther's exposition of the meaning of the Ten Commandments in his Large Catechism will serve as an illustrative case study because it makes explicit the inherent ethical import of his anthropology. For Luther, God's relationship with humanity is primary and determines the kind of relationships and societies human beings ought to create with one another.

For Luther, the meaning of the first commandment, "you shall have no other gods," extends far beyond the worship of religious idols or relics. It means that human beings are "to cling to [God] with all our heart" and not replace a love for God with a love for other things, such as "money and possessions."[19] Because we exist in utter dependence upon God's grace, we must put our ultimate trust in the divine—not in any human or other finite goods or powers. Only when we strive to trust God to this degree are we able to put our priorities, values and relationships to others in any semblance of proper order. For Luther, this first commandment fundamentally conditions the other nine as their source and guide. Simply put, our relationship to God informs our relationship to neighbor.[20] This theological explication of humanity's dependence upon and intrinsic relationship to God gives birth to a vigorous social ethic.

To illustrate, Luther draws a broad arc of responsibility in his commentary on the fifth commandment, "you shall not kill." He writes,

> [T]his commandment is violated not only when a person actually does evil, but also when he fails to do good to his neighbor, or, though he has the opportunity, fails to prevent, protect, and save him from suffering bodily harm or injury. If you send a person away naked when you could clothe him, you have let him freeze to death. If you see anyone suffer hunger and do not feed him, you have let him starve.[21]

For Luther, in addition to proscribing murder, this commandment *prescribes* life-supporting actions. Christians have the positive obligation to ameliorate human suffering and need. When they fail to do so, they have sinned as much as those who actively kill someone. In a related vein, Luther rails against those persons and businesses that charge interest, "gentleman swindlers and big operators," who control the markets and profit off the misfortunes of others.[22]

According to Luther, we fail to fulfill the commandments because we fail to trust who God is and what God has done for us. In this failure, we turn in upon ourselves—selfishly and anxiously clutching at whatever we can to make us feel secure, powerful, and satiated—rather than turning outward to face our myriad neighbors to whom we are accountable. Simply put, we fail to love our neighbors because we do not know who we are and to whom we belong.

In summary, Luther's theological anthropology does not necessarily lead to quietism and complacency in the moral life. It did not for Luther. The fact that we human beings are utterly dependent upon God for salvation justified by God's grace and loved unconditionally does not free us from attending rigorously to the needs of this world. White Lutheran ethicist Cynthia Moe-Lobeda makes the point eloquently: "If Christians are to *be who they are*, they will not run from suffering at the cost of failing to serve neighbors in need. Christian moral life entails not escape from worldly life and the suffering entailed in seeking the well-being of all, but living fully in that life."[23] Put more bluntly, we are not free to sit apathetically on our justified behinds. If understood rightly, Luther's anthropology insists that human beings must be deeply engaged in the moral life—for the sake of the well-being and healing of all. Indeed, if human beings are to be truly human, we can do no less.

What might Luther's theological anthropology mean specifically for healthcare ethics? At its best, this vision first calls attention to the fact that we human beings depend on something greater than ourselves for life—whether we call it God, grace, love, providence, or something else. Second, it emphasizes that we, by virtue of the *very structures of our being*, are accountable to one another. Relationality is not an elective to be chosen or not. It is not a question of whether or not we choose to be in relation to another, but rather if we will honor the relationship that already exists between us. Ultimately, human relationships are not sealed by contracts, consent forms, insurance coverage, or court decisions. A sacred bond binds us in mutual responsibility to one another. Sophia, one of the women with breast cancer with whom I spoke, commented, "We are here [on the planet] to take care of one another, right?"[24] Human beings can create all kinds of priorities to order their lives, can make anything the most important goal or moral anchor. Yet Luther calls us back to a pivotal theological and social norm by which to measure the quality of our relationships and structures: In our hospitals and clinics, are we loving others as much as we love ourselves? Are we treating every patient as our neighbor to whom we are both related and accountable?

Before moving into the twentieth century, I want to signal what I find to be the limits of Luther's theology. So far, this summary of Luther's theological and moral anthropology represents him at his best. While it is faithful to the spirit of Luther, it is important to acknowledge that his writings are not free of contradiction. Luther's anti-Semitism was used by many Lutherans in World War II as justification for the Holocaust, both by those actively engaged in it and those who did nothing to stop it. Also, while Luther departed at times in important ways from patriarchal views deeply embedded in Christianity, he did not free himself from them to affirm unequivocally the full humanity of women.[25]

Luther's failure, ironically, consists in neglecting to see particular human beings in certain of his writings through the lens for which he so passionately advocates in others. Even as Luther took much information from actual worldly relationships and realities for his theological understanding, he nonetheless failed at crucial junctures to see all particular human beings as fully human. At times, Luther failed in the actual application of some of his most searing and poignant theo-ethical insights. Thus, even as I acknowledge my theological inheritance from Luther, I cannot endorse any of it uncritically. His theological anthropology is not sufficient in itself to address present sociohistorical contexts.[26]

By being critically aware of Luther's limits, we might become attuned to our own. Acknowledging that Luther excluded some in his attempt at theological anthropology could prompt us to double-check our own endeavors. Theologians and religious ethicists continually need to ask ourselves, Who is being left out of my vision of humanity? Whose identity is glossed over, over-simplified or poorly understood? My reading of white feminists first opened these questions to me by making it apparent how poorly the majority of western theologians have understood and appreciated the lives of women. In particular, the work of white feminists complexified and deepened my appreciation of embodiment and relationality for the doing of theology and ethics.

Twentieth-Century White Feminist Theology: Embodiment and Interdependence

In significant ways, Luther's anthropological vision resonates with key theological convictions in contemporary white feminist theologies.[27] However, white feminists made a groundbreaking contribution by uprooting androcentric, individualistic, and universalized conceptions of the human being (and the divine) as implicitly or explicitly "man."[28] One of the founders of contemporary feminist Christian ethics, Beverly Harrison, writes,

> I submit that a theological tradition that envisaged deity as autonomous and unrelated was bound over time to produce a humanism of the sort we have generated, with its vision of "Promethean man," the individual who may, if he chooses, enter into relationship. Where our image of transcendence is represented to us as unrelatedness, as freedom from reciprocity and mutuality, the experience of God as living presence grows cold and unreal.[29]

Harrison contends that this limited and flawed vision of God has had worrisome consequences for an experience of God. And as human encounters with God "grow cold and unreal" so may their relationships with one another.

In the latter portion of the twentieth century, white feminists made bold and brilliant contributions to theological anthropology that emphasized mutuality, embodiment, sensuality, and interdependent relationality.[30] What follows cannot summarize all of these contributions. Instead, I will highlight just two themes that carry pertinent moral weight for this project: Embodiment and mutual interdependence. Both bring us closer toward an adequate understanding of the significance of particularity for theology and social ethics.

Carter Heyward represents one of the most sustained and provocative white feminist voices to lift up embodiment and mutuality as integral to theology. She eloquently argues that human knowing (epistemology) is grounded in the embodied senses and feeling—in the utter physicality of the human being:

> The quality of our intelligence is embedded in feeling connected to one another. Our feelings are evoked and strengthened sensually by touching, tasting, hearing, seeing, and smelling with one another. Our senses and the feelings that are generated by them become primary spiritual resources. In knowing one another through our senses, feelings, and intelligence . . . we come to know God.[31]

Human knowledge is situated within human bodies.[32] This knowledge includes not only knowledge of self and the material world, but also includes real knowledge of God. The intellect, the ability to reason, develops with visceral experience and in relation to others. Human knowledge—emotional, intellectual, spiritual, and moral—is inextricably rooted within human bodies.[33]

Given the primacy of the body for epistemology, Heyward contends that the body (both female and male) needs to be reclaimed and redeemed in theology. A recovery of the female body can be made especially poignant if one considers that across historical times and cultures, the female body has been a primary target of violence and oppression. Her body is the one that has been most controlled, sold, beaten, objectified, legislated, eroticized, malnourished, raped, overworked, and otherwise brutalized.[34] Heyward's work, along with that of other white feminists, is strengthened to the extent that it pays attention to actual bodies. Their descriptions of sensuality, *Eros*, and embodiment are often beautiful, but in elaborating them in general terms, and without locating them in *particular* female bodies, they can ring hollow. The same is true for their insights into relationality.

A second argument that has become a cornerstone in white feminist theology is the claim that all human beings are intrinsically relational creatures. Beverly Harrison states this point plainly: "To speak of the primacy of relationship in feminist experience . . . is, above all, to insist on the deep, total sociality of all things. All things cohere in each other. Nothing living is self-contained; if there ever was such a thing as an unrelated individual, none of us would know it."[35] We exist in myriad relationships with other human beings, with God, and with all of creation. Heyward contends that we are persons *only* as we are persons in relation. "[T]he experience of relation is fundamental and constitutive of human being. . . ."[36] No knowledge of the self is possible without knowledge of the other and of the inherent relations between and among selves. One cannot truly know another without embodied contact and communication with the other(s). Human beings come to know one another in the deepest sense of truly hearing one another's stories only as they labor, love, play, and struggle together.[37] In short, to be human is to exist and function in relation to others, including the nonhuman aspects of creation.

Furthermore, when speaking of relationality, Heyward continually emphasizes mutuality. For Heyward, "[M]utuality is not merely reciprocity. . . . It is a process of relational movement . . . in which two or more people are struggling to share power between/among ourselves. . . . It involves learning to stand and walk together and to recognize and honor the differences we bring to our common ground."[38] Mutual relation necessarily involves the sharing of power. Human beings become and fully live into who they were created by God to be as they grow in ability to experience and create relationships that are based on mutual interdependence, respect, care, and dignity.[39]

Given this mutual interdependence, human beings have the responsibility to create justice within actual communities and societies. Again, theological anthropology is also moral anthropology. Heyward maintains that it is possible to achieve such mutuality because the very power to do so is divine.[40] God is the sacred power that originates and makes possible right relationship within creation. The human self participates in this power to the degree that it seeks such relations.

Thankfully, white feminist theologians have dug up much of the once taken-for-granted root of western theological and philosophical anthropology, which tends to see humanity in individualistic and male terms. Due to these labors, it is no longer second nature for theologians and ethicists to assume that the anthropology operative in Augustine, Aquinas, or Luther, especially with respect to gender, is true or adequate for present understanding. In addition, Womanists and other feminist scholars of color have courageously critiqued the subjective racial and socioeconomic assumptions hidden within it.[41]

Another View of White Feminist Theology: Mary McClintock Fulkerson

Indeed, these white feminist insights, while important, are not in themselves adequate for safeguarding the dignity of all persons within human relations and systems. More work remains to be done. Unexamined assumptions based on whiteness, socioeconomic class, and ethnic/national identity found in theological anthropology need further examination and rooting out; and white scholars need to do our share of the tugging. Succinctly put, white (especially affluent and/or well-educated) persons must no longer be the frame of reference for understanding what it means to be human.

To illustrate, Mary McClintock Fulkerson critiques her white feminist colleagues who, in the name of inclusion, fail to attend adequately to difference:

> It is not just that we (women) are different, and that the variety of subjects who represent different races, classes, and sexual preference need to be assembled in the creation of theologies that will reflect a rainbow of multiplicity. This liberal narrative implies that I can tell what difference is by looking at other women and judging them on the basis of my experience as an oppressed woman who finds liberation through certain strands of the Christian tradition. The processes of recognizing and respecting difference are more subtle and problematic than that, and the inclusionary logic does not get at these complications.[42]

We white feminists cannot simply include others at *our* table. For true right relation, Fulkerson argues that dominant groups and voices must be transformed by the others they had originally sought to include. Seeking a larger discussion is not enough; the very terms of the discussion, and the process by which they are determined, needs to shift. Speaking as a middle-class, white woman in the academy to other white feminist academics, Fulkerson explains, "The empowering of the other from a theo/acentric grammar requires. . . . us to be transformed by the other and to resist, where we recognize it, our domestication of the other."[43]

Fulkerson makes a strong argument for judging the adequacy of one's descriptions of one's own identity based on the kind of others they create. She strives to hear fully the stories and self-descriptions of others without subsuming them as justification for her own story or sense of self:

> [W]e need to narrate our stories in such a way that they enable the stories of the other to teach us. Identity is not something we have and then share or use as a basis from which to define the other. In fact, we discover from poststructuralism that our identity is rendered by the others it creates. . . . The implication of this for our work is . . . that our positing of story and identity should always be subject to criticism, particularly by the other it creates. Constructively, the test for our rendering is whether our story—our remembering of Jesus, if we are Christian—opens up the worth of the other.[44]

If theologians or ethicists are to tell any kind of truth in our descriptions of human subjects, the full humanity and worth of the ones described must be thoroughly apparent. It is not sufficient to "tack on" the stories of women visibly different from the one speaking or writing.

In contrast to white feminist theologians who seek to describe an essence of human identity, Fulkerson resists such a project.[45] Instead, she emphasizes practices. Noted above, Fulkerson offers this measure for Christians in assessing the adequacy of practices: "whether the story, our remembering of Jesus, opens up the worth of the other." Rather than articulate an essential self as the basis for prescriptive norms, Fulkerson turns to cultivating affinities and commitments between human persons.[46] Feminist theorists, theologians, and ethicists would do well, according to Fulkerson, to work at forming a sense of common projects or commitments rather than searching for a common identity. Her vision for white Christian feminists in particular involves critical attention to the connections between beliefs, practices, and communities.[47]

Fulkerson pushes white Christian feminists to consider critically the profound relationship between truth claims and the communities and contexts in which they are embodied. However, one serious weakness of Fulkerson's work is that she offers very little by way of what these commitments and affinities might look like. She does not describe them in detail beyond references to respect for the other and working for the well-being of the other. Moreover, she proposes little by way of articulation of processes by which such commitments and affinities may be cultivated. Interestingly, one concrete means that Fulkerson does offer is the practice of storytelling.[48] Yet she leaves this idea at the level of general affirmation.

White feminist theologians committed to the liberation and flourishing of all people must continually push themselves to be ever more constructive and concrete. As Moe-Lobeda notes, "Theological constructs . . . do not issue in moral power for social transformation if not embodied in practice."[49] Even theological work, such as Fulkerson's, which is informed by critical theory (e.g., postmodern, postcolonial, critical race theory, or other schools of deconstructionist thought) and which showcases practices as pivotal to adequate theological reflection falter if they do not articulate possible means for embodying such practices or offer descriptions of their active presence in the lives of actual moral communities.

To sum up, the limits of twentieth-century white feminist theological scholarship are twofold: (1) They offer descriptions of human identity that, while important correctives to androcentricism, have not incorporated sufficient attention to other crucial differences among human beings; and (2) When they do articulate a concern for particularity and an emphasis on practices that create mutual understanding and solidarity across difference, the work is often left at a theoretical level. Certainly many white feminists are active in their communities—churches, volunteer projects, and social service organizations. However, they do not always bring this work to bear directly upon their academic work.

At critical junctures, Luther failed to perceive and defend the full humanity of Jews, women, and peasants. For its part, white feminist theology has critiqued sexism and patriarchy, but it has not always attended adequately to racial, ethnic, cultural, and socioeconomic differences among women. However, even with these limits of method and perspective, both Luther and white feminist theologians have also articulated pivotal theological and ethical norms. Taken together, their specific insights into incarnation, finitude, neighbor-love, embodiment, relationality, and *imago dei* constitute a fundamental set of theo-ethical assumptions that I carry forward. I cannot leave them behind because they have been, in large part, the conceptual impetus for engaging in ethnography. Moreover, they still function as central convictions within my liberationist theological anthropology.

Indeed, the problem is *not* in having preconceived theological and ethical claims per se, but rather in *how/if* they have been tested. In general, theologians and ethicists hold themselves more accountable to the academy than to other human beings. Consequently, our theological constructs, many of which have strong merit, sometimes ring hollow because they were crafted in relative isolation. Simply put, it is my conviction that a theological anthropology formulated primarily by individual theologians sitting at their desks and computers will not be able to address social realities or the complexity of human beings adequately. Fulkerson contends,

> While many women of color may have non-middle-class communities and histories that give them such sensibilities, many of the rest of us do not. Even though feminist theology rooted in activism works to highlight such relations, the point is, these constructions of us are incidental to qualifying as a theological scholar. The formation of "thinkers"— theologians . . . would require a very different set of processes if our qualifications were judged in relation to our capacity to hear or receive from the other. The continued approbation of reality as God's requires from us the capacity to see grace in the lives of those who speak of God's ways under the adverse conditions we rarely or never live in.[50]

Indeed, concrete work with people in other vocations and life circumstances is as crucial to feminist theo-ethical scholarship as is work with other academic disciplines. Fulkerson's insight suggests that institutions of higher learning may very well need to rethink thoroughly the process by which scholars are formed. For example, perhaps more service-learning and other opportunities for learning "in the field" are needed across majors and departments.

Pushing the Boundaries of Theology: Insights from M. Shawn Copeland

Numerous liberation theologians have called privileged communities, including academia, to account for their failure to confront the realities of those marginalized by human configurations of power. For example, liberation theologians have contributed sophisticated and scintillating theologies by theorizing out of the experiences and the social, political, and economic contexts of the impoverished; those who have suffered at the hands of white colonialization or apartheid; and those who have been despised and left to die due to their sexual orientation or HIV status. What these groundbreaking theologies share is the understanding that in order to achieve adequate theological knowledge, or to see human responsibility accurately, an individual and/or community must be in solidarity with the most vulnerable and oppressed. Concrete involvement (praxis), which grows out of this solidarity, serves as an important moment for theoretical understanding (reflection). The dynamic back and forth of this dialectic between action and reflection is constantly at work—faith (re)forming praxis and praxis (re)forming faith.

Roman Catholic Womanist theologian, M. Shawn Copeland, is a member of this large and diverse body of liberationist thought. Many of her insights discussed below are echoed by others; however, she, more than many, takes theological anthropology as a centerpiece for articulating what has to change in how theology is both theorized and held accountable. Thus, I draw upon her work in this area because it reveals both what needs to change in theology and how theo-ethical norms and solidarity are nonetheless possible.

While concurring that action in solidarity with the most vulnerable creates new understanding, Copeland also emphasizes that before the most adequate expressions of solidarity are possible, there must be profound understanding. She cautions white feminists in particular who may be inclined to jump too quickly into identification with others through a superficial call to "sisterhood" or solidarity. Before issuing a call to "feminist unity," structural power differences must be directly confronted and undermined.

Akin to Heyward, Copeland appreciates that the relational and interdependent aspects of humanity must be explicit within any adequate theological anthropology. However, she adds that there must also be room in any understanding of the self and of bodies of selves to be seen—in their *difference*, on their own terms, for their own sake—as full human beings and moral agents. Copeland explains, "[D]ifference carries forward a struggle for life in its uniqueness, variation and fullness; difference is a celebrative option for life in all its integrity, in all its distinctiveness."[51] To work collaboratively for mutual right relationship, the profound depth of differences between and among human selves must be acknowledged.[52] Copeland agrees with white feminists that the subject of anthropology may no longer be the western, white, educated, rational man. She continues that it must not be a white, middle-class, educated, western woman either.

As already noted, too often white feminists have failed to plumb the depths of differences that permeate humanity. Copeland argues that feminist theologies "require differentiated understandings and pluri-voiced speech."[53] A nuanced appreciation for difference is crucial for appreciating particularity and for respecting others as they themselves define their own identity. At root is the imperative for women—in every racial, socioeconomic, and cultural context—to be seen and understood as full human beings in and of themselves, as ends in themselves. To be fully human is to be loved as a full person *in and of oneself* (even as this self is *also* inherently interrelated with other people and all of creation).

Beyond this caution to white feminists, Copeland makes a vital contribution to theological anthropology. Specifically, she contends that the only viable anthropological subject is the one situated among the bodies and persons of the most despised. In this move, the standard of who or what defines humanity is thoroughly particular. Copeland readily acknowledges that this standard is not a universal description of what all human beings experience. Yet she eloquently and powerfully argues,

> [Feminist theologies] use logic to debunk stereotypes; to expose ideology; to demystify systems, structures and processes that divide and oppress. These theologies take up their stand for truth at the feet of poor white, yellow, red, brown, black women. From this point of departure, critical feminist theologies insist that truth is never independent of cultural, social and historical conditions. For these theologies, the search for truth is motivated by the deepest concerns of all those who transgress the definitions of so-called "acceptable" women—especially poor women and lesbians who embody "indecent difference." Thus, the experience, insight, understanding and judgment of poor, oppressed and marginalized women stand as normative in any critical feminist theological formulation.[54]

All feminist theologians—however light or dark their skin—are accountable to those most vulnerable due to structural inequalities. They "take up their stand for truth at the feet of poor white, yellow, red, brown, black women." These feet show feminist (and other) theologies where to start walking and how to assess the adequacy of their theo-ethical norms. It is permissible and indeed necessary to ask *any* theologian what his or her Christology, soteriology, or eschatology contributes to the lives of actual human beings living on the margins of a society.

Liberationist theologies, exemplified here by Copeland, offer a distinctive theological anthropology to social ethics: Given present national and global socioeconomic and political realities, the only viable anthropological subject is the one situated among the bodies of "the exploited, despised, poor woman of color."[55] Rather than holding up an abstract ideal of what a person can be, essentially is or ought to be, Copeland challenges theologians and ethicists to understand the meaning of human being-ness in light of the actual experiences of the ones most vulnerable, objectified, and likely to be disregarded.

Theological and ethical definitions of what it means to be human will only approach adequacy if they include explicit, substantive respect for these persons.

The implications of such a shift in subjectivity are weighty. Foremost, this shift includes an implicit awareness of embodied particularity while still making a case for solidarity and a common humanity. Copeland's revised notion of the anthropological subject addresses people—not only in their "otherness" *but also* in their shared humanity. Moving from the particularity of poor, exploited women of color makes a claim regarding humanity in a larger, even universal, sense. In this theological anthropology, any human self is *only fully a self* to the degree that it is cognizant of its accountability and interconnectedness to this particular human subject: "From the perspective of the new anthropological subject—exploited, despised, poor women of color—solidarity is basic to the realization of *humanum.* . . . "[56] Thus, to be fully human, one must be in solidarity with the needs and requirements for the humanity of "exploited, despised, poor women of color." Differences are not erased, yet in solidarity with this subject there is a basic claim to a common *humanum* grounded in right relation between and among human communities.

Moral claims, therefore, are assessed by the degree to which they enable or diminish the full humanity of the most marginalized along with the degree to which they work toward or against right relationship among different peoples. In this vision, theology is not divorced from ethics. The theological entry point is inherently a justice entry point. The requirements of the most vulnerable within a society are the normative starting point for an adequate understanding of what justice means in human relations. In short, ethicists, sociologists, chaplains, healthcare providers, and theologians can only arrive at an adequate sense of dignity and personhood in the context of healthcare when they take seriously the experiences and voices of those most marginalized by societal/structural inequalities.

To a degree, Copeland's theological anthropology turns the enterprise of theological anthropology on its head. Rather than beginning with a completely abstracted notion of the human being and then overlaying it on all persons/peoples, this theological stance begins with a more concrete subject and then assesses adequate understandings of the human being and related requirements for human flourishing against this particular standard. The move is away from universal theory and toward exploration of actual lives in order to understand what it means to be human in actual contexts.

Having said this, it is also true that Copeland's articulation of the human subject is still theoretical. It depends on assumed theo-ethical norms such as justice, interdependence, and the belovedness of all human persons. Moreover, dependent upon the particular issues and persons a theologian or ethicist is responding to, this definition of the human subject needs greater specificity. In the case of the present work, the embodied referent for humanity is found in Black and Latina women with breast cancer. What is important to see is that Copeland is willing to put her norms in dialogue with the experiences of actual persons straining and suffering under various forms of oppression. She understands that, ultimately, arriving at an adequate understanding of what it means to be human is possible only through encounters with particular persons and communities who have been left out of, or obscured by, theoretical formulations. Only by listening to such persons will theologians and ethicists learn what concepts like *imago dei*, relationality, child of God, neighbor-love really mean in actual relations and lives. In other words, while the norms may transcend time and space, they do not necessarily look the same in every context. Moreover, they may need to be informed, altered, or corrected by norms that are discovered through particular listening and engagement.

Poetic sentiments about loving another as much as one's self or neighbor-love need teeth. They need to be enfleshed—surrounded and undergirded—by the knowledge that comes out of concrete relationships, especially with those who are in some way vulnerable—those who are fighting to live, to be seen, heard, understood, and loved as ends in themselves. Ivone Gebara explains,

> To love the other as oneself has to be understood in concrete situations in which each individual, whether among community, friends, family, or work associates, is ethically obliged to place himself or herself within the skin of the other. A mutuality takes hold and transcends any principle or judgment deriving from already established dogmatic laws. We have to construct among different groups provisional agreements, always capable of revision, in order to allow the common good to be effective, not just a beautiful expression stated in a document, like the Universal Declaration of Human Rights, that lacks any force.[57]

What it means to love the neighbor as one's self only becomes real in the particular. It is discovered experientially and must be continually open to revision. The most meaningful descriptions of neighbor-love begin with the particular to see what it looks like in a concrete moment. From here, the task of the theologian and/or ethicist is to articulate both the norms they brought with them to the encounter as well as the norms they discovered in and through collaboration with others.

In summary, theological descriptions of the human self are adequate only if they substantively attend to several aspects: To radical particularity and difference, to the sensual body, to communities as well as to persons, and to power dynamics that stand between human beings. Finally, any description of the self must always be tentative and self-critical of its inescapable limitations. To recall Gebara's words, at its best, a theoretical elaboration is only a "provisional agreement" among different people, never the final word.

White Lutheran feminist theologian and ethicist, Elizabeth Bettenhausen, once put this last point to me this way: "To come up with a set anthropology makes no sense. How is the defining process of who is human always held accountable? How do operative anthropologies affect lives today? Is your anthropology, *are you*, only held accountable to other academics?"[58] Indeed, a given definition of what it means to be human is not the only matter of concern; instead, the process by which it is constructed is of vital significance. If theologians and ethicists are in conversations—wide and ongoing—with others very different from ourselves, then together it is possible to develop normative notions of what it means to be human and of what constitutes adequate respect and attention to human needs. At their best, theology and ethics are collaborative endeavors. It is not difficult to see how such convictions make the case for qualitative modes of study, such as those found in ethnography.[59]

A Place and Role for Ethnography

Ethnography is one possible means by which to make these methodological and theo-ethical commitments concrete. I have come to realize that if I am serious about starting with the particular while also paying attention to structural inequalities, then I must step away from the familiar territories of classroom, library, and computer desk and step into conversations with women very different from myself. Their knowledge and experiences ought to inform any theo-ethical conclusions that I might draw. Moreover, they ought to be truly present and represented at the tables of healthcare discussions and policy debates.

Four main topics within qualitative methodology merit attention. First, I note salient differences between quantitative and qualitative research methods. Second, I articulate four general, underlying methodological commitments that informed how I approached the fieldwork component. Third, I describe the specific shape of the fieldwork itself—summarizing basic information with respect to the people with whom I spoke and how I collected and analyzed the information. Finally, I conclude by relating and analyzing the first (and unexpected) site of research: The IRB approval process.

Research Design: Qualitative versus Quantitative Methodologies

Most scholars across disciplines would agree that all theories or truth-claims must somehow be tested within lived realities and observed events. However, there is wide diversity in the methods proffered. Some researchers, often in positivistic sciences such as medicine and other natural sciences, favor deductive reasoning to the exclusion of any inductive approach.[60] In deductive research, one begins with a theory or proposition and then moves to explore actual events, interactions, and lives. This method is useful to quantitative studies in which one wishes to test a hypothesis using large, randomized data collections and surveys. For example, if one wishes to test the efficacy of a new cancer drug, a deductive method will be essential to the work. Operating with a reasonable hypothesis, based on findings from prior research, the researcher can test a large population using blind trials and a control group. If the sample size is large enough and replicated in other research, the researcher will be able to make a fairly objective claim regarding the drug's usefulness and potential harms (barring any undue influence from the pharmaceutical company sponsoring the new drug, as was seen in the tragic case of Vioxx).[61]

In contrast, the purpose of qualitative research, in an inductive approach, is to describe in textured detail what the researcher learns from his or her immersion in a particular context. This method seeks neither to quantify a given reality nor compare it to another. Instead, an inductive approach begins in the street or in the hospital room and observes what is there. This learning then informs any subsequent formal analysis. Hypotheses grow out of work in the field. Only after digging deeply into a small section of the ground does an inductive approach move to a higher vantage point to survey a larger scene.

The present fieldwork has utilized a qualitative, ethnographic method.[62] It has not sampled the opinions of large numbers of people; it used no questionnaire. I do not claim that any one story represents "all Black women" or "all Latinas." There is no such thing as *the* "Black" or "Latina" experience. None of the persons who spoke with me are to be understood as "the voice of women of color with breast cancer." They speak for themselves, not their race. Finally, this research does not deny that the experiences voiced by the participants may also be shared with members of other racial and socioeconomic groups.

Unlike quantitative studies, this qualitative approach foregrounds the stories of a few individuals that may shed light on larger dimensions of human experience. I have attempted two things: (1) To listen well to these particular persons, without manipulating what I hear to simply confirm my assumptions; and (2) To describe well the experiences and insights of a case study of people who are members of social groups that directly confront (and often bear the brunt of) healthcare quality disparities.

One critique that quantitative researchers often make of qualitative work is that its sample sizes are too small. In a quantitative study, it is not uncommon for hundreds or even thousands of people to be enrolled or interviewed. In stark contrast, many qualitative studies work with a few dozen or even fewer participants. Some ethnographic studies limit themselves to focusing upon one person in depth. In this case, I interviewed 14 people. The size of this sample makes it all the more important to emphasize that I do not claim that the experiences or views of any of the participants adequately represent those of an entire community or professional group.

Yet, it is also important to note that even as the sample size may be relatively small in some circles, it is rather large for theologians or Christian social ethicists. Far too few ethicists and theologians attempt this kind of research at all. My hope is that reading this work will inspire others to attempt similar ventures in their own scholarship.

A desire to hear from Black and Latina women in their own languages and voices lies at the heart of this endeavor. It is imperative to learn from the experiences of those who most directly confront healthcare quality issues. Even as they cannot speak "for everyone" who shares similar racial and/or socioeconomic backgrounds, listening to their stories and perspectives may still nuance understanding of what quality healthcare looks and feels like to those in need of care. In short, this work is simply one attempt to listen to women who are, or have been, acutely vulnerable and who are generally at risk within society's practices and systems. They know what it is to be both physically and emotionally compromised by breast cancer as well as what it means to contend with discrimination, prejudice, stereotypes, and structural inequalities in social goods such as healthcare, education, housing, and employment. The purpose of ethnographic fieldwork, then, is to create a vehicle for such listening.

Methodological Commitments: An Ethic of White Listening

Fundamental questions quickly surfaced as I set out on this path: How can I (a white, relatively privileged, academic) be a credible listener to and recorder of the experiences of these women? Why should they speak with me at all, let alone reveal such intimate information? What kinds of practices build trust between white theologians/ethicists and communities of color—the very ones to whom many of us hope our research will be of service? How ought dialogue be structured in order for the process and all of the participants to maintain their integrity? The following discussion addresses these pivotal questions. Specifically, it explores four fundamental methodological touchstones that informed how this fieldwork was done.

These commitments form the methodological backbone of this qualitative study. In addition to articulating why I structured this research in a specific way, these insights specifically offer suggestions to other white researchers, theologians, and ethicists contemplating the incorporation of qualitative study into their own research projects. I offer them as constitutive of an ethic of white listening. Hopefully, attention to them may facilitate the shaping of white scholars into responsible listeners when working with communities of color. They are not foolproof guarantees that white scholars will not "muck it up," but they may help. They can be described under the rubrics of inductive learning; seeking collaborators; and the need for both reflexivity and accountability.

Inductive Learning

Sometimes, the best way to learn is to first admit that you know nothing. Rather than testing a prior assumption, an inductive method seeks to discover what is there when one has limited assumptions of what one will find. Ethnographer James Spradley explains the distinctiveness of the inductive approach in this way:

> Western educational systems infuse all of us with ways of interpreting experience. Tacit assumptions about the world find their way into the theories of every academic discipline—literary criticism, physical science,

history, and all the social sciences. Ethnography alone seeks to document the existence of alternative realities and to describe these realities in their own terms. Thus, it can provide a corrective for theories that arise in Western social science. . . .

Ethnography, in itself, does not escape being culture-bound. However, it . . . says to all investigators of human behavior, "Before you impose theories on the people you study, find out how those people define the world."[63]

Ethnography, as Spradley describes it, intentionally attempts to displace the "expert's" theory or knowledge and, by association, the "expert" herself. It does so in order to describe a reality, a person, or a people *well*—namely, in their own terms. An inductive, ethnographic method may help to chasten a researcher's assumptions and heavy-handed theories.

Mindy Fullilove explains that part of the distinctiveness of qualitative methods is that in using them, the researcher does not impose a weighty agenda. The process is not about asking a list of questions, but *searching* for the questions. She describes it as "feel-forward research." The researcher needs to discipline herself from having too many preconceived ideas.[64] One must get into the work without predetermining in stone what is relevant or irrelevant, where the information is to be found or not, and what the "right" and "wrong" questions are. Instead of flying through an interview with a clipboard, an inductive method puts the researcher in the position of groping for the questions—not knowing from where the meaning might come—and staying open to being surprised.

Practicing this kind of discipline can be immensely helpful. And it is of particular import to white scholars. Racial power dynamics and the active presence of a particular social and material history are inherently operative whenever a white scholar works with communities of color.[65] An inductive method may, at least in part, correct broad generalizations and stereotypes made by white scholars—anthropologists, sociologists, physicians, scientists, or ethicists—that reduce (consciously or not) complex realities and human identities to woefully inadequate observations.

Inductive methods may help some white researchers avoid mistakes of both our forebears *and* contemporaries. It is interesting to me that when acknowledging the presence of flawed and/or racist assumptions along with shameful abuses of power enacted by white researchers, white people often cite examples that reside comfortably in the past, such as the notorious eugenics of Nazi doctors. Less often do we remember and discuss the white assumptions and brutality that made tragedies like the Tuskegee Syphilis study possible. Even less often do white persons in general make the connection between white assumptions and the 41 shots fired at Amadou Diallo.[66] Assumptions can be lethal.

In light of current realities, white scholars in the United States have the responsibility to teach, confront, and own both historical and contemporary manifestations of racism particular to our own context and nation. The significance of inductive learning, then, extends far beyond the boundaries of a particular research project. Indeed, taking up inductive modes of inquiry may not only chasten heavy-handed research preconceptions, but they may also help white scholars to recognize and resist their noxious presence in other areas of society as well.

Twenty-first century white theologians and ethicists interested in social and racial justice have the work cut out for us—both in terms of constructively owning this history and in building relationships with darker skinned communities. An inductive mode of study incorporated into the work of Christian theology and social ethics constitutes one way to help us resist presumption in our theories and interpretations. Rather than co-opting people's stories or describing them so that they fit into our view of the world, inductive learning represents one viable way to acknowledge and critique our preconceptions at a methodological level.

Seeking Collaborators

Much of quantitative research, along with some qualitative research, uses the term "human subject" to denote persons participating in a given study. This choice of terminology is not value-free. How the researcher identifies the people with whom she is working signals a particular kind of relationship. For example, one might study or work "on" a subject. Other possible terms such as "collaborator" and "informant" imply a different sort of relationship. Spradley highlights the contrast:

> Social science research that uses subjects usually has a special goal: to test hypotheses. Investigators are not primarily interested in discovering the cultural knowledge of the subjects; they seek to confirm or disconfirm a specific hypothesis by studying the subject's response. Work with subjects begins with preconceived ideas; work with informants begins with a naïve ignorance. *Subjects do not define what is important for the investigator to find out; informants do.*[67]

Language matters. Is the participant your teacher or an object of study? Hopefully, and most likely, a white scientist who uses the term "subject" does not think of or treat the individuals with whom she is working in any way similar to a lab rat. Yet the choice of terms may indicate whether or not one thinks that the participant has a role in helping to define what is important to learn. This choice, and the ethos invested within it, can make a real difference to participants and researchers, even if on a subconscious level. If participants feel their insights and experiences are genuinely valued by the researcher, they are more likely to trust the scholar and to teach her more of what they know.

Moreover, how a researcher conceives of the role of the people with whom she speaks can make a great difference, not only in rapport-building, but in re-situating the claims and importance of the researcher herself. The key in this kind of work is that the researcher is not the expert but the novice. She needs to be taught by the people with whom she works. This attitude decenters the authority and presumptions of knowledge or expertise on the part of the researcher. Rather than becoming defensive, rationalizing, or flat out denying what darker skinned people tell us about the contemporary appearance and dynamics of racism and white privilege manifest in society, lighter skinned scholars need to listen seriously to this testimony. This is a realm of experience that we ourselves have not personally confronted.

In this vein, "collaborator" is a helpful term because it emphasizes that the researcher needs to partner with the individuals interviewed. The goal of this kind of qualitative research is to learn from an engaging conversation with someone who has direct knowledge of and experience with something that the researcher does not. To have an insightful and meaningful conversation, one needs to be emotionally present, rather than attempt to be an authority. (In fact, trying to come off as an expert usually guarantees you will *not* have a good conversation.) Researchers need collaborators in a way that they do not need subjects. Collaborators are colleagues, not subordinates. They not only contribute information about something but also help to construct the questions, the method, the frameworks, and operational definitions.

A caveat: While honoring the fact that participants have much to teach, it is imperative that this awareness is not used to deny or overlook the power dynamics inherently present in the collaborator/researcher relationship. A white researcher, doctor, or theologian in the United States is not in the same social position as a research participant of color. Even if she respects the persons as collaborators, she does not face the same risks they do; moreover, she will benefit more directly from the research than they will. As a matter of course, IRBs mandate that consent forms state explicitly that participating in the research will not benefit the subject/informant/collaborator.

In speaking about this reality, Mindy Fullilove eloquently commented, "There's no benefit to them. It's a gift. You're working with a gift that is their lives. We are nothing without our informants. We stand on their shoulders and it's a burden on them."[68] Her words echo and reverberate in my heart. Some of the women with whom I spoke may die of cancer. One already has. My research cannot change this fact. I am not facing mortality in the same way. Speaking with me will not change or heal any of the hurt they have experienced. Researchers, and particularly white researchers, must not forget that there is a cost to participants of color in speaking of their experiences. Sadly, these experiences often involve hurt, betrayal, violence, and/or disrespect by white people. It is lamentable that I, as a white researcher, need to be taught about such things by persons of color in the first place.

Certainly, white researchers, doctors, theologians, and ethicists may very well know some rather important things and have particular expertise. Yet we need the knowledge of others as well; and we need it in a way that does not simply fit into, accent, or nuance our frameworks and paradigms, but in a way that displaces and (re)forms our knowledge. Though we may have significant medical, scientific, or theological expertise, we will never know more about the values, cultures, and personhoods of others than they themselves do.

Consequently, for any exchange or project to be authentically interracial and collaborative, a truly diverse coalition of energies, knowledge sources, and input needs to be present from the ground up. White scholars cannot simply set the table and then invite others to come and dine. In my work, I have come to realize that Black and Latina women have helped me learn the questions I need to ask. Even now, the search will continue. As I go forward, I will continue to search for the right questions and my collaborators will continue to help me articulate them.[69]

This insight is especially important because white people (especially those who are highly-educated and/or are from middle- and upper-socioeconomic classes) are generally accustomed to a certain "authority" and agency in carrying out our lives and work. Many of us take for granted that we will be treated with dignity, that our rights will be respected, that we will be heard.[70] We also tend to assume that we are knowledgeable, rational, skilled individuals. Many of us are socialized by white privilege and white identity to do so. Much of this socialization must be *un*learned in order to learn while doing qualitative ethnographic research. Even more importantly, it must be unlearned if we are to become fully human.

Lest the above be taken to mean that white theologians, ethicists, and researchers simply need to "go talk to people of color" or engage in "voyeuristic tourism" and call it practical study, I need to reflect upon two additional insights that speak to the concrete mechanisms and kind of engagement needed. Qualitative research methodology is anything but monolithic. Numerous approaches fall under its umbrella. Thus, it is important to further specify the particular kind of qualitative study that is helpful to the project of white listening and responsibility.

Reflexivity

Pierre Bourdieu has made vast methodological contributions to the fields of anthropology, ethnography, and sociology. Though these cannot be discussed here in their entirety, one particular insight is especially pertinent to the present work. Bourdieu, among others,[71] has elaborated a reflexive method of study for these disciplines. Stated simply, reflexivity means three things: First, conscious awareness of assumptions the researcher brings to the field; second, self-reflection on the part of the researcher as part of an academic culture; third, a mutual give and take between a researcher and collaborator in such a way that not only do the researcher's actions/ideas affect the collaborator, but the collaborator's actions and information also fundamentally affect the researcher as well.

According to Bourdieu, sociology that fails to reflect critically upon itself as part of the research will not learn much at all:

> Ordinary sociology, which bypasses the radical questioning of its own operations and of its own instruments of thinking . . . is thoroughly suffused with the object it claims to know, and which it cannot really know, because it does not know itself. A scientific practice that fails to question itself does not, properly speaking, know what it does.[72]

Bourdieu understands that work that lacks reflexivity often reproduces itself—its biases, discourse, and presumptions—rather than learning from the contexts and persons it wishes to engage. This insight does not mean that researchers are supposed to become "blank slates" when doing qualitative field research. Instead, it means that they need to know that they have biases and assumptions and that they need to question them. Part of this questioning means that the case study itself is able to speak back to and alter these operative assumptions or norms.

A reflexive method holds itself accountable by being attentive to the way researchers situate themselves in the field study. It does so by being attentive to various biases that may get in the way of fully seeing and hearing the collaborators in their own voices and right. Loic Wacquant identifies three types of biases with which Bourdieu is concerned. First is "the social origins and coordinates of the individual researcher" (e.g., race/ethnicity, socioeconomic class, gender, cultural background, sexual orientation). Wacquant believes this bias to be the most obvious and easy to correct through self-critique.

However, Wacquant thinks the second bias is not as often interrogated, namely, the specific location the researcher occupies within the academic field. Bourdieu and Wacquant maintain that the fact that sociologists and other academics are producing their work in order to advance careers in some form or other is not often addressed in a self-reflective way with respect to their research. All academics are competing for jobs and grants and this can shape how they/we write, for whom they/we write, and ends served by their/our work. The results can become solely self-serving if this reality is not held up to critical self-reflection.

Wacquant credits Bourdieu with being the most original in his thinking in terms of a third meaning of reflexivity that confronts academia even more directly. According to Bourdieu, in academic culture there is an "intellectualist bias which entices us to construe the world as spectacle, as a set of significations to be interpreted rather than as concrete problems to be solved practically. . . ."[73] When such a bias is present and unchallenged, academics—even in the name of liberation or social justice—may fall into the trap of simply writing about people, without contributing to their lives in meaningful ways. What may be a vexing intellectual question for an academic could mean life or death for a person living with the problem. For example, white academics often do not directly live with the same harsh realities of substandard education, a lack of food and clean water, the pervasive presence of AIDS or cholera, or widespread violence that poor people and/or people of color living around the globe do. To add insult to injury, scholarship can be, intentionally or not, condescending to the ways of thought, being, and acting of the communities and contexts it seeks to engage. This danger is particularly important for white scholars because so much intellectual discourse and theory have been produced by white folk, often either directly or indirectly *about* others.

Particularly for white theologians and scholars committed to racial justice, reflexivity means self-critique at these precise points: As a white person with assumptions and from a particular social location; as an academic trying to stake out a career and name within a specific field; and as part of an intellectual culture that tends to objectify others and create theories about them without helping to solve actual problems.[74] A rigorous and ongoing commitment to critical self-reflection, as an individual and also as one located within a larger academic culture, is one way to test assumptions and to evaluate them based on what is learned through actual dialogue and work with people who may be, in ways obvious or not, different from the academic.

A methodological reflexivity is also helpful because it emphasizes the dialogical relationship between the collaborators and the researcher. Collaborators ought not simply answer the specific question asked, as if they were circling the correct response on a survey. The best interviews are the ones where collaborators trust enough to not limit their feedback to brief, narrow answers to the particular questions posed. Collaborators are often the ones to identify the best questions. Thus, a real conversation—a flow back and forth—is needed between the researcher and the collaborator, which can only happen when there is adequate trust and accountability present.

At its best, reflexive, qualitative research decenters and tests preexisting theory and assumptions and evaluates them based on knowledge gained inductively in a case study. The scholar's assumptions and theories are offset by the experiences and evidence in the field. This kind of listening and reflexivity means that white scholars cannot simply go into the field to extract what they want and then leave. I ought to be affected by the experience and these effects need to be evident in my research. Reflexivity implies a return. To be a responsible scholar or listener, I need to be informed and (re)formed by what I see and hear. I also need to be aware of my responses—emotional, intellectual, physical—to the stories and persons to whom I am listening. The issues and persons with whom I work ought to influence me in fundamental, and hopefully transformative, ways. Good qualitative research (and I would add substantive cross-cultural dialogue) necessarily involves a cost to myself as a white person—a real investment. It costs these women of color to speak; it ought to cost me to listen.

Accountability
Most likely any scholar who engages in some kind of direct research with human beings will become well acquainted with an entity known

as the IRB. This is the most formal way in which scholars are held accountable. IRBs are charged with ensuring that human participants involved in research are not violated, that they are protected from unnecessary harm and unethical studies, and that they are informed of their rights and of the purposes and procedures of the study. While receiving IRB approval is a rigorous and important process, it alone does not suffice to ensure accountability between the scholar and the people with whom she is working. Indeed, there is more to accountability than compliance with IRB mandates. Above all, research is accountable to those interviewed or studied in some other way.

By accountability, I want to identify four distinct traits. First, any scholar engaging in qualitative fieldwork needs to make real commitments to some kind of follow-up and feedback loop with her collaborators. Vigorous guards against misappropriation and misinterpretation are essential. Perhaps collaborators might have the option of reviewing transcripts of interviews and conversations. In this way if the researcher missed or misinterpreted something, changes can be made before the project progresses any further. Minimally, participants ought to be invited to hear or read the findings at some point. Some people may not wish (or be able) to read anything, but they would appreciate hearing an oral presentation, perhaps given to a group. Later, if anything is published, collaborators not only ought to be acknowledged somehow, but they also ought to receive a copy.

The exact nature and degree of reporting back may vary depending on the number of people with whom the researcher works and on the collaborator's age, health status, availability, interest level, and other variables. Yet the principles of opening one's work to critique by collaborators, honoring and acknowledging them for their wisdom, and contributions and transparency within the research findings are constant. This kind of relationship does not mean that the researcher will necessarily change an observation or interpretation with which a given collaborator does not agree. It *does* mean that a researcher's findings and method will be less likely to overinterpret or misrepresent others if she shares her work and solicits feedback. This kind of engagement embodies, rather than simply writes about, respect.

A second form of accountability speaks to the nuance of description. Whenever a researcher sets out to engage someone or something, her first task is to describe it well, in detail, and with regard for the person or situation's complexity. If the analysis overgeneralizes or essentializes individual or communal identities, making them into caricatures, the scholar is guilty of objectification. In this event, not only does the quality of research suffer dramatically, but a kind of violence is done to the participants, even if the researcher refers to them as "colleagues." When white scholars describe persons of color in such a way that they become identified as the representative of "*the* Black experience" or "*the* Latino identity" (as if there were any such thing) they violate the complexity intrinsic to any community and individual person.

Third, accountable research considers the collaborators first. It considers their physical, emotional, and social well-being, especially if they are members of communities who are in any way vulnerable within the larger society. Special attention needs to be given to a collaborator's particular interests, needs, and sensitivities. Is this person at risk of deportation? Is she in any kind of pain? Do her immediate needs conflict with the researcher's agenda? If so, her needs come first. No research is ethical if a collaborator's dignity is violated or her privacy not protected. Collaborators need to understand fully the reasons for the research and what the researcher hopes to accomplish. They also need to agree to help without any pressure or even subtle coercion. It is not justifiable to impose upon anyone, even if the researcher is convinced that she has much to teach her/him. No one ought to serve simply as a means to another's career enhancement.

A final aspect of accountability is this: The research ought to matter in some way to the positive transformation of society. At the risk of sounding brash, I argue that scholarship ought to be accountable to pressing needs and issues within society. There ought to be some connection between the intellectual work and the shaping of the world. Otherwise, too many trees are being cut to produce paper. Granted, some links may be more direct than others. Still, it is possible for scholars, and morally incumbent upon us, to articulate why a given theologian, theological notion, ethical formula, or qualitative field study matters to those outside of the discipline or outside of the academy.

Collaborators have the right to demand that the researcher answer the questions: To what ends? Why is this research important? The researcher's questions and topic ought to correspond in some way with the palpable needs of people in a given society. Spradley suggests,

> One way to synchronize the needs of people and the goals of ethnography is to consult with informants to determine urgent research topics. Instead of beginning with theoretical problems, the ethnographer can begin with informant-expressed needs, then develop a research agenda to relate these topics to the enduring concerns of social science. Surely the

needs of the informants should have equal weight with "scientific interest" in setting ethnographic priorities. More often than not, informants
can identify urgent research more clearly than the ethnographer.[75]

Starting with "informant-expressed needs" implies that some kind of
relationship is present between the researcher and the particular pop-
ulation(s) from whom she hopes to learn. Research will not stumble
upon the needs or the right questions unless researchers are in dialogue—over time and in a sustained manner—with the communities
they hope their work will serve. In a sense, the collaborator, not the
researchers, drives the questions of the process.

Furthermore, no researcher has unlimited time in which to accomplish her work and use her gifts. So she needs to choose wisely. Given
the constraints of time, energy, and resources to commit to a project,
the choice of which project to pursue ought to be strategic. By strategic research, I mean research that ultimately matters to the actual lives
of human persons and communities and that will hopefully enhance
the quality of real lives and futures.[76]

One might argue that this is a subjective call, dependent upon the
interests and biases of a researcher. Certainly any given scholar is more
equipped with particular skills and interests to explore some topics
more than others. However, I think it is reasonable to assume that
regardless of the field—whether microbiology, economics, history,
medicine, law, art, business, or theology—there are always choices to
make about what specific questions and issues to commit one's self.
All disciplines have ways of touching upon contemporary social and
moral questions that shape the well-being of life on this planet.

Given the relative privilege and high standard of living of white
scholars in the United States and Europe, I think that it is not only possible but also imperative that we ask ourselves, regardless of our disci-
plinary field, questions such as these: What am I creating or
contributing to? What do I ultimately hope to achieve with my life's
work? How does my work help to enlarge and enliven human imagination regarding how we might more fully thrive together? What
larger purposes—ecological sustainability, civil or human rights, or
advocacy for those left out of "bottom line" equations, et cetera—are
being served by this work? In the wake of tumult and tragedies in New
York City, Afghanistan, Iraq, Israel, Palestine, does my work contribute in any way to interfaith dialogue, or to intercultural and international understanding, or to peace endeavors? Might my work in any
way matter to an African child living with HIV? These questions are not

meant to be judgmental, but rather to serve as a tool for self-reflection. At its best and most fertile, intellectual work makes meaningful connections between scholars and others—across disciplines *and* vocations.

This discussion of the contributions of inductive learning, collaborators, reflexivity, and accountability outlines the contours of the methodological approach I have taken in doing ethnography. Beyond this general level, it is important to introduce the fieldwork itself and articulate the specific methodological steps taken. In addition, I will share the insights I gained through the process of petitioning an IRB for approval.

Fieldwork Overview and Methodological Steps

In the course of research, I have been asked a few times (and interestingly, especially by white professionals and researchers) why I chose to interview Black and Latina women. Some have wanted to know why I did not design the project to include conversations with white women or with women of additional racial-ethnic backgrounds. These questions were posed the most sharply by members of the IRB.

In response to this inquiry, it is important to acknowledge that my decision to focus upon these two general groupings of women stems from both analytical and personal reasons. On the analytical side, I reflected upon the fact that Latino and Black populations comprise the largest communities of color living in this country. As seen in chapter 2, they also have the highest rates of uninsurance. Both have been underrepresented in medical and healthcare research. I also reflected upon the fact that I speak Spanish and might be able to learn from women who have encountered language barriers and whose reflections in Spanish might enrich any English-based understanding of their experiences. Finally, both Blacks and Latinos confront systemic racism in myriad forms and sectors of U.S. society. On the personal side, the preface of this text noted my background in healthcare. As a chaplain and budding ethicist, I directly witnessed how communities of color are sometimes particularly vulnerable in hospital settings. In addition, I accompanied, and lost, a dear friend to cancer. This specific experience was the impetus for the focus on women with breast cancer.

From June through December of 2003, I interviewed a total of 14 people. Eight were Black and/or Latina women who have had, or currently have, breast cancer. In addition, I interviewed six healthcare providers.[77] I met the women with cancer primarily through women's cancer support group networks. The healthcare providers work at, or are affiliated with, a New York City area hospital. As it turned out, none of the women with cancer had ever been patients of this particular hospital. As previously explained, this work foregrounds the experiences and insights of women of color with breast cancer. The knowledge of the healthcare providers is used to supplement the information offered by these women. Specifically, these latter perspectives illumine a bit about the institutional context in which care is often delivered.

Three of the conversations were in Spanish and the rest were in English. In addition to the actual in-person dialogues, I gave each participant the option of reviewing the interview transcript. In two cases, I asked follow-up questions via email or telephone. Additionally, I met a second time with the three women with whom I spoke in Spanish to review the transcript and to ensure that I had not misunderstood or misinterpreted anything that they had said.

In order to process all that I heard from these collaborators, I took several distinct steps. First, I wrote copious field notes in a journal immediately after each interview. In my notes, I wrote down as many exact quotations as possible. I paid attention to comments that surprised me and also to any emotions and reactions that surfaced in me. Later, I listened to each recorded conversation before composing or reviewing the transcripts.[78] I listened to each recording again as I corrected and cleaned the transcripts. I went back at various points to portions of the recordings in order to refresh my memory not only of what they had said, but also of *how* they had said it—their emphasis, tone, and the emotion evident in their voices. With respect to the transcripts and field notes, I read over each numerous times and took separate notes about them in order to flesh out both unique perspectives of each individual and also common themes that surfaced across individual experiences.

For an additional check, I shared a bulk of the content of the interviews with colleagues. In particular, I met regularly with members of a qualitative methods writing group[79] in order to nuance my identification and analysis of the themes that emerged. This is a racially and culturally diverse group of women and men (gay and straight) who are all actively doing their own qualitative research for degrees in public health, education, social psychology, among others. I was the lone theological and social ethicist in the group. I showed my work to them at critical points and asked them to comment on the themes and analysis I was developing. They raised important questions and critique and helped me see more than I initially had. They also helped me to devise a coherent organization for the presentation of the fieldwork data. Finally, they were instrumental in helping me to navigate the IRB review process.[80]

I have learned a couple of important things with respect to method from doing this fieldwork. Venturing into the unknown territory of ethnography has enriched my understanding in many ways. Not only have I gained insight into what it can mean to be a woman of color with breast cancer, but I have also learned a lot about the complexities of doing ethnographic research. In an effort to be self-reflexive, I would like to highlight briefly this methodological learning before elaborating upon what I have learned from the collaborators in the next chapters.

Perhaps the most basic learning of which I am now acutely aware is this: It takes great care both to understand fully and to describe people well—as they are—without making them into idealized versions. I was surprised by how much time it takes to reflect upon even one of these individuals. Fullilove once remarked that in "listening carefully and reporting it accurately [one discovers] 90 percent of the meaning" to be found by doing qualitative research.[81] Moreover, it takes a lot of material. Fourteen ethnographic interviews yield rather tall piles of paper. These conversations converted into over 500 pages of transcripts, not including field notes. Part of the challenge and quest has been to discover the best way of presenting the material so that it illumines without overwhelming.

Working with two languages complicates and enriches this responsibility of listening carefully and reporting it accurately. During the conversations in Spanish, there was significant repetition. I often asked for clarification and would reflect back to the women what I thought they were saying to ensure that I had understood. This experience of working in my second language reinforced the awareness of how much attention and effort it takes to make sure one really gets it right. The complexity of working with two languages for these interviews mirrors, albeit on a microscopic level, some of the language issues encountered by care providers. However, what is also critical to understand is that such intensive listening is not only needed *across* languages but within the same one as well. Indeed, the awareness brought out by working in Spanish also served to remind me *to slow down in the English conversations as well*—to not assume too quickly that I had understood exactly what the English speakers meant either.

In short, this fundamental task of understanding and describing another accurately and faithfully is not to be underestimated. It can be all too easy—especially in a situation where the researcher does not share the same racial-ethnic or socioeconomic background as those she interviews—to settle for truncated understandings and to describe people in ways that impose labels upon them. I have tried not to take short-cuts. For ethicists and care providers alike, the difficult but honorable challenge is to show in our descriptions, reports, and analysis that we genuinely see who others are, rather than reduce them to superficial facts or accessible and convenient caricatures.

This point ought to be brought to bear upon any context in which the main responsibility of one's work involves attending to other human beings. A sobering comparison may make its significance plain: Each of my conversations lasted between 40 and 85 minutes. In rather stark contrast, after initial intakes and diagnoses, it is common for a clinic doctor's visit to last ten minutes and for an in-patient hospital visit on rounds to be even shorter. Now, add the dimension of different first languages. Ten to 15 minutes does not allow for much repetition on either part. How do both patients and care providers ensure that they fully understand the other and have communicated all their questions and comments to the other? Efforts to build trust and relationships are realized only through hard work; at worst, they are fraught with thorny complications. There are no express lanes on this road. It takes considerable time, focus, and commitment to get to know people and to really hear them. Now consider those who have dozens or hundreds of people in their care. How can there be consistent regard for each person? It seems nearly inevitable that the needs of some will rise above the needs of others. The question is then, Which wheels get the grease?

I want to underscore that it is a gift that each of the collaborators spoke with me. I do not take their candor for granted. They received no compensation for their time or effort. I tried to stay aware of a valid question that any of them might have as they considered me: Why should I reveal anything to this white woman? How do I know she will be a credible and trustworthy listener to me? Why is this worth my time? I am not naïve; I am sure that none told me absolutely everything that they have witnessed or know. Yet I am astounded at how much they did share—both the providers and the women with breast cancer. They all took significant risks in speaking with this stranger. It is important for researchers, healthcare providers, and ethicists to honor that which people reveal to us, while not permitting any successes to make us overly confident that we have achieved a full, complete story of another's identity, life, experiences, or feelings.

The IRB Approval Process

With respect to the IRB, perhaps I was guilty of naiveté. I assumed that the largest hurdle would be building trust and rapport with women of color with breast cancer so that they would speak with me. I must confess that I had not given as much thought to the process of receiving a second tier of formal permission needed to do ethnographic fieldwork. Specifically, I miscalculated the degree and kind of involvement of the IRB.

Researching and writing any book in theological and social ethics is an adventure that involves twists and turns that can never be fully anticipated. It can get even more unpredictable when one goes beyond textual sources to learn from actual persons facing difficult realities. Fullilove was essential in pointing out to me the reality that sometimes important learning happens when one thinks she is on the way to the learning. It is important to not miss the insights that happen along the way, even if they fall outside of what one initially identified as the focus of the research.

In the eventual course of the actual interviews with Black and Latina women with breast cancer and healthcare providers, I noticed the emergence of four themes present in varying ways and degrees in each of their stories: The interplay of racial and socioeconomic assumptions; the imbalance of power dynamics in the patient-provider relationship; the role and necessity of advocates and self-advocacy; and the impact of bureaucratic processes and financial bottom lines. These themes will be elaborated upon in the next chapter. However, in reflecting at the methodological level with respect to this IRB experience, I realize that these themes had already begun to appear before I had even one conversation with a collaborator. Experientially, through a prolonged process of receiving approval, I learned a fair amount about bureaucracies, the imbalance of power dynamics between the IRB and myself, the power of assumptions to shape the field of visibility and intelligibility of a person and her identity, and the necessity of advocacy and self-advocacy in such a situation. So it is important to pause and reflect upon this learning from the "unexpected research that took place before the research."

One caveat merits a word: In significant ways, my experience with a particular IRB mirrors the dynamics articulated by the women of color with cancer as they discuss the effects of the systems and practices they have experienced in their own patient-provider relations. However, in important ways, my experience bears *no* resemblance to theirs. First and foremost, my life was not at stake. Also, my exchange with the IRB, while longer than anticipated, lasted for a lesser period of time and involved far fewer encounters than any of these women have had with care providers during the course of their illnesses.

IRBs came into being in the wake of scientific horrors such as experiments done on Holocaust victims during World War II and the Tuskegee Syphilis study. To test a new drug, treatment regimen, or device, one needs an IRB's authorization. Moreover, any academic research that wishes to interview people usually needs IRB approval—especially if one intends to publish the findings in a medical, sociological, or anthropological journal or text.

IRBs, then, are very important organizations. They are commonly affiliated with a hospital and/or university. Specifically, they make sure that informed consent will be properly acquired from subjects, that participation will be wholly voluntary, that risks to participants are minimized, and that their privacy and confidentiality will be protected. Finally, IRBs are concerned that the selection of subjects be equitable. This emphasis has come out of the increased awareness that women and communities of color have often been shamefully underrepresented in clinical trials.[82]

Individual IRBs are given a significant degree of autonomy in how they carry out their responsibilities and define the boundaries of appropriate protocols. Because they are not a single institution, but rather numerous individual ones, each has its own character. Thus, they are not at all uniform in their perspective, experience, or interpretation of the fundamental criteria for a responsible study.

The particular IRB to which I submitted my research proposal had not before encountered a qualitative or ethnographic study. They routinely review quantitative medical, scientific research (e.g., drug therapies, treatment regimes, devices, research with human tissues). They are an influential IRB, affiliated with both a hospital and a university; they review at a minimum hundreds of protocols each year.

This IRB is also rather large in terms of its membership. According to their membership list published in June of 2002, this specific committee consists of 25 members (one is Ad Hoc). At least two IRB staff persons also regularly attend the full committee meetings. Furthermore, a lot of degrees sit around the table, specifically in the field of medicine and positivistic sciences. Of the 25 committee members, there are 17 MDs, 3 PhDs, 2 Pharm Ds, 1 MDiv, 2 JDs, and 1 R.N.[83] The exact ratio of men to women is not easily identified from the membership list, but a fair estimate would be that 14 or 15 are men and 10 or 11 of the members are women. I met in-person with this committee on one occasion in order to answer some of their questions and concerns regarding my research. The vast majority of the members appeared to be white.

Why does this information matter? The demographics of the committee membership along with the fact that they had, as a committee, no prior experience with a research proposal of this nature meant that there was a considerable leap in mutual understanding that needed to be made. The majority were senior practitioners of medicine or scientists. They were highly sophisticated with regard to medical and clinical psychological studies; they were not at all sophisticated in qualitative research methods. In fact, it was completely new to all of them, except for the relatively new dean of this IRB. Given this chasm in worldviews, in hindsight, it is not at all surprising that they denied approval of my initial submission. This information also matters in the context of the power this entity holds with respect to the researchers who submit proposals to it.

Eventually, after four months, one in-person conversation, and dozens of pages of explanations to their questions, I was granted approval. During this time, I was asked to respond to one three-page rejection letter, and later, to another four-page letter asking for further clarifications and changes. In addition, the dean of the IRB advocated for the value of qualitative research and sent my proposal to independent reviewers at another IRB in another state to get their assessment that helped this IRB comprehend the validity of this project. One of the committee members told me that this degree of time and attention spent on one protocol was incredibly rare, in part because of the large number of submissions this IRB reviewed every month.

Clearly, my proposal stirred things up—provoking emotions and deeply held beliefs of some committee members. Indeed, while I was ultimately granted approval, the vote was not unanimous.[84] The process was so intense that I commented to a colleague that it seemed easier to get a protocol approved to test a new drug or to do experiments on human tissues than to get approval simply to ask people how they feel. It struck me as incredibly ironic that the IRB perceived my research to be far more invasive and dangerous in a sense than to ask people to submit to new drugs, experimental procedures on their bodies, or to have their tissues sampled. Perhaps on some level they believed that such a study was dangerous *not* to the participants, but to the hospital's reputation because it might open up the institution to invasive critique.

The text of the two letters, first the outright rejection and later the follow-up after my in-person meeting with the IRB, are both fascinating. They reveal the great distance in understanding between the culture of this IRB and the basic perspective and claims of my research. In the rejection letter, the first point stated the following:

> As the study is presented it seems to imply an inherent bias. Are black and Latina women singled out and presumed to have a lack of care? Would it be more accurate to have a Caucasian control group? As currently written, the study may have the appearance of being offensive to the subjects and to [this] Hospital. It is suggested by the Committee that seeking guidance from someone with expertise in qualitative research would be helpful.[85]

These comments merit a bit of exegesis. First, the committee did not approve of the small numbers I proposed to interview or of the fact that I was selecting two specific racial-ethnic groupings at the exclusion of others. Taking the perspectives and experiences of a few people of particular races was seen by key members as inherently biased and thus invalid research.[86] Ponder the weight of this viewpoint: The experience of one person, or of persons within particular social groupings, is not valid. What does this (un)conscious assumption communicate about how the IRB, even with its concern to protect the rights of research participants, actually values human beings? The story of one is not valid. It must be measured against a control group. In particular, it was suggested that I compare the experiences of darker skinned women to those of lighter skinned women. The implied message (whether intended or not) is clear: The stories of darker skinned women by themselves are not worthy or sufficient for reflection.

Second, this sentence in the extract quoted above also merits a word: "As currently written, the study may have the appearance of being offensive to the subjects and to [this] Hospital." It was never made clear to me how Black and Latina women might be offended by this study. I did understand why care providers might be hesitant to speak with me. Unwittingly in this comment, the IRB revealed that one of its central concerns may very well be not only the protection of research participants, but also the avoidance of offending those in authority at the hospital. While not explicitly acknowledged, I think there was a fear that my research would embarrass the hospital, even though no names (of participating individuals or institutions) would be made public.

Third, the last sentence indicates that they assumed I knew nothing about qualitative research. Undeniably, it is their job to challenge researchers and make sure they have ethical research methods that do not harm subjects. Yet I had demonstrated in a couple of places on the protocol that an expert in qualitative research was working closely with me. I had also given a lengthy explanation of the rationale for this particular kind of study, which showed familiarity with qualitative methodology.

Also in this rejection letter, the IRB committee noted that they did not like the use of the term "Black" and suggested instead the use of "African American." They deemed it might be offensive to some readers and advised me to "ascertain what is the most accepted descriptor." I subsequently explained that I used the "Black" because not all women of African descent identify as African American (some identify as African, or Caribbean or Puerto Rican, etc.). I explained that "Black" is a general descriptor and its use is an attempt to be as inclusive as possible—to attract as many potential participants who fit under its general umbrella. I also clarified that in speaking with actual persons, I would ask how they defined themselves and from that point on, I would use this terminology in describing them.

One other major concern of the IRB is important to mention. In their rejection letter and in subsequent letters and exchanges, the committee continually expressed strong reservations that this project might cause participants significant emotional or psychological distress.[87] Consequently, as a condition for reconsidering my protocol, they insisted on very detailed and specific measures to ensure that appropriate referrals for emotional support and counseling would be readily available to participants. In doing the actual interviews, I was careful to give a handout listing counseling and referral sources to each of the collaborators. Many expressed relief that their actual names, or the names of hospitals and doctors, would not be used. However, none expressed an interest in the counseling/psychological referral handout—either before or after the conversation. In fact, at the conclusion of the interviews, all of the collaborators smiled, expressed that they had enjoyed the conversation, were glad to help, et cetera. While I do not definitively know if anyone experienced distress after the interview, I do know that none has expressed any kind of regret or distress in subsequent conversations/contacts.

After the initial rejection, I met with the institutional sponsor of this research, a chaplain in the Department of Pastoral Care and Education who also sits on the IRB. Together, we later met with one of the IRB staff persons to discuss the issue. Then, I reworked the protocol to respond to their list of 18 concerns. Finally, I asked to meet in person with the IRB so that they could field their questions and concerns to me and so that I would have an opportunity to clarify things directly. In preparation for this meeting, I submitted a revised protocol and a lengthy cover letter detailing my responses and changes to each of their numbered points.

Meeting with the IRB was fascinating. They do not often meet with researchers. It was a packed room with a long table. Each seat was taken, but someone got up to give me a seat near the door. My conversation with them lasted approximately 20 minutes—an eternity for them to dwell upon just one protocol. I learned later that a heated discussion about my protocol ensued after I left. It intrigues me that the first and weightiest objection was not brought up while I was in the room; namely, why I was interviewing so few women and why only Black and Latina women without a control group. However, I learned from the chaplain and the dean of the IRB that this topic became the center of the debate as soon as I left. One white woman in particular, who holds a PhD in psychology, was the most adamant in her rejection of this research. Yet she uttered not a word or question in my presence.[88] Debriefing my meeting with the IRB committee and their discussion that followed my departure, the chaplain told me that my protocol had raised fundamental questions for them with respect to what constitutes science and research: "These folks have not had basic assumptions challenged within the bioethical model. . . . It's a clash of cultures. It's not something they can validate because it's not how they confront truth and power in a very sophisticated biomedical model."[89]

I cite this experience not to deride the IRB but to emphasize the gap that may exist between a theo-ethicist's perspective and that of the medical/scientific establishment. One cannot take for granted that others will share the view that women of color are able to speak truth in their own right and out of their own experiences—without comparison to others—about human personhood, dignity, and adequate healthcare quality. The IRB did not initially understand that prioritizing a few particular voices was not a denial of the significance of others.

The western scientific mentality generally esteems neutrality, blind samples, objectivity, and research that can be "generalized"—able to be replicated in other contexts and thus made "universal" in its findings. This research openly violates these rules. It claims, at the outset, a subjective stance and denies that there are any wholly objective stances with regard to these issues. Everyone is socially positioned in ways that inform how they view and value these questions.

Rather than comparing Black and Latina women's experiences with white women, or comparing the experiences of every racial-ethnic grouping, this study has sought to develop a thick description of experiences of a few individual women.[90] The point is not to tell every story, but to tell a few with care and attention to detail. Indeed, while not telling us absolutely everything there is to know, one story can still convey a great deal of information about what good care and respect look and feel like. This study aims for rich description, not exhaustive analysis. This is the heart of qualitative, ethnographic research.

What took four months for the IRB and me to come to a shared (for the most part) understanding is this: One basic function of qualitative research is to gain insight about what constitutes adequate respect and care from members of social groups who experience systemic inequality and discrimination in U.S. society. In other words, Black and Latina women who have had a cancer diagnosis and who have sought medical care may have distinct perspectives that would benefit larger discussions focused on improving healthcare quality.

To say this does not mean that darker skinned women will report experiences to which no other persons can relate. Indeed, the experiences that they have may resonate with people of various racial-ethnic and socioeconomic groups. As I wrote to the IRB in one of the protocol revisions, the purpose of this research is not to argue that "[t]hese women experience things that no others do or can relate to," but rather to contend that "[t]hese *particular* women, who on historical and societal levels are often not listened to and who are under-represented in research, have something important to say and ought to be heard." They are—as is every human being—ends in themselves.

In the process of receiving IRB approval, I learned valuable lessons not only about these entities, but about power relations as well. Initially, there was no assumption on the part of the committee that I, a white academic in Christian social ethics, might have well-thought out reasons for proposing this study. There was no assumption that this kind of qualitative method was valid. The burden was upon me, a person with relatively little institutional authority, to prove that my approach was both significant and valid. They assumed that I had not thought about the matter of using "Black" instead of "African American." Even though I stated explicitly on the protocol that I spoke Spanish and translated the consent form and ad into Spanish myself, the committee missed this information, asking in the follow-up responses if translators would be utilized. In short, I had to prove that I had something important to say and that I knew what I was doing. They, in contrast, were in a position to either formally acknowledge my knowledge or not.

While my experience cannot be equated with the experience of women of color with cancer, there is a connection that I find interesting. Black and Latina women with breast cancer have to negotiate healthcare systems that have significant power and discretion in listening to them or not. If I (a white, educated, and extroverted woman) had so much difficulty in being heard by the IRB, how difficult might it be for women of color to be heard by healthcare institutions?[91] Certainly, many women are very articulate, determined, and proactive advocates for themselves and know how to find the right doctors, insist on being taken seriously, be persistent, and direct their treatment. Some have great support systems that also assist in the advocacy. However, this is weighty, often exhausting, work to take on in addition to fighting cancer. And given the fact that they are ill, not all women are able to maintain this level of involvement and advocacy on their own behalf. Some do not have solid support systems in place. In these troubling scenarios, I fear that many women may fall between the cracks and fail to be heard. They may not even be given the acknowledgment that they have something important and valid to say.

Conclusion

The use of both theological language and ethnography in this book is in the service of imagination. Qualitative fieldwork may contribute to fleshing out the meaning of theo-ethical norms that are relevant for how human beings ought to regard and treat one another. This kind of research may also critique and revise these norms using the insights and norms that are discovered in the voices and experiences of collaborators. For its part, theo-ethical language can, with thick description, actively contribute to honoring the worth of every human being. Knowing that one matters, that one counts, is a basic human need. This knowledge is food for the human heart. Theology is a discipline uniquely gifted at articulating why each life matters and how each is cherished beyond comprehension.

The relationship between the two is like this: In doing ethnographic research, I did not attempt to create a theological "blank slate" within my mind. Rather, I tried to acknowledge consciously that I hold certain theo-ethical convictions (e.g., neighbor-love, *imago dei*, the intrinsic interdependence of all life), and to open them to (re)formation by others different from myself. Some collaborators may not share them or may even dispute them. Similarly, they may work with very different anthropological and theological understandings that come from particular cultural and faith traditions.[92] As liberationist theologies have long understood, such engagement will enrich my understanding both of others *and* of these concepts because of the active interplay between praxis and critical theo-ethical reflection.

Healthcare systems, practitioners, and ethics can be enriched by both theological ethics and qualitative research. Other people ought to play a part in holding academics, healthcare providers, and policy makers accountable for what we posit in terms of anthropology and how human beings ought to be treated. In what follows, I will demonstrate the sorts of insights available to those willing to engage in theological and ethical reflection on the particular stories of collaborators in a qualitative research project; in this case, the particular stories of Latina and Black women with breast cancer and healthcare providers.

4

Listening

After being submerged in theological, sociological, and qualitative methodological texts for so long, it was refreshing to come up for air. Conversations with people became the oxygen I needed. Rather than reading and writing, I listened. This shift in my learning method was essential for my growth both as a scholar and as a person. Over the course of six months, I met 14 fascinating people. While they have different areas of expertise and sources for their knowledge, all know a significant amount about healthcare quality. At the time of the interviews, all of the women with breast cancer had received their cancer diagnosis within the last five years. Five of the six healthcare providers work predominately with cancer patients—as an oncologist, social worker, nurse, or nurse case manager. The sixth is a third-year medical student.[1] Taken together, the collaborators had many and varied experiences and perspectives. None of their perspectives simply confirms another.

This chapter begins with the women with breast cancer. After briefly introducing each to the reader, I highlight four themes that emerged in the course of the interviews and then retell the stories of three particular women in more depth in order to bring these themes to the surface. The chapter concludes with analysis of these themes and draws upon additional insights from the collaborators. In particular, the voices of the care providers are introduced at this point. What is striking about this second tier of interviews with the caregivers is the way in which several of their testimonies reflect similar themes and concerns as those of several of the women with cancer.

All names have been changed. Hospital names will not be used. Seven of the eight women with cancer chose their own pseudonym, while only two healthcare providers chose to do so. I was glad when participants offered their own fictional names. It was another way to respect their voice and identity, rather than impose either upon them.

Eight Introductions

The women with breast cancer range in age from 33 to 67 years old. Seven of them explicitly express a Christian faith. One has Christian roots in the Black Church and notes that although she does not attend anymore, she has a belief in a higher power than humankind. The women vary in how they describe their racial-ethnic backgrounds. Two identify as Black and two as African American; two identify as Latina; one prefers the term Hispanic (of these three, one specifically identifies as Puerto Rican and two as Dominican).[2] Finally, one woman identifies as Black Puerto Rican, underscoring the fact that one can be both Black and Latina.

One woman first had cancer of the cervix and uterus in the 1980s before having subsequent diagnoses of breast cancer in the 1990s and in 2003. For the others, breast cancer was their first diagnosis. They have received cancer care at several different sites—private specialty hospitals, public hospitals and clinics and teaching hospitals. Together, they offer vivid snapshots of a wide spectrum of U.S. healthcare. Seven are presently insured: One has Medicaid; another has Medicaid and Medicare; five have employer or school-based insurance. One woman had lost her employer-based insurance and was uninsured at the time of the interview.

Before drawing out relevant themes that emerged from these conversations, I would like to introduce these women to the reader. Each woman deserves attention in her own right, as an end in herself. Having acknowledged this commitment, however, I must also admit that what follows represents only a small fraction of each woman's story. While it may be impossible to be exhaustive in describing the breadth of anyone's personhood and experience, it is still possible to describe faithfully salient aspects of each. What follows is an informative glimpse into the windows of the lives of eight women who have simultaneously faced breast cancer and U.S. healthcare systems.

Hannah Jacobs

Hannah Jacobs is 44 years old.[3] She has run marathons and 5 Ks since the late 1970s. She emphasized that she is very selective about the persons with whom she shares personal information. "I'm a great listener. And I listen to them before I open myself up, you know, to a person. But then, you know, as time go on, I start to open up . . . I'm very selective of who I share my information with. . . ." When she began speaking about her life, and especially about her faith, she came alive with energy and enthusiasm. As she spoke, she conveyed self-confidence—a firm and peaceful centeredness in who she is. She wants to be known first and foremost as a born-again Christian woman. "You know, I know who I am, and I know God has a plan and purpose for my life." She is also African American. Hannah is married and has three children. She commented that her husband and children have been wonderful sources of support, understanding, and strength throughout her diagnosis and healing. She works for a large, successful company and says that she has excellent health insurance. She was treated for her cancer in New Jersey.

Hannah was diagnosed with breast cancer in December 2000. She went in for a yearly checkup and mammogram. Hannah had not noticed anything unusual in her breast before the mammogram. The mammogram showed a calcification clustering, so she had a biopsy. Her doctor, whom she has known for ten years, caught the cancer very early and referred her to a breast specialist who is also an African American woman. Hannah glowed with praise for this specialist and emphasized that they have an excellent, even personal, relationship. This physician gave her three options: Lumpectomy, chemotherapy, or mastectomy.[4] Hannah choose the mastectomy because she did not feel she needed chemotherapy and she knew that if she had the lumpectomy there was no guarantee that the cancer would not come back to that breast. She was hospitalized for just 24 hours. Hannah has had no radiation or chemotherapy, nor has she taken Tamoxifen—an oral preventative drug often prescribed to women who have either had cancer or who are deemed to be at a high risk for breast cancer.

Even as Hannah is reserved, she knows how to find the doctors that she will trust and has been able, with the help of her insurance coverage, to be selective in choosing them. She makes her decisions based on her comfort with a given doctor's personality and observed skill level, not on her/his race. "I don't choose doctors based on their race. I choose them based on. . . . have people recommend[ed] them to you and, you know, I just—You could get a certain—when you see them, you know, you know right away if that's the one, if there's a connection or not." I found it interesting, however, that Hannah acknowledged that in the past ten years, she has chosen three African American physicians as primary physicians for her and her family.

Yet, Hannah was firm in her position that she does not think that racial dynamics have much to do with the quality of her doctor-patient relationships. When I asked her whether she thinks that racial assumptions/dynamics can get in the way—if they can filter how others see her or not, she adamantly replied, "It doesn't get in the way. It doesn't get in the way. It doesn't get in the way. I can fit in anywhere, really. I really don't have any problems fitting in anywhere I go. I mean, not so much fitting in, but I can—I'm, you know, I can adjust." Indeed, Hannah emphasized a couple of times that she is able to build rapport with people of various racial backgrounds.

Throughout Hannah's description of her life, perspective, and identity, I heard a strong refusal to allow race to define her—in her own or another's eyes. "I know who I am and *Whose* I am." (Emphasis hers.) She expressed that God is "colorblind" and that she tries to be as well: "I know I'm Black. I know I'm African American. But I would, for me, today, I want people to see me as a born-again Christian woman, somehow who—see Christ in, not so much as color. God is colorblind. And that's how I like to be, also."

However, Hannah did emphasize that she thinks that health insurance can significantly influence people's ability to access good quality care. In particular, she expressed concern for the lack of public health/hospital outreach to certain communities regarding cancer prevention and detection:

> There's some women out there who need healthcare who don't have insurance. I think that there should be more awareness of places to go for those treatments. A lot of times the information's not reaching, you know, the Black and Latino community. . . . I'm reaching out to them because they're not going to come to those places. I don't know, what are their—are they advertising enough? . . . [A]re they doing their part? I don't know. But they're not reaching the Black and Latino community. And they're right there in the community, and they're not reaching them. They're not bringing them in for their yearly mammogram.

While Hannah had nothing but praise for her healthcare providers, she did raise concerns regarding how well the established clinics and hospitals are serving Blacks and Latinos who reside in their neighborhoods. In this regard, she did see that having members of a given racial-ethnic or cultural community reaching out to its own people serves a vital purpose. In a related vein, she also noted the fear of possible costs keeps many uninsured women from seeking care:

> [N]ot everybody is as fortunate to have, you know, insurance. . . . And that's why they're not coming in for their mammograms, because they're worrying about the cost. . . . They don't have the money. They

don't have insurance. . . . For the most part, you know, they're just thinking about keeping food on the table. You know, and for a woman, she's the last person she's thinking about. . . . She's thinking about her family.

Hannah commented that through her volunteering and cancer support and education outreach, she has encountered many women who focus on taking care of everybody else, to the exclusion of themselves—that providing and caring for the family is their primary focus.

Wanda Kelly

Wanda Kelly is a soft-spoken 38-year-old woman.[5] She squeezed in speaking with me before a busy work day, after having dropped off her son an hour early in order to meet me. Wanda was polite and candid in her responses. She both complimented her care and critiqued certain dynamics that she has observed by working in and around healthcare for several years. Wanda describes her racial-ethnic identity as African American. She also identifies as an active Christian. Wanda works in cancer outreach to other women of color. She communicates dedication and energy for this vocation. Wanda is married and has a son.[6] She has experienced cancer care in two different New York City clinical settings.

Wanda was diagnosed with breast cancer in September 1999. She noticed a nipple discharge and went to have it checked out at a city hospital. The first breast specialist she saw recommended that she have a mammogram and a sonogram. Wanda said that technician who saw the discharge on the film at the time of the tests said, "Oh, that's nothing." Wanda thought this was an inappropriate statement to make given that the doctor had not yet seen the test. The results came back negative. The discharge stopped for about a month, but then restarted and Wanda went to see a different specialist at a different hospital. Following additional tests, she was diagnosed with breast cancer. One of Wanda's siblings worked in the first hospital and helped connect her with a specialist there. After receipt of the initial negative results from the test done there, Wanda decided to consult another site of care. She knew someone who worked at the second hospital, which specializes in cancer. Through this contact, Wanda was able to connect with a second breast specialist.

Wanda said she was surprised by the cancer diagnosis. She had always heard about lumps as being warning signs but not about a nipple discharge. She was also much younger than most women are when they get breast cancer. She had insurance through work then and still does. Her insurance did not pay for all the costs incurred at this second hospital, so she paid the difference in order to go there. Wanda had a mastectomy, followed by six months of chemotherapy. At the time of our interview, she was taking Tamoxifen, which she would do for two more years.

Wanda has been very pleased with her care at this second hospital and with her breast specialist (a white woman). After giving the diagnosis, this doctor handed Wanda all of her paperwork and films and encouraged her to get a second opinion at another hospital. Wanda did so because she had a friend who had had breast cancer and knew of a very highly respected surgeon. Wanda chose to go back to this second hospital and breast specialist that had given her the cancer diagnosis. She continues to see the same doctors there for checkups and feels that they have always been compassionate, thorough, skilled, and encouraging of her own agency.

María de Lourdes Maldonado

María is a 67-year-old mother and grandmother.[7] She smiles often. We spoke in Spanish, which is clearly her first language and clearly *not* mine. She was patient with me and gave full answers to my sometimes grammatically impaired questions. María came to New York 34 years ago from Puerto Rico. She defines her racial-ethnic background as Hispanic. She finished the sixth grade in Puerto Rico, but then her mother died and she had to quit school in order to take care of her family.

She has had breast cancer twice in her life and has experienced care in two different settings in New York City. María told me that she lost faith in the first hospital. She most recently had breast surgery in 2000. María speaks with pride when she explains that it was she who first found the cancer both times through breast self-exams. She has both Medicare and Medicaid health insurance. She occasionally volunteers to speak to Latina groups about breast cancer detection as well as her own experience. Her story is given more attention below.

Luz Hernandez

Luz Hernandez is a 44-year-old Spanish teacher for a New York City primary school. She is married and has two children, one of whom is autistic.[8] Luz is a vivacious woman, overflowing with exuberance. She freely expresses a range of emotions and is open about sharing her experience with others.[9] Luz also has a generous spirit—she insisted on buying me coffee before the interview. It did not matter to her that she was doing me a huge favor by taking time out of a full weekend to speak with me.

Luz described herself as "a feisty woman." With respect to getting good medical care, she commented, "A few people have to have your back, but one thing I tell you is that if you sit back and wait here, you don't get anything. You have to be determined." Luz is self-confident and assertive in many areas, not just around her cancer diagnosis. For example, she worked exceptionally hard to complete her education, including holding down three jobs simultaneously to cover her expenses. She now has a Master's degree in education. Her strength and determination to succeed and to thrive (not merely survive) flow directly from her deep love of her family and from her passion to live. She has had to advocate for herself in gaining access to good quality care, even as she has had insurance throughout the course of her illness. Despite the poor care she initially received, Luz expressed no bitterness.

Luz describes her racial-ethnic identity as Dominican but noted that she most intimately understands herself as African Caribbean—explaining that she is a mixture of white, Latino, African, and indigenous roots. Luz is also an evangelical Christian. Luz's first language is Spanish, but she also speaks English well, although learning the language did not come easy for her. In our conversation, we spoke in both English and Spanish, jumping from one language to the other in order to enhance a particular understanding or description.

Luz was diagnosed with breast cancer in 2002. Initially, Luz saw a Spanish-speaking Latino physician who assured her it was not cancer, even before doing a biopsy or mammogram. Upon doing a physical exam, he told Luz, " 'I don't feel anything, but since you are over 40, I will send you to have a mammogram.' " They did a mammogram that did not reveal anything conclusive, only a small shaded area. Luz was not convinced that there was no reason to worry. She asked the doctor to remove the little ball she felt. The doctor agreed to do a lumpectomy in his office. Upon doing so, and *before* having any lab report, he told her, " 'It doesn't appear malignant, don't worry. I will give you the results within a week.' " Nine days afterward, he called her to come into his office. After realizing that it was cancer, the doctor reassured her again by telling her and her husband that it was not a serious cancer and that she only needed a "clean-up," not a full mastectomy: "When they told me the news in this moment, [my husband

and I] started to cry . . . And we said, 'And now, what do we do?' The doctor told me, 'This is nothing, what you have is small. They will clean up the spot.' They made the preparations to send me for a clean-up, not a mastectomy, but a cleaning of the area where there was cancer."[10] As Luz recounted this part of her story, her eyes welled with tears, still not believing that he had been so wrong (and so wrong to reassure her without any hard facts based on tests) and that she had had to wait so many days to get the results.

The doctor made arrangements for her to have pre-operation appointments ("pre-ops") at a city hospital with which he was affiliated. However, after experiencing what she described as a slow, ineffective, impersonal, and careless healthcare setting, Luz decided to seek care elsewhere. Luz emphasized that this first hospital is where many people in Manhattan go who do not have much money or good insurance. She related her knowledge of two sisters who both had had breast cancer, but they lacked insurance and had gone there. Both had "clean-ups," not full mastectomies; neither received radiation or chemotherapy. Both died. "The poor dears, two *Mestizas* . . . the two small, young [sisters] died of cancer. And the one was told that she was O.K. and that they had cleaned the area. And the sister, the same— they cleaned the area and did not give her chemotherapy, they did not give her anything. [They both died.]" Knowing of these outcomes in the cases of these two women of color made Luz all the more determined to seek care somewhere else.

She called for two days trying to get into another hospital that has a well-respected cancer center. They told her that they had no appointments and that they would not accept her particular form of insurance. Luz did not give up.[11] Instead, she contacted a friend who has a sister-in-law that works in the cancer center as a nurse for one of the senior cancer physicians. Upon hearing about Luz from this nurse friend, this doctor at the center called Luz at home and told her to come in and that he would accept her insurance. From this point on, Luz glows about the quality of the care she received. It turned out to be an aggressive cancer. She had a mastectomy followed by almost seven months of chemotherapy. All within three days, she had her first appointment with the specialist (a conversation that lasted 25 minutes), another mammogram, a sonogram, an ultrasound, an initial cleaning of the area, and a radical mastectomy.

For Luz, racial bias or a lack of understanding across cultures was not an issue in her care. In fact, she strongly preferred the white male doctor over the Latino physician. In contrasting the two doctors, Luz explained the following:

> [E]ven though he spoke the same language, he was not like caring because he didn't understand my feelings. For example, you know that what you are telling me is from you, it's not from medicine. It's not like you have tested this and know that this is a fact. You just see a worried person and you are going to tell me something to make me feel better, not something that is medically correct. When I sat down with [the second doctor] he told me, "your cancer is aggressive. It's a bad cancer." He told me. He told me the truth about my cancer.

Luz preferred the white specialist both because he was skilled in getting and interpreting all of the medical facts quickly and because he was thorough and honest in his examinations and conversations with her.

More than racial dynamics or having good cross-cultural understanding, what made the difference in the quality for her care, Luz thinks, was money and insurance. "It is not the color of [one's] skin. That no. It is money and the way in which you present yourself. . . . These days a change is occurring in society and the greatest change is the money that you have—at least in the United States." Indeed, Luz repeatedly emphasized the strong role money and the economics of healthcare plays in determining the amount and quality of care a person receives.

I commented that I thought that having a connection that helped her gain access to a caregiver and setting specializing in cancer treatment was also very significant. She responded,

> I, with my cancer, I called the office [at the specialist's hospital], I called that office so much so that—my friend says to me, "No, I am going to call my friend who is a nurse" so that she could help me. So then, she called and that is how I got an appointment. The doctor called me himself. [Because] I had gotten tired of them telling me, "No, we can't accept your insurance here; we cannot treat you here." Yes, at first, I had this response for two days and my friend told me, "No, you cannot go to any other hospital, come with us. I am going to call this nurse." And the nurse is the one who helped me. And she says to me, "Don't go to any other place, come here and I will talk with the doctor for you." She herself talked to him and he called me the next day. And the doctor told me "the nurse spoke with me" and that I should come there.

Overall, Luz credited her friend's assistance, her insurance, and her own determination with the fact that she was able to access such speedy and high quality attention, which in turn, she feels strongly, saved her life:

> Here in the hospital where they treated me I did not need chemotherapy in general, but just in case there were some cells that were still there, they gave me six months of a mild chemotherapy. If I had said that my finger nail hurt, they would have come to find out what was wrong with that finger nail. You see what I am saying? But not all hospitals are like this and it could be because of race—the two sisters were Black—the two that died of cancer. It could be due to race or something else. . . . I think that the economy has a lot to do with [the quality of care].

She again noted that the two sisters had been treated at a public hospital whose population is predominately poor and/or uninsured.

Marcela Rodriguez

Marcela Rodriguez is 33 years old.[12] She is married and has two small children. She was soft-spoken during our conversation. She also has a sense of humor and laughed occasionally. She showed much hospitality, inviting me to her home and serving tropical juices that she blends from a variety of fresh fruits. Marcela identifies herself as a Christian. She expressed several times that she is profoundly grateful to God. For example, she gave thanks and credit to God for the fact that chemotherapy did not make her too ill and that she was able to secure childcare for her two small children during her illness. She emphasized that she felt God's steady accompaniment, which was especially important to her given that all of her family, except her husband and two children, live in the Dominican Republic. Overall, Marcela has a solidly positive outlook on life. She did not complain about any of her life circumstances, some of which seemed to me to be challenging. She gravitates toward seeing the good in people and in situations—even in ones that are far from optimal. Marcela's generosity and understanding for others' limits impressed me.

Even as she is not an overly critical or confrontational person, Marcela nonetheless knows how to look out for herself. She learned of the opportunity to enroll for emergency Medicaid after the events of September 11, 2001, and took advantage of it. Prior to this date, she had been uninsured. A couple of times during the course of her illness, there was a danger that her Medicaid coverage would be discontinued, given that she had only received the "emergency" version. So she had to work hard—filling out additional paperwork, going to the Medicaid office, having appointments—to do all she could to make sure the coverage continued. At one point in the process of diagnosing her cancer, she thought the doctors were taking too long in scheduling the tests and deciding upon a treatment plan. So Marcela took all her information to a second hospital to get the diagnosis. She then went back to the first hospital for treatment because it is significantly closer to her home.

Marcela describes her racial-ethnic identity as Latina. She has lived in the United States for seven years, coming from the Dominican Republic. She speaks Spanish and just a little English. Similar to María, Marcela was patient with my Spanish and gave full answers to my questions. She elaborated upon terms and expressions with which I was not familiar. She has not noticed any racial discrimination or different quality of treatment for Medicaid patients. She said that language issues have not been a problem for her because her husband or a friend has translated for her. When she has gone to appointments alone, she said that she can make herself understood and can understand enough of what the providers say to her.

Marcela was diagnosed with cancer in December 2001. "I received the news the 17th of December of 2001. That date I will never forget." She found the lump during a self-exam, while she was nursing her four-month-old son. At first, the doctors thought it might be the milk in her breast. "They did a lot of tests on me because they did not believe that a person my age could have [cancer]." She did not think that what she had found in her breast was a side effect from nursing. "Because it bothered me a lot, it hurt. . . . They told me to return [later] and see if the pain went away. When I came back, I told them that it had not gone away and [the doctor] send me for more analysis— she sent me to have a sonogram and later a [biopsy/aspiration]."[13] Marcela was assertive in following up and in having more tests done. She has undergone several stages of treatment. First, they gave her chemotherapy, then she had a lumpectomy. A month later, they decided a full mastectomy was needed. This operation was followed by more chemotherapy and then radiation. At the time of our interview, she was taking Tamoxifen. Marcela has had three different doctors for her cancer in less than two years. No one gave her a full explanation of why they left. None spoke Spanish with any significant facility.

In describing her doctors, Marcela commented that "[t]hey had enough patience. Patience and understanding—are the two things that one most needs. . . ." In fact, when I asked her if they were not in too much of a hurry, she exclaimed, "No, I think the one who was in a hurry was me!" It was then that she explained that at one point she felt they were taking too long in the process of getting tests done, so she went to another hospital with all of her records, had the tests done, and then came back to the first hospital for treatment. She laughed a bit in telling me about this experience:

> I went to [the first hospital] and from there they told me that it was a tumor but they did not know if it was cancerous. So then what I did was to go and since they gave me an appointment and I found them to be very slow, I went to another hospital. . . . So then when they [at the second hospital] told me all that I had, then I already knew what I had and so I took everything and came back [to the first hospital] . . . I simply had their opinion, but not another and so I told myself, "Well, I will go and [the second hospital] will tell me what I have and at the same time I will get another opinion."

Marcela struck me as a very astute and determined woman even as she was very unassuming, soft-spoken, and kind in her demeanor during our conversation. She was both very understanding and complimentary of her care providers. Yet, she also took a lot of initiative to seek out additional information and to help herself navigate a complex network of healthcare systems.

Even as she did not think that it negatively affected her own care or understanding, Marcela did note that language is an area where there is discrimination in healthcare for some people. More than simple racism in society, Marcela identified language barriers as an important issue. To illustrate, Marcela commented,

> I think that it has gotten better, racism has gotten a bit better. Because also what happens principally here, what helps racism is when a person does not know the language. . . . Because sometimes when one does not know the language, they don't try to talk to the person. And there are persons who do not understand. . . . [I]f one does not know the language perfectly, yes, things change.

Again, it is important to underscore that Marcela had nothing but appreciation and gratitude for the care that she received as a woman with breast cancer, who speaks almost no English, and who was insured only by Medicaid at the time she received her cancer care.

Interestingly, there were times when I found myself bothered by certain events that she herself was not. When I asked her if she had translators whenever she needed one, Marcela responded,

> Yes, I tell you all that was necessary. The only [she starts to laugh] the only thing was when the change of doctors . . . You know when there are moments in which the time comes when the doctor has to be changed because that one goes to another hospital . . . . Yes, and so, another comes, another doctor is placed. [She laughs]. But, yes, always what I have needed has been there.

And in terms of translation, she explained, "Well at first, my husband always was with me and as he speaks English, well he always went with me and at least could help me. And then later I went out, I went trying. Sometimes I looked for Ana [a cancer support network person] so that she could serve as interpreter. And from there on, I helped myself. . . ." In listening to Marcela, and in reflecting on my own assumptions about and reactions to her story, I realized that while I might be angered by some things, I cannot assume that they are significant issues for the person seeking care. Indeed, I cannot assume that "my agenda" equals hers. For example, while I was frustrated by the numerous changes of doctors and the lack of translation services provided, Marcela focused on the fact that her doctors gave her very good care and that she was, at the time we met, free from cancer.

Slimfat Girl

Slimfat Girl is a tall, dignified woman who, at the time of our conversation, had not been diagnosed with cancer for very long.[14] She struck me as a private person, yet she was very direct and forthright in what she did choose to share. She conveys an inner core of strength to which she clings when various external attacks threaten and test it. For example, she has had to brush off the comments of others that "put you in the ground before your time" along with callous assumptions of people who do not know her.

Slimfat Girl describes her racial identity as Black. She is in her mid forties and has four children.[15] Her immediate family is very important to her. She works in an accounting department and was on medical leave at the time of our meeting. Slimfat Girl has health insurance through her employer. She was raised Roman Catholic and still considers herself Catholic. She expressed that God "has always been there" for her throughout her life.

Slimfat Girl was diagnosed with a fast-growing breast tumor in May of 2003. The cancer had spread to eight of her lymph nodes as well. She recently had a mastectomy and was now undergoing chemotherapy (for a total of 12 weeks) to be followed by six weeks of radiation. She did not like her first doctor (a white male) because of "his manner." She later added that he was "abrupt." So she has a different one now. She said that she likes her current doctor (a white male) who is a "people person" and has especially appreciated the care she has received from Mike, the nurse who administered her chemotherapy. When I asked her if she sees any signs of racism in healthcare, she replied, "I don't see it. I can't say that I do. I mean, I get the same treatment, and I thank God for that, with my insurance helps. I get the same treatment as everybody else."

Slimfat Girl conveyed the fact that she was very much still adjusting to this new reality in her life:

> So the good thing is that they caught it all [the tumor], but it got in my lymph nodes. So that's why I'm taking, like, heavy does of radiation, because of the seriousness. Out of 19 lymph nodes, I think it was in eight of them. So they don't know whether it got into my bloodstream or not, so that's why I had to take this heavy doses of chemotherapy. Which is, like, 12 weeks of chemotherapy. And then I have to go for six weeks of radiation on an everyday basis. And [my doctors are very good]. And they said, you know, "This is beatable, you know, this is beatable. You're going to be fine." So the point is that I have to lose my hair, you know, I've got to go through different changes, you know. And in the long run. . . . I think I'll be O.K. . . . I deal with it on a day-to-day basis, I can't predict what's going to happen tomorrow. But for today, I'm still here.

She expressed that the adjustment is hard on many levels. She was still getting used to not having one breast, to not having hair for now, and to not feeling good physically. She shared that the cancer diagnosis has been hard on her relationship with her boyfriend:

> And even 'til today, I'm not the same person that I used to be. I'm not the same person. . . . You know, because of what I'm going through, I think people look at you differently, you know . . . I have my life, which is the most important thing. You know, I thank God for that much. But it's not like I still have both of my breasts. You know, I lost all my hair. I had very long hair. All that's gone. . . . My relationship with my boyfriend has suffered a strain because of this. And I'm hoping we can bring it back to where it used to be.

At the time, she said that she was not going out as much, not laughing or smiling as much, not being as social as she had been before the diagnosis. Indeed, cancer can have far-reaching effects on one's life and sense of self—well apart from the most immediate physiological ones.

Sandra Gavin

Sandra Gavin is a quiet and assertive woman.[16] She told her story with great detail and recollection. Sandra is 56 years old and has four adult children. She is divorced. Sandra describes her racial-ethnic background as Black, but she also notes she is a mixture of Native American, African, and white ancestries. She noted that she grew up in the Black Church but that she no longer attends.

Sandra has the most formal education of any of the women I interviewed. When we spoke, she was pursuing a PhD in nursing education, which she subsequently completed. She has worked as a nurse and as a hospital administrator, so she sees and understands both the interpersonal and systemic levels of healthcare. She has also witnessed the gamut of healthcare settings: Managed care sites, a choice in care sites and providers due to employer-based insurance, public clinics and hospitals due to being uninsured for few months, and regaining choice through student health insurance coverage.

Sandra is a resilient woman who has faced four diagnoses of cancer since the early 1980s. She was first diagnosed with cervical cancer in 1980–1981. Two years later, uterine cancer appeared and she had a full hysterectomy along with chemotherapy and radiation. Sandra was first diagnosed with breast cancer (on the left side) in the early 1990s. In January 2003, she noticed drainage from the right breast and was again diagnosed with breast cancer. Sandra has been on a wild journey in just 12 months, going to three different doctors in three very different care settings. This tale receives sustained attention below.

Sophia Andre

Sophia Andre is a sharp, thoughtful, courageous woman.[17] She is 41 years old and has an eight-year-old son. She has also been the primary caregiver of her 92-year-old grandmother who is blind, has Alzheimer's, and lives with her.[18] She defines her racial-ethnic identity as a Black Puerto Rican woman. She identifies herself as Christian. Sophia exudes both inner strength and warmth. Her presence draws you in. She has a great sense of humor. She speaks plainly and with conviction. She conveys both self-respect and humility. While she indicates that she knows how to protect herself—how to guard her feelings/reactions, she was very open during the interview. She may not want to show everyone her emotions or dwell on them, but she does not deny their presence within her.

Sophia has a localized regional recurrence of stage three metastatic breast cancer.[19] She was first diagnosed in 2000; the recurrence was in March of 2003. While she lives in New Jersey, she is from New York City and has received all of her cancer care in New York at a hospital that has emphasized cancer treatment and research. When she was first diagnosed, she had good health insurance through her employer. However, she had just been laid off before the recurrence was diagnosed and was uninsured at the time of our conversation. The same care providers have treated her for both cancer diagnoses. When we spoke, she was on a payment plan. Her story appears below.

Emergent Themes and Three Stories

Before delving into the core themes which surfaced in the stories of these eight women, it is important to note three general observations. First, some were more critical of their healthcare providers than others. In a related vein, some overtly identified the role of systemic problems and issues around race, class, and the structures and limits of U.S. healthcare provision, while others focused more on the level of individual provider personalities and sensibilities. All identified the significance of socioeconomic factors and insurance, although some dwelled on this point more than others. It is also important to emphasize that none reported wholly negative experiences. Indeed, everyone glowed about at least one of their doctors and/or nurses. In fact, even those who were the most critical of aspects of their care still found doctors and care settings in which they are comfortable and pleased. Simply put, their experiences and degrees of satisfaction are just as complex and multilayered as the healthcare systems are themselves.

Second, none scapegoated the healthcare systems or providers—even those who encountered very disturbing practices. To varying degrees and with different foci, all emphasized their own responsibility, agency, and power to affect their care. They each noted how women themselves need to take the initiative to get checked out, to insist on follow-up, to search out second opinions, and to take risks in sharing their information and personhood with their providers. Their conceptions of self and of survival strategies have a central place for their own agency.

Finally, in listening to each of these women, I was struck again and again by the complexity of their lives. Each has had to contend simultaneously with much more than cancer. Furthermore, the nightmare of cancer in their lives reaches far beyond the physical, emotional, and financial realms: It takes a serious toll on their children, their relationships to their husbands and boyfriends, the logistical management of household tasks and budgets, and their friendships.

To illustrate: In addition to caring and advocating for her children, especially her autistic son, Luz worked full-time during her chemotherapy so that she would not lose the income and risk losing insurance. Sophia remained the primary caregiver for her live-in grandmother as well as her son. Slimfat Girl and her boyfriend struggled with the adjustment to the cancer diagnosis, and she learned to guard herself against the insensitive comments of others.

Moreover, a couple of the women had to fight to either access or keep medical coverage. Even as they have been critically ill, Marcela and Sandra in particular have had to run to various offices (Medicaid and student health insurance offices) to secure insurance. And Marcela did this much on her own without the benefit of English fluency. Even as both Sandra and Marcela were feeling ill, or were having serious symptoms, they hustled from appointment to appointment, filling in paperwork, making calls, et cetera, in order to gain or retain access to insurance—whether private or public in nature.

In short, these women worked simultaneously on many projects and on many dimensions of their lives. When cancer came, it was added to the already existing demands, pressures, and challenges of work, home, and budgets in addition to complicating them and adding new ones. Nothing let up—no one came in and took off the pressures of the previous demands. Life just got more complex for them, and they took on more and different challenges in addition to the prior responsibilities. These women kept busy and kept moving. Over the course of their lives, they have become experts at, as Slimfat Girl put it, "dealing with life on life's terms."

In addition to these general observations, through the process of reflecting upon and analyzing the interviews, four central themes emerged. They surfaced again and again in the fieldwork, even if they did not appear with the same prominence in every individual conversation. These themes include the interplay of racial and socioeconomic assumptions; the imbalance of power dynamics in the patient-provider relationship; the role and necessity of advocates and self-advocacy; and the impact of bureaucratic processes and financial bottom lines.[20]

The discussion that follows focuses on describing the social, economic, racial, cultural, and power dynamics that these women have encountered through the process of having cancer and seeking care.

In searching for a way to best explore these themes, I ultimately decided to begin by relating the journeys of three women—Sandra, María, and Sophia—in which the themes are interwoven throughout the narrative. To begin my analysis in this way corresponds with the way the themes first came to my attention—embedded within stories of particular lives. However, the analysis moves beyond this level of discussion. The concluding section of this chapter synthesizes these themes, integrating additional insights of providers and other women with cancer. These additional voices will help to amplify and nuance each theme's scope and significance. In the next chapter, these four themes will be picked up again in conversation with the women's theo-ethical insights.

Sandra Gavin: Following One's Gut and Getting Answers in a Healthcare Labyrinth

Sandra is no stranger to cancer; by 2002, she had faced it three times. Then one January night in 2003, Sandra noticed bloody drainage emanating from her right breast. This story tells her experiences over the course of seven months, in which she sought out care from three different doctors in three very different care settings. All three of these doctors are white and Jewish; one is a woman. Of the three doctors, Sandra only felt comfortable with one. What follows is a brief charting of her journey.

Upon noticing the drainage, Sandra immediately called a friend in another state who is a nurse and "a great diagnostician." This friend told her to call a doctor the very next morning. At this comment, Sandra was terrified. She had no insurance. She said, "I was so scared because I just knew I was going to die," meaning that she was scared not only because of the symptom or the serious tone in her friend's voice, but also because of the likely combination of having cancer while being uninsured. Sandra feared that such a mixture would be lethal. She had been laid off from her job as a hospital administrator two years earlier. And instead of taking another job, she decided to draw unemployment and work on her dissertation to get out of school. She had insurance for the first few months through the Consolidated Omnibus Budget Reconciliation Act (COBRA),[21] but then let it go because it cost $450 a month—a mighty chunk out of any student's budget. In a tragic irony, Sandra let her COBRA go the same month she discovered the bloody drainage.

Feeling the urgency in her bones and thinking quickly, Sandra called another friend, also a nurse, who works in a public clinic in New York City. This nurse knew of a doctor who commanded respect among the nurses and who treated breast cancer. Her friend helped Sandra get an appointment. Of this first doctor, Sandra reflected, "[H]e was a nightmare . . . He scared me more than the cancer did, really." To begin, he belittled her for letting her insurance coverage lapse. "[H]e never let me forget that I did something stupid." His words cut especially deep given the fact that she already felt ashamed for being educated and a nurse and yet letting her insurance go.[22] They intensified the shame Sandra inflicted upon herself.

Beyond chastising her, this doctor also suggested delaying treatment. Sandra quoted him, a surgeon, as advising her to leave and find insurance before pursuing any treatment. She recalled the encounter in this way:

> He says, "And I can't cut corners for you. The hospital won't allow me to cut corners for you. So you need to get a job. You can wait three months. Just go and get a job and some insurance." . . . Now, we haven't done any biopsies or anything, so we don't know . . . We just did a slide. And we know we have atypical cells. We know that I have a bloody drainage. That's it. O.K., but in the meantime, I'm supposed to get a job, wait three months. He tells me, "You have time, you can wait three months. And then we can do everything O.K., because the hospital is not going to let me do everything that I can do for you."

Stark words. However, having dropped this advice in her lap, the doctor did not offer a solution to the conundrum of what he would do if, after finding a job and waiting the three months, Sandra's new insurance refused to pay for a preexisting condition and she could not afford to pay him out of pocket.

So instead of taking this advice and going away, Sandra stuck with him. She was afraid to walk away, to start all over—afraid she would not be able to find other care and that she would die. "What kept me going to the first doctor was a fear of dying and not knowing exactly what I had." Sandra did not want to let time slip through her fingers without getting a diagnosis and doing something about the probable cancer in her breast. Ultimately, this first doctor did a biopsy that confirmed that she had cancer. He then began to propose a plan for surgery.

However, Sandra became increasingly uncomfortable with him, in large part due to the fact that their professional relationship quickly devolved into a protracted confrontation. Sandra noted that they did not have discussions or consultations but rather "arguments." She went so far as to say that she felt she was in a "bad marriage." She would come to his office with questions after having done research online because she wanted to know what he thought and if he could clarify certain things she did not understand. She thinks he interpreted this initiative as a challenge to his knowledge. His responses demeaned her, and he would often raise his voice. She quoted him as saying, "Well, you're a nurse. You're a doctoral student." He even corrected the way she pronounced clinical terms. Given his abrasive responses, Sandra did not find being a nurse (or being known as a nurse) to be an advantage in this case.

Sandra left this surgeon and clinic. Ultimately, she could not consent to his surgery plan because she did not feel comfortable with him. However, it is important to note that Sandra stuck with him for two months, out of fear of not finding access to other care in time. What emboldened her to walk away was remembering that she was eligible for student health insurance. In fact, as a full-time student, the student plan was mandatory unless she had proof of other insurance.[23] In past semesters, she had always waived the student plan because she was either employed or had COBRA.

Enter doctor number two. After an initial consult with a doctor at the student health services, she received a referral for this second doctor, a white female surgeon affiliated with a different hospital. Sandra liked the first visit with her. She found this physician to be nice and pleasant, if a bit distant. However, Sandra did not like the setup of her office. The doctor did not see patients in a hospital clinic, but instead she had her own set of offices situated near the hospital. Sandra noted the examining room and offices were "beautiful," but they were overly "sterile" and "impersonal." Even more important, she did not like a "time-saving" procedure in place there: A nurse acted as a "screener," asking her a series of questions before she saw the doctor. What the doctor had heard from the nurse did not reflect the full or accurate information Sandra had given her, so Sandra ended up repeating herself. Sandra described the situation this way:

> You were placed in this beautiful examining room. She has this beautiful set of offices [on the Upper West Side]. . . . And so you're placed in a room by this nurse who looks very nice, you know, done, and it's like she's just so neat, and the place is so sterile and everything. And you go

into the room, and [the nurse] comes in, and she sits with you and asks you a lot of questions. And I never really liked that. I always find it too impersonal. You know, where you're dealing with two different people, O.K. So [the doctor] came in and she asked me questions. And sure enough, like I thought, half of what I had said had not been conveyed, and I had to go through this, you know, all over again. And then that, it just—it annoys me. It, you know, provokes kind of anxiety, you know, within me because then now I'm wondering what else is left out.

Sandra added that the doctor did not explain the recommended procedure with much detail. She commented that it would have helped if the surgeon had drawn a picture while explaining the procedure. The examination lasted at the most eight minutes.

In all, from Sandra's description, it gave me the sense that everything in the office's appearance and functioning was "perfected." The setup was carefully crafted to be neat, attractive, impressive, professional, and efficient. Unfortunately, a discernable problem was a gaping absence of genuine human connection. Still, the experience was certainly better than the "bantering" so common to Sandra's exchanges with her first doctor. So she made a second appointment to take place shortly before surgery.

The second visit did not go well. Between visits, the surgeon had changed the procedure that she was going to do. Sandra was surprised and had many questions. Sandra quoted the doctor as saying "Well, you act like you've never heard this before." The brisk dialogue turned icy. The doctor's manner became brusque. Sandra lamented,

I started asking her questions because now we're scheduling surgery for I think the following Thursday. And I don't know how I annoyed her, but we had an argument, you know. . . . [S]he tells me, "I'm a surgeon. I don't know. I don't know the answers to those questions. Well, if you want to wait, then you wait." And, you know, I'm just saying, "Well, if you don't think, based on the reports and this and that, that it's this serious at this time, do you think I should wait?" "Well, sure. That's up to you." You know, but so now I'm feeling, you know, like, well, what did I say, you know, what did I do, you know, why is she being so mean and so detached?

Sandra knew the answer to her own questions; this doctor also felt challenged by Sandra.

And I wasn't challenging—I'm—my voice is pretty much the same all the time. I hardly raise it or lower it for pretty much anything. So I didn't feel like I had said something, you know, to cause what happened. . . . But

I couldn't go to surgery with knowing that I've had—I have not had the answers, and that we've had this kind of, you know, conversation that wasn't good.

Ultimately, Sandra reflected, "Both doctors had me crying in their office. And I just couldn't get answers. It seemed like when I asked questions I had a more difficult time with them than if I just sit there, docile, and, you know, listened and just let them do their job. That's how I felt. And so I left." In both cases, the surgeons grew impatient and noticeably irritated when Sandra asked questions. Sandra felt caught. She knew that she had cancer and needed surgery. Yet she could not consent to surgery after having such combative exchanges with the persons who would be performing them and without having her questions answered (or even respected). What may have been an annoyance or disruption in the doctors' schedules was a potentially life-threatening gamble for Sandra.

These two doctors had recommended procedures with the same end result—the removal of the cancerous tissue and duct system, but they had proposed different methods for getting at the duct system. The first doctor had proposed a surgery that would have cut nerve endings and made her nipple become inverted. Thus, she would have had no sensation in the breast and the breast would have had no cosmetic touches to lessen the change in its appearance. Sandra commented, "I just felt like this man is going to just chop my breast off, and it was going to be this horrible, horrible thing left, and that he just didn't care as long as he could do the surgery." Even as she knew she could not sit on this situation indefinitely, her intuition kept her from deferring to either doctor's judgments and recommendations.

Sandra felt trapped in another way as well. She explained that after this visit with the second surgeon, she went back to the doctor at her student health services clinic who had made the initial referral. The health services doctor was upset with Sandra for not going ahead with the surgery with this second surgeon because she very much liked her and felt comfortable sending students to her. Sandra felt the doctor's frustration, but Sandra stuck to what she felt strongly; namely that "you have to really be comfortable with a doctor when you're about to have something as serious as surgery, and the follow-up, you know, the chemotherapy. You want to be able to talk to him, you want to be able to know that he's there for you. And I didn't feel that, you know." This difference in opinion between Sandra and the health services physician left Sandra in an awkward and vulnerable position. She was not in sync with a primary person able to make referrals to surgeons. Sandra explained the snare in which she felt caught: "So now I'm feeling like I have to hide, you know. I've really got to now just go on my own, find myself a doctor, and find a way around, you know, this doctor [at health services], so that I can get a referral. Because you can't do anything without a referral at health services."

Despite feeling entangled by these power dynamics, Sandra had to focus on the most essential matter: Treating the cancer. Knowing time was against her and feeling that she did not have other options, Sandra contemplated returning to the first doctor. Just before she did, something unexpected happened. Her chiropractor, whom Sandra has known and trusted over several years, happened to learn from a mutual acquaintance that Sandra was having some personal difficulties. The chiropractor called Sandra at home and convinced her to share the nature of her problems. Upon hearing that she had cancer, he immediately gave her the name of a surgeon with whom his own mother had just had breast surgery.

Enter doctor and hospital number three. Sandra called and was flabbergasted to receive an appointment for the very next day. She acknowledged that she had to wait four hours to see this third physician. But even more, she was impressed with how many women in the clinic reception area were waiting for him and praising his care: "I felt at home for some reason, you know, just looking around that office and seeing these women, it just—and to hear them talk about him, and them being willing to wait that long to see him."

This full waiting area contrasted with the previous clinic and office settings where Sandra did not encounter nearly as many people. She explained,

I couldn't believe all the people that were sitting there waiting for this doctor to come in, the women. And, you know, I was impressed with that because the other offices I had gone to, I didn't see patients sitting around waiting for a doctor. I didn't see—the lady doctor, there were maybe one or two patients on the second time I went. The first time was one patient. And maybe she does that, staggers her patients, I don't know. And the [first doctor], his office, as well, pretty vacant, you know.

Interestingly, Sandra preferred a crowded office where the patients all spoke fondly of the doctor, than one that was the model of professional décor and elegance.

Also contrasted with the "perfection" and efficiency of the second office, this one was fairly chaotic. Sandra observed that this doctor had one secretary and "not all the fancy file cabinets, just charts stacked, I don't know what kind of system, and how [the secretary] remembers everything, but she did." Despite the tardiness and clutter, these signs of life, enthusiasm, and focus on patients already told Sandra something important.

When Sandra finally met the doctor, she was overwhelmed by his compassionate and thorough attention. "When you went into his room, they didn't just take you in there and sit you in there, didn't ask you questions and go away. You were—you went to the room and then he came in, and he talked to you. He had this very soft, soft voice. I mean, just—it was just so soothing. . . . And he explained, Aana, he explained everything . . . He was truly kind. He was considerate." This surgeon reassured Sandra about the procedure, he drew pictures, and he answered every one of her questions. He proposed a method for removing the duct system that, unlike the other two prior proposals (especially the first), would leave the nerve endings in tact and would leave the nipple in place and erect. Thus, it would not traumatize the breast tissue as much in terms of sensation or cosmetic appearance as the other methods would have. Sandra explained the difference between the methods and attitudes of the first and third doctors regarding the procedure:

[The third doctor told me] "Well, you won't have to worry about [the nipple being flat] because we do a little tuck behind the nipple so that it'll still be erect,"—because that's one of the complications, you know, that the nipple is flat and inverted. And, you know, things that probably you shouldn't be worried about, but in terms of image, you do think about them. You want to know, you know, if it's going to happen, and [if] there's nothing that can be done about it, then yes, you accept it. But the other doctors, you know, it's like you had to accept it, you know, "This is the complication, your breast is going to droop, and there's nothing we can do about it." And the first doctor, "The nerve endings, they're going to be cut. You're not going to have any feelings in the breast." This [third] doctor, "We don't touch your nerve endings, you know, we go around the nerve endings, we remove everything, and everything is fine." O.K.? The [first] doctor, he would do the biopsy this week, then next week they would—he would remove the duct system, they would send that out to the lab. "Next week you come back and we remove your whole breast." . . . I was a basket case because, I mean, why all these steps? How do you think I'm going to be to come back in one week for you to remove my whole breast? Why wouldn't you do all that at the same time? You know? So these are the kinds of things that I just couldn't get answers for. I was just—I was just totally floored, you know, at the differences between doctors, you know, and their whole philosophy on, you know, how they do things.

Sandra finally relaxed. She had the surgery shortly thereafter followed by chemotherapy.

Sandra persevered in finding a care provider who both respected her and in whom she trusted in spite of the continual onslaught assailing her self-confidence and self-esteem. Bearing internal shame and fear along with the vulnerability of being ill and temporarily uninsured, she managed to keep moving. Having such serious symptoms and yet refusing to settle for unsatisfactory care took a lot of courage.

María de Lourdes Maldonado: ¡Hágame Caso! (Pay Attention to Me!)

María's story represents a struggle to be taken seriously by care providers. She negotiated the dynamics of two languages and an inattentive staff. With the aid of her daughter, she was ultimately able to find a care setting in which she was comfortable.

María's first cancer diagnosis was in 1983. Her second diagnosis of cancer came in 1996–1997. She was treated at the same hospital up until 1999. She had trouble dating the second diagnosis because when she found a lump she went right away to the hospital's breast cancer clinic. However, she explained her frustration that the doctors did not do anything about the lump, other than order a few very basic tests. They thought that the lump might be a "little sac of water." She was not satisfied with this explanation. María said that she kept "going and coming"—(yendo y viniendo) to the clinic, appointment after appointment, for over a year. After the biopsy, she left the hospital for another site of care.

The doctors at the first care setting finally performed María's biopsy in 1999–2000. Afterward, María returned to the clinic with her adult daughter to learn the results. The doctor came and sat across from María and her daughter. He told her that she had cancer. María started to cry. He responded in English by saying, "Don't worry, you didn't die before, you won't die this time." "That cold," ("Tan frío") María told me, still not believing his lack of tact. She said her daughter became very angry and exclaimed to the doctor in English, "How are you going to talk to my mother this way!? Don't you have a heart, so inhuman?!"

The doctors wanted María to sign a form right then, presumably saying that she had been given a diagnosis and had consented to a treatment plan. María refused. She did not trust them. She told them that she would seek out a second opinion elsewhere. With the help of her daughter, she was able to get an appointment at another hospital known for its cancer care. When the doctors at this second hospital operated, they found not one but two malignant tumors. María blames the first hospital for losing time in attending to her—for not paying much attention to her—"*No me hicieron caso.*"

María also observed in this first setting that each time a different doctor saw her and that instead of bringing her full chart, they often only brought with them "two or three little pieces of paper" ("*dos or tres papelitos*"). She explained that the doctors who saw her were often students and that they did not speak much with her or spend significant time with her. In fact, she noticed that they would schedule as many as ten patients for the same appointment time slot. The doctors were English speakers. So, either her daughter came with her to help with translation or she went alone, saying that she is able to understand a fair amount of English on her own.

Other aspects of the clinic environment bothered her as well. María complained about the support staff at this first hospital clinic. Over the course of her visits, she noticed that many of the staff did not treat the patients with very good manners. In particular, she found the receptionist to be "nasty" and oftentimes bad humored. María noted the irony that "if it weren't for the patients, they would not have work. Their jobs depend on patients so they should give them more respect."

Having a different doctor each visit certainly complicates the process of getting a full medical and social picture of a person, not to mention building a relationship and trust with the patient. At an even more basic level, it may interfere with the communication of important information. For example, after the first surgery in 1983, María's doctors put in a breast implant. However, during all her visits, both routine and after she felt the lump in 1996, no one ever told her that the implant needed to be changed after five years. She has had it for 20.

María much prefers the hospital where she now goes for her care. The same oncologist sees her every time and takes more time with her. Here she has not had translators either, but she says it is O.K. because she speaks enough English and they don't explain things too quickly. Instead, they explain things little by little.

María acknowledges that she prefers to speak in Spanish, that it is more comfortable. However, I found it interesting that neither María nor the other two Spanish-speaking women expect their providers to speak their language or to have translation services. Marcela, for example, hardly speaks any English. They seemed accustomed to bringing their own help with them or to making do on their own. Unlike a stereotype I sometimes encounter, which assumes that Latinos won't learn English or that they expect others to learn Spanish, these three Spanish speakers each communicated the effort they have made, or their earnest desire, to learn English. I expected them to be more frustrated and angry about the lack of language competency and services provided. I certainly was. It struck me how understanding and patient they were with this part of their care.

In terms of the first hospital, María said that the problems stemmed from a combination of "*el racismo, brutalidad, y una falta de consideración—de todo un poco.*"[24] She saw discrimination in the fact that they looked at her differently than an "American"—meaning someone born in this country. She also noted that they seemed to give more attention to whites and Americans. María thinks that they did not pay as much attention to what immigrants were saying and that the doctors assume Latinos are less educated or less intelligent than others.

We cannot know what her providers were actually feeling or thinking. Moreover, it is quite possible that they held overtly egalitarian principles while also having unconscious assumptions or biases that influenced how they related to her. What we *do* know is that regardless of their conscious attitudes and even good intentions, María did not feel respected and came to not trust them. Her perspective and feelings matter because they are evidence of an important lack of connection between her and her doctors.

In short, María did not feel believed or heard, even as she had a history of breast cancer. She was eloquent in saying that while she may not express herself with as much fluidity as others, she does not speak so crudely either. "I know how to express myself in my own words" ("*en mi palabra*"). María told me that she wants to be seen "not only as a patient, but as a woman, as a Latina." In this statement, I heard a plea for providers to give consideration and respect to the particular— to this woman, this life—in front of them in any given moment. From all that María said, it is clear that she knows a lot about her body, about cancer, and about healthcare systems.

Sophia Andre: One Woman's Quest to Not be Abandoned

Of all the women with whom I spoke, Sophia shared the most time and was extremely candid. She took a lot of risks with someone she had only just met. I left our conversation feeling deeply grateful and also a bit off balance. Some of what she said surprised me; all of it enriched my understanding. Most of all, her insights left me feeling humble.

Sophia Andre taught me much about the travails and hurdles one may go through in seeking care and in getting care providers to know who one really is and to become invested in a particular life. Her story lifted up with vivid detail each of the four aforementioned themes. In particular, her story illustrates the dramatic interplay of racial and socioeconomic assumptions held by others about her. While it is possible sometimes to distinguish a racial stereotype from one more related to socioeconomic class, many times they are very much enmeshed in how they work in relation to and restrict a person of color. Specifically, I will discuss two examples of stereotypes that Sophia has confronted—one more racially based and the other more socioeconomically—but their interrelationship will be apparent. Moreover, in these two illustrations, the need for advocacy, the imbalance of the power relations, and the dehumanizing elements of the healthcare bureaucracy will also come into view.

The first story speaks to the stereotype of emotional volatility. One of the first things Sophia told me was how great all her doctors are—that they work as a team, that "excellence precedes excellence," that they discuss her case weekly as a group, and that they really care about her as a person:

> I've heard horror stories with treatment. Maybe it was because I had the insurance, or maybe it's just because I got into a sympathetic situation, a place where people are sympathetic to your plight. Because [my first doctor] just works in a place where it's a whole team. So it's like excellence precedes excellence. So my doctor referred me to [my breast specialist] just automatically, [who] in the same place, got me my oncologist. My oncologist got me my radiologist. And they all got together, the nurse practitioner, and they automatically put me in a support group, gave me—they gave me an itinerary of everything I was going to do while I was on treatment for all those months. And they took care of me.

In particular, Sophia noted that she has had a strong relationship with her breast surgeon since close to the time of her diagnosis. "She's been great . . . I don't even have to see her by appointment. She just sees me whenever."

I was glad to hear this and assumed at first that she meant her experience had been like this from the beginning. However, Sophia went on to describe the process of relationship and trust-building that took place between herself and her doctors. She explained that at first, most of her doctors, with the exception of her breast surgeon, did not see her—the real her, but rather their own assumptions about her. This was especially clear around the showing of emotions. She explained how she often felt that they were careful and a bit distant—not wanting her to "go off" on them. So they would be very professional, very cautious in their manner.

It is not hard to imagine that having such a serious diagnosis would cause a lot of emotions to erupt in a person. Yet Sophia felt that she needed to be very careful in how she expressed her emotions so that her providers would not be put off in any way. She went so far as to stop her sister from accompanying her on appointments to the cancer center because her sister would sometimes raise her voice in fear, sadness, and anger regarding the severity of the disease and in an attempt to advocate for Sophia. Sophia explained that her sister's emotions and defensiveness did not help her. She said,

> I told her, "You know what? You forget how people can think, and how we have a responsibility, because they might not know any better, to change that . . . just for ourselves." Because we have to do this, we have to get better. And I told her, "These people are treating me, Letty, and I can't have you coming in here ranting and raving every time that you see something goes wrong. Because your ranting and raving is different from somebody else's ranting and raving. It feels different. And we can't have that—I can't have that. I can't deal with your emotional outbursts because it's not to my benefit. And I'm the one that's going to get treated. And I'm the one who has to come to this Center." . . . And in meantime, I've got all these megabytes running all over my body.

Sophia feared (or knew) that Letty's emotions, their expression, would be interpreted by her care providers differently than mine would be as a white person. Thus, it was not safe or helpful for Letty to come and advocate for her sister. Instead, Sophia went alone.

Sophia continued to describe how her relationships evolved over time, how she built a relationship with each of her doctors, the nurse practitioners, and other key staff at the center. It took time and a lot of appointments. She explained that people were always nice, that they would not ever say anything overtly racist or biased, but that nonetheless she could feel that how they were looking at her *limited her*—limited who she was or could be in their eyes. "They don't dislike you, and they don't think bad of you. They just limit you. They just automatically believe that you can't—that you're probably on a certain level.

And they are surprised if you're any higher." When I asked if she meant educational level, Sophia said yes, and also added, "in terms of your standard of living, in terms of etiquette, speech, mannerisms." She also added that at first, many of her doctors and nurses seemed overly cautious with her. She explained,

> Like when they first told me what kind of treatment I was going to have and everything, you know, and when things don't go right, I feel like they expect me to attack them. . . . [L]ike they expect you to do that, I don't know, that ghetto thing. Like "What do you mean I can't see him?" . . . [L]ike the minute I open my mouth, they, like, tell me to relax, or they're taking a step back.

As mentioned above, a significant exception to this experience was the breast surgeon. Sophia liked her breast surgeon (a white woman) and felt a strong connection with her from close to the very beginning of their relationship. And even since then, they have gotten closer over time to the point that now Sophia does not need to make an appointment to see her—she may just go in when she wants to and the doctor will make time for her. Sophia credits this strong relationship to the fact that they have a common understanding. Sophia thinks her breast surgeon might be gay and she knows that she has adopted children. So, she says that they have a mutual understanding regarding their respective, potential sites of stigma—"You know, I see her like, you don't judge me; I don't judge you. That's how I see her." Sophia thinks that this way of seeing and approaching one another helped them both to relax and really get to know and like each other.

Sophia also felt limited by the lighter skinned women in her cancer support group. They expressed surprise at a darker skinned woman having achieved beyond a certain educational level. They were surprised that Sophia had private health insurance and told her how lucky she was. She also felt stereotyped for being a single mother and was quick to point out to me that there are white single mothers too. Sophia's words:

> I'm not saying that [the white women in the cancer support group] weren't sympathetic and that we weren't going through the same thing or whatever. But they're like, you know, like one girl, she said, "Well you're *very, very* lucky to have healthcare. You're very lucky that you have such good insurance." And I'm like, "Why am I more lucky than you? What are you saying, I can't get a job that could give me good insurance?". . . And things like, well, "You know, you're a single parent."

I'm like, "I'm not a single parent because I'm Puerto Rican. There's a lot
of white women who are single parents." I mean, just don't assume
things so much. (Emphasis hers.)

Assumptions can put a lot of distance between people, even when they
are going through similar health crises. Yet given the stakes, the perceptions of her care providers matter the most. Sophia was crystal clear that she needed her doctors to care genuinely about her—as a person, an individual—so that they would advocate for her, not just give the care that they are responsible to give, but to try in earnest—to not give up on her. "I tried hard to get them to see *me*." The power dynamic is palpable. These people, in her mind, have her life in their hands. She needs them to like her, to not be threatened by her, so that they will care for her. And she felt it was her burden, her responsibility to change their minds—to show that she was not like their stereotyped impressions—that she would not "go off" on them. "[T]hey think that my way of reacting to anger is, you know, to come out and start cursing them or start fighting with them, or start twitching my head. Which actually I do on a normal basis anyway...." She explained that she thinks they expect her to prove that she is different from their perceptions of Black Puerto Ricans.

Sophia recognized the injustice of this reality—that white people get emotional too, but are not stereotyped in the same way. At having to reassure white doctors that she would not be overly emotional, she expressed that people of color have to convince their doctors that

> [w]e're not going to start knocking things off the counter, and "What do you mean I've got cancer, you cock-a-doodle-dandy doctor, you know, you're full of shit!?".... I'm not saying that doesn't happen every now and then. But you know what, anyone has the ability to go off.... The only difference is that maybe people of color might knock things down, where you know, white people just, will send you—will sue you! [she laughs].

Sophia did sense a real change over time in her relationships with her doctors. They stopped being careful—stopped the calm, rational distant professional persona. Instead, they began to tell her exactly what they were thinking, not mincing words. She acknowledged that she feels like a person now in their eyes. "After, like, three or four years, now they see me for who I am. And they don't want me to be sick.... Now they're rooting for me, like, and when I speak, they're concerned with what I have to say. You know? They depend on what it is I have to say for their knowledge, which they never would have done before." Sophia feels they are invested in her life and are not afraid of her or of any emotions she might express. And she thinks they came to this out of a group effort, that she too let down some of her defenses and let them see more of her—of her life, and of the various challenges and fears that she lives with every day. "I think it's a team effort. I think it's me not being so—not being so quick to assume, and then them not being so quick to assume as well." She later added that she thinks it made a difference that she let them know things about herself every now and then, for example, that she was caring for her grandmother at home.

One concrete turning point in their relationship came, she thinks, when she decided to do a clinical drug trial. They pushed her to do a chemotherapy trial because they thought it might do better than the traditional chemotherapy regimen. In her words,

> I knew that they weren't scared of me anymore, or worried that I was going to have an outburst, because at the end of my treatment, like the last two chemos, I told them I didn't want to do it. I said, "This is it. I cannot do this anymore. I'm stopping." And they put me in a conference room, and they told me—they were not scared of me. And I know that before they would have been, like, well, "You know what, we can't make you," this and that. But they were like, "You know what, you have to do this. You have to do this." And my [oncologist] said, "You *are* going to do this. And if you don't think that you can do this on your own at home, then we will admit you right now until you've finished treatment and you will stay in the hospital until you finish. But you *are* going to finish treatment." (Emphasis hers.)

They all applauded her when she finished. "I know they were really proud of me when I finished treatment."

In speaking about the decision to go with the clinical trial instead of the standard treatment, Sophia explained,

> I said, "This Taxiter [the chemo drug being tested], can it do me, can it do any worse?" They said "no." So I said, "It's either going to do the same as the other medicine or better?" They said "yes." So, I said, "Then, I want the clinical study." And I think that also kind of changed their minds a little bit, like I wasn't so starched. Like whatever it takes to get me better. *Whatever.* They didn't tell me that the Taxiter, now we find out, is a better drug, but that the side effects are worse. They didn't tell me that. Another thing they didn't tell me is that—because my doctor told me I must finish all the treatments when I said I didn't want to do it

anymore—and they clapped at the end—he didn't tell me that most people do not finish this chemotherapy because it is that bad. (Emphasis hers.)

I find it both interesting and disturbing to learn that in presenting her options to her, Sophia's oncologist told her that the drug trial would either do the same or better than the other chemotherapy treatment. If it was an experimental drug trial how did he know this definitively? Furthermore, he expressly *did not* tell her that the side effects would be worse or that few people had actually finished all the rounds of the drug. Are these not basic components to "informed consent" mandated by all Institutional Review Boards (IRBs)?

The second story speaks to the role of socioeconomic class and insurance in Sophia's life. When she was first diagnosed in 2000, she had private insurance through her employer. Once her doctor felt something, the doctor moved quickly to do a biopsy and to refer her to a breast surgeon. Sophia went to a care center that specializes in cancer treatment. In February of 2003, just before her diagnosis of a recurrence, Sophia and all of her 3,000 coworkers were laid off. Her company folded after 70 years of business. She found another job within two weeks, but during this time she also learned of the recurrence. Her employer failed to offer anyone COBRA and she had not had time to do anything about it. So when I met her, she had no private insurance and no Medicaid, only unemployment. She was on a payment plan for all her medical care and said that her doctors have assured her that they will not stop treating her. They put her on chemotherapy again right away, which was donated by a pharmaceutical company.

I commented how good it is that she has such a solid relationship with her care providers. She replied, "Well, this will test to see how really solid the relationship is, won't it?" She is convinced that people who have to go to public clinics are at a disadvantage in their care. She tries not to, but she admitted to worrying that they will stop treating her at some point—that money will become an issue. "And the doctors would like to have you think that they don't deal with [the financial end of care]. 'Oh, I don't deal with that. Talk to my people about that. I'm only concerned with your care.' But that's not true. . . . [T]hey want to know how you are going to pay this." As it is, she constantly—before each new test or procedure—gets calls from the accounting office asking about her insurance:

> "Hi, we notice that you have an appointment for an MRI on this date. We were just wondering, because your insurance papers [do] not

match—your insurance information doesn't seem to be coming
through. How are you—how are you going to pay?" Every time I have
an appointment. Before the appointment . . . Every time. I'm like,
"Here we go. This is first things first."

Again and again, Sophia has to explain that she does not have insurance
and that she is on a payment plan.

She explained that one thing that doctors, desk clerks, accounting
people, et cetera could do to make her feel more like a human being is
to attend to her physical needs and ask how she is doing—check her
out medically—before checking to make sure that the finances are in
order. "[The doctor or nurse] will look at your chart. They'll look at
the bottom of your insurance, and they'll go—once they see everything's clear, then they slap it closed and then they go, 'Well, what
seems to be the problem?' " [Sophia laughs]. Sophia went on to
explain that whenever she goes in, she—and other patients of color—
have to go to the accounting/financing office first before they see the
doctor. She has observed that sometimes white patients get to bypass
this step (they do it on the way out instead) and see the doctor first.

Again, Sophia expressed the burden to change provider and staff
assumptions: "I think they kind of expect us to change their
minds . . . I think they expect us to make them believe that we're not
going to go off on them, or that we're not going to stick them with the
bill." She wished the finances would not come first but said they
do. She thinks that if you are a new patient, they will want to put the
finances in order before they invest themselves in you, in your life.
She commented, "It's like they're afraid to get personal with you
because then if they like you, they don't know how to turn you
away. . . . Money really messes it up and the assumption that we don't
have the funds."

In terms of advocacy, Sophia has turned her doctors and nurses into
her allies. Sophia has become her own advocate and has built the kind
of relationship with her care providers so that they will advocate for
her—make a case to the drug company, for example, as to why they
ought to donate the chemotherapy to this specific patient. Another
example is that her oncologist got her onto another experimental
treatment based on antibodies that was so encouraging that there was
a three-year waiting list. Sophia is convinced that over time, having
your providers care about you to this degree makes a difference—it
means that they will go the extra mile, make a few more calls, work to
find a way to pay for the treatments. "I don't want them to leave me.

Like ever . . . I want them to care about me always. I don't want them to discard me." What she wants most from her doctors is for them to not abandon her.

Additional Thematic Discussion

Sandra, María, and Sophia have shared a great deal of insight into healthcare quality and systems by telling me their stories. The themes highlighted above are clearly evident in each of their experiences. However, additional attention to each theme is needed in order to tease out even more their respective meanings for healthcare quality and ethics.

The Interplay of Racial and Socioeconomic Assumptions

Through the conversations, one realization that crystallized regarding racial and socioeconomic assumptions is how they can sneak up on a person from all sides. I had been on the lookout for them in provider-patient interactions; I had not anticipated their appearance in women's cancer support groups as well. I should have known better given the fact that I have studied the feminist movement in this country and how so many lighter skinned women have alienated darker skinned women due to our failures in race and class analysis. Why was I surprised when Sophia made it clear that having cancer does not necessarily purge such assumptions in white women? And while white healthcare providers may be more careful in the things they directly say to a woman of color's face (due to diversity trainings perhaps), white women with cancer may not be as reserved or cautious.

Sophia was not alone in such encounters. Slimfat Girl felt very uncomfortable by the remarks and attitude that she received from a white woman at the first cancer support group she attended. According to Slimfat Girl, the white woman seemed annoyed that Slimfat Girl had brought her daughter with her to the meeting. She then went on to make comments throughout the meeting that indicated that she assumed, in turn, that Slimfat Girl did not have a job, insurance, or a home computer. In her words,

> I went downtown . . . So I went to the first meeting. My daughter came with me . . . There was the [white] lady sitting beside me [who] had a problem with my daughter being there . . . So now we in the group, so

every time she said, "Well, I'm bringing my daughter next time . . ."
And I'm like, "Why is she saying all of this, O.K.?" So, we're talking.
This lady assumed I did not have a job, O.K.? She said, "Well, maybe if
you had a job . . ." I said, "What makes you think I don't have a
job?". . . So then the next statement, she . . . is saying her doctor is the
one who wrote the paper on this, that, and something else. So she said,
"Well, if you had a computer . . ." I said, "What makes you think I
don't own a computer?!"

Slimfat Girl resented this woman's presumption and condescending tone.
It bothered her so much that she never went back to this group. Instead,
she found a Latina support group in another neighborhood. There they
speak in both Spanish and English. Despite the fact that Slimfat Girl does
not speak Spanish herself, she said that she feels at home and accepted
there. Both these stories from Sophia and Slimfat Girl vividly show how
important it is—how basic is the need—to feel understood, respected,
supported, and seen for who one truly is. And they reveal how enervating
it is to one's spirit when one is not. Not surprisingly, rather than risking
the hurt, it is easier for some to put up proactive defenses or, when possible, to seek out care and places where it is less likely that the defenses
and explanations of oneself will be needed.

For example, Luz offered insights into heading off negative assumptions before they take hold in others. It is true that Luz did not identify racism as a negative force restricting the quality of healthcare.
Instead, she focused more on the socioeconomic causes of disparities.
However, she nonetheless commented that she thinks it matters how
one presents oneself when seeking healthcare. I took this to mean that
it matters if you dress up for appointments, speak articulately, look
professional, et cetera. In response, I remarked that when I go to a
doctor's office, I do not have to worry that they will initially assume
that I am uninsured or a "welfare mother." Luz agreed with this point
and then she recalled that long ago, her mother told her that she had
"three strikes against her: Being Black, Latina and a woman." Luz's
only recourse, her mother reasoned, was for her to get as much of an
education as possible. Luz's attention to the way she presents herself to
others and to getting an education are ways to counteract any preexisting and generalized assumptions present in society (and potentially
in a provider's mind) that have designated one's Blackness, femaleness,
or being Latina a "strike."

The healthcare providers of color with whom I spoke also perceive
the power of racial and socioeconomic stereotypes. In particular, Lucy
Bristol, a nurse with 23 years of experience in oncology, articulately

spoke of this reality.[25] She is also pursuing a Masters degree in nursing education. Lucy describes her racial-ethnic identity as Jamaican, but also added, "I just see myself as a nurse—a Black woman who's a nurse." I asked Lucy what she sees as the biggest barriers blocking high quality care for people of color. Her answer was simple: "Insurance." Yet she went on to agree that even people of color who do have insurance still wrestle with negative stereotypes. As evidence, she explained that

> [b]ecause of [stereotypes] you have patients who will tell you, they will come in, and they're already angry. And the first thing that happens, they will tell you, "I'm not on welfare." They'll verbalize that, you know, "I'm not on welfare." And you say, "Well, I didn't assume you were." But this is how they want to make sure—they, like, create some identity so that they don't get inferior care. So they establish that right away. They start telling everybody, you know, "I'm not on welfare." Or they'll tell you, "I have insurance." You know, this is their way of protecting themselves because they know what they're up against. I mean, they'll come in with that attitude, so that it has to come from somewhere.

Lucy has witnessed many cancer patients who, for various reasons, enter the hospital with lots of defenses and anger. What is interesting in the case of patients of color is that they not only have such walls up because of their feelings around cancer per se, but also because some anticipate being stereotyped as having no means—as being a financial burden on the hospital. Lucy's words recall Sophia's sense that she and other patients of color live with the burden of proving that they will not stick the provider with the tab. Along these lines, Slimfat Girl and Hannah also made direct references to not wanting to be seen by providers as a "bill" or conversely a "paycheck."

Certainly, all patients are at risk of being reduced in the provider's mind or institutional tracking to their insurance status. And the way many hospitals function can be alienating to patients of all racial and cultural backgrounds. Yet when I started to say to Lucy that it is not easy to be ill and hospitalized no matter who you are—no matter the racial or socioeconomic background—she jumped in:

> But if you have a language barrier, or if you are a person of color, the odds are up against you even more. And you see it. You see the patients who get more . . . the squeaky wheel gets oiled. . . . [L]ike here, they cater to, like, you know, clienteles of all types. And they have the very rich, and they have the very poor. And you find the people with money,

they get treated differently. It might not—sometimes it's consciously. And sometimes it's subconsciously. But it happens. You see it.

She added, "I've heard doctors refer to patients as welfare patients, you know, because of their skin color and they just don't respond to them the same way."[26] Lucy's remarks make it clear that while cancer and hospitalizations are a heavy burden for anyone to bear, racial and socioeconomic assumptions can add additional weight for some.

The presence and significance of these interlocking assumptions can be seen, conversely, in their absence. Hannah's vivid and impassioned description of her love and appreciation for her breast specialist (who shared her racial-ethnic background) exemplifies what is possible when such assumptions are *not* in place initially. Hannah's experience speaks to what is possible in a relationship when a patient does not have to break down or translate her personhood and experience in order to get her provider to see her and take a concerted interest in her particular identity and situation. Recall also that Hannah had excellent insurance coverage. All her providers knew up front that the bills would be paid.

Two caveats are needed: First, it is important to acknowledge that Hannah does not think that race makes a difference in terms of her healthcare providers. Even as she has chosen three African American physicians in recent years, she was very clear that she does not pick her physicians based on race and that she has always been pleased with her chosen providers: "I don't have any negative comments with the nurses and doctors that came through my path. Even through childbirth . . . I had great, you know, obstetricians." Hannah is confident that she is able to build positive relationships with people, regardless of their racial or cultural background. Instead, she thinks that a lack of health insurance is the real barrier to quality care.

Second, not all patients and doctors who share the same racial-ethnic background have this experience of trust and connection. Luz certainly did not have this kind of affinity with the Latino doctor. In fact, she strongly preferred the white male specialist (both because of his medical knowledge and skill and the way he interacted with her) to this first doctor. Indeed, this quality of connection cannot be taken for granted to exist in any and every race-concordant professional relationship.

Still, it is important to understand another main point with respect to these assumptions: They have discernable effects. They do not simply remain at a conscious or unconscious level of ideation; their presence bleeds into actual practices, relationships, and consequences.

They are not ill crafted yet benign thoughts with no implications. They act out. Lucy offered an illustration of how provider assumptions can come into play[27]:

> I had a patient once who was from the islands. And the doctors thought she was confused. And she wouldn't eat hospital food. But I used to speak to her daughters. They would bring her food. So I knew she was eating. But [the doctors] didn't take the time to find out. And they just kept saying—we're on rounds and they're saying "This woman is confused." And I'm going, "But she's not confused." And she was, like in her seventies. So they . . . look at her age. She had a very heavy dialect, which they didn't understand, so they automatically assumed she was confused. And they didn't take time to talk to the family.
>
> So then this went on for a couple of days. And then one day I came in, and they wanted to talk to her daughters because they wanted to put a PEG[28] tube in because they're saying she's not eating, . . . and I'm saying, "Why are you putting a PEG tube in this woman?" Which would mean she'd have to go to surgery. They'd put in a permanent feeding tube, which she didn't need because she was eating. But she would only eat the food they brought from home. So I said to the doctors, "Well, did you bother to ask?" And I said, "First of all, she's not confused. You might not understand her dialect, but she is speaking English. She's not confused. And her daughters told me, as long as she's been sick, she will never eat hospital food. She's used to eating her island food." So, you know, it's things like . . . that that's frustrating. [The doctors] come in on rounds, and five minutes they're there, and they assess the patient, and they make these medical decisions without really—but then, they don't do that in all cases.

When Lucy alluded to situations when doctors do not make decisions without consulting more thoroughly with the patient and family, she was referring to the cases in which there is an active family presence. This point will be picked up below.

Antonia Morales is a third-year medical student.[29] She defines her racial-ethnic identity as Puerto Rican and speaks Spanish. Already at this early stage in her career, she has noticed staff making assumptions and gave two examples with respect to family configurations and sexuality. In one case, staff assumed a young Mexican woman was a teenage mother of four children because they had come in with her to the hospital. In reality, she was in college and they were not her children. The other example she gave was of a young African American girl, perhaps 16 or 17, who had come in with a urinary tract infection. The staff assumed the girl was sexually active. When she vigorously denied it, they doubted her and decided to give her condoms anyway. They may have been justified or not in doubting her. What Antonia understands is that stereotypes around Black sexuality are potent. So if the girl had not been African American or had a higher educational level, they may have been more likely to believe her claim to virginity.[30]

Beef Stew also sees how assumptions act out on the oncology floor. She is a nurse case manager who identifies as African American.[31] However, she added that her ancestry is more complex: "If you really want to get down to it, I'm a Black Italian Native American." She firmly believes that prejudicial racial/class stereotypes are still alive and well, but they are more hidden than in past eras. She gave these examples of the subtle way they manifest:

> [I]t's just more undercover. Now you can't say it in open discussion. Now you have to wait 'til you get into a locker room, and you're talking to your buddies; and, you know, then it's out. . . . [J]ust because you don't see it doesn't mean it's not there. I don't see air, but I'm breathing, so I know it's here. . . . [A]nd it doesn't have to be verbal . . . When you go into a patient's room, and there's no contact isolation, but you're going in there, and you're putting on gloves anyway. What are you putting on gloves for? There's no contact isolation. Versus the . . . person who's Caucasian, and they're on contact isolation, but you're going in there like it's gravy. And then you're going to come out, and then you're going to infect all of us. You know what I'm saying? And one could say, "Well, maybe that's just a breach in the fact that they don't know the difference between contact iso"—no, no, no. No. No. You know when you don't want to be around somebody, you're going to put up barriers. Versus someone that you're comfortable with, you're not going to put up barriers.

Beef Stew reinforces an important point: Stereotypes do not have to be spoken to exist or to have unsettling effects on human behavior. The simple act of putting on gloves when you do not need them sends a strong message. She added that she has also seen staff with an attitude of being "terse, abrupt . . . standoffish, very mechanical, like an assembly line, to those patients" as contrasted with the attention and effort they make for the "VIPs" that come into the hospital.[32]

Indeed, negative postures and dismissive practices can be communicated in many ways: By body language and eye contact, by the presence or absence of touch, by how hurried or distracted one seems while another is speaking or by a cool, professional demeanor that communicates distance, self-protection, and disinterest. It is true that this communication is complicated by the fact that different cultures interpret body language and gestures in different ways. For example, a given manner style may be too formal for one patient who prefers someone more casual and friendly; however, another patient may expect this formality, which gives her or him more confidence that the care provider is a skilled professional. Yet, even as it is important to acknowledge that the same action can be interpreted differently by different people, still it is also true that there are many indirect ways to convey discomfort, dislike, fear, disrespect, or a lack of empathy and compassion. Lucy noted that she has seen hospital staff displace darker skinned patients who are about to be discharged out to the solarium to wait for transportation while lighter skinned patients are allowed to wait in the room.[33] Whether whispered or not, assumptions and stereotypes bellow and reverberate through actions.

The Imbalance of Power Dynamics in the Patient-Provider Relationship

The conversations impressed upon me the reality of the lack of mutuality in the patient-provider relationship. Again and again, I was struck by how compromising it is to be ill and to have to work so hard to develop rapport with doctors so that they will do everything possible to save your life. These women need their care providers in a dramatic way that is not reciprocal. They need their care providers to see them, to listen, to understand not simply because that is what human beings owe to one another in general as human beings, but because their lives are at stake. Slimfat Girl spoke poignantly about the emotional and traumatic nature of having cancer, of how much it interrupts one's life, and of how destabilizing it can be. Simply put, cancer puts one—even the most strong and courageous woman—in a position of acute vulnerability.

Sophia's story rings in my ears and pierces my conscience. While both Sophia and her providers may all have taken risks in building their relationship, the undeniable fact remains that Sophia took such risks as a woman of color with cancer and that they took risks as predominately white, relatively healthy care providers. The power dynamics make the risks unequal. From positions of relative vulnerability, women like Sophia make sacrifices—such as being part of a brutal clinical drug trial—in addition to making other significant efforts in order to get their providers to take an interest in the particular person—to be seen as unique and important individuals worthy of investment. Sophia felt the burden to change—to break through—her provider's assumptions. While having to make such extra effort may have been a pragmatic necessity, it seems far from just.

Sophia was not alone in this vulnerability. As María was putting up with doctor appointment after doctor appointment, her tumor was growing all the while, to be soon joined by another. Recall also how nonchalant Luz's first doctor was in reassuring her that the lump was not malignant, and when the biopsy revealed that it was, that it was no big deal. In the best construction of his attitude, one could argue that he was trying to keep Luz from worrying. However, to Luz, his attitude was disrespectful because it did not take her concerns and emotions seriously.[34] Even more disconcerting to Luz—what truly dismayed her—was that the doctor took such a cavalier stance without the facts to back it up. He was not worried, but his life was not potentially on the line; hers was. And if Luz had listened to him, she would have had a minimal "clean-up" of the breast tissue instead of aggressive treatment, which would have meant, she feels strongly, that she would no longer be walking this earth.

Though not perturbed by the power her doctors exerted in relation to her, Marcela related an experience that makes the inequality apparent. Following the initial chemotherapy, Marcela wanted to have a full mastectomy instead of a lumpectomy. She said that up until the day before the surgery, her doctor (a white woman) kept trying to get her to reconsider, saying that the chemotherapy had reduced the tumor a lot, that Marcela was young and should give this less aggressive surgery a shot before giving up her breast. In her words,

> I wanted them to [remove the entire breast] the first time. And [the doctor] told me, "No, you are very young, you cannot do that, give it a 'chance.' You don't know if with the first operation it will be enough." I said, "No, I want you to remove it all." She tried to convince me. . . . Still, the day before the operation, she insisted with me that they not remove all of it. I said, "O.K. fine, but I know that you all will have to operate on me another time." That is what I said to her . . . And that is what happened—they operated on me and one month later, another operation. So then, she did not violate my decision because I did not let her convince me. Because I was aware that they would have to do a second operation.

Certainly, this doctor was well intentioned. She saw a young, attractive mother and wanted to save her breast if possible. Even as Marcela finally agreed, she knew she would need the mastectomy eventually. Marcela turned out to be right; a month later they did a full mastectomy and reconstruction. I asked Marcela if she was angry about being pressured. She replied, "In a certain way, yes, it bothered me." She acknowledged the power imbalance by saying that the doctor has a lot more medical knowledge than she does and a lot more experience with cancer, so how could she really argue? However, in looking back on this incident, Marcela focused on the positive. She said that even as she had been initially annoyed, it all turned out for the best because, initially, she had not known about the option of reconstruction:

> Look, what I also thought is that this is very good because—it was good because—for the first operation I told her that if she is going to remove the breast that I did not want reconstruction because I did not know anything about reconstruction. I simply wanted that they take off the breast period. If she had done this when I had told her, she would not have done reconstruction. But the second time then when they did take the breast, they did reconstruction.

Marcela reasoned, if she had had the full mastectomy right away, she would not have had reconstruction because she had not yet learned anything about the procedure. Indeed, Marcela credits doctors with being the experts in this area. She emphasized that patients need to cooperate, work with their doctors, in order to achieve the best results possible. She explained,

> If a person has the ability to accept and to fight—to fight together with the doctor—the doctor is going to help you. But if you do not give this opportunity, the doctor, what can he do—for the more that he tries, the more that he wants to help, he will not be able to help because you do not want him to help. Understand? So I arrived to that hospital, I did not know anything. At first I felt a little depressed. But I said I have to survive. I have to fight and go on. So they want to help me, I don't know anything about medicine. I simply looked for orientation—[information] about which I did not know—information with people who had been through this. That is what I did. So, one accepts the help of the doctor that he is going to give and that same way they also are going to respect your opinion and you can all discuss things.

Marcela repeatedly emphasized the importance of accepting the expertise of the medical experts, being cooperative. In addition, she also continually stressed the power and responsibility patients have to take care of themselves. Indeed, Marcela was also strong enough in herself to not feel intimidated by her doctors. In fact, recall that when they did not work fast enough, she took her records elsewhere to get the tests done and then reported back to them with the results.

In short, I cannot tell Marcela's story in any way that denies her own agency in relation to her doctors, even if there is a power imbalance. She accepted the expertise and advice of her doctors. She worked with them. She accepted the limited translation services and did the best she could to understand. But she made her own decisions. She took responsibility for her own quest to survive. Still as I continue to reflect on her story, even if Marcela does not give this imbalance much weight and while she may not agree, it seems to me that when someone is, or is considered, an expert it may feel daunting or scary to go against the recommendation—especially when the threat of death hovers near. Perhaps the truth lies somewhere between our two perspectives.

The Role and Necessity of Advocates and Self-Advocacy

Sandra identified that what was most helpful in terms of safeguarding her dignity was having others who helped her navigate the healthcare maze—friends who are nurses, other nurses she met while a patient, the chiropractor, and other women with cancer. Nurses and nurse friends helped Sandra find out where to register complaints—who the Director of Nursing was in a particular place, for example. At the first hospital and clinic setting, sometimes Sandra's nurse friend would call ahead to the hospital and alert someone that Sandra was coming in for a test or procedure. This same friend was the one who helped Sandra get into see the first doctor, whom the friend viewed as skilled (even if intimidating). Sandra explained that even this negative experience with the first doctor was helpful. Experiencing it and being able to confer with her nurse friend during this time helped Sandra to learn what "I needed to ask, to do and when I needed to move on."

In addition to a network of healthcare provider contacts, friends and acquaintances who have faced cancer also served as pivotal reality checks for Sandra. Those who shared their own experiences helped Sandra understand the complexity of what she herself was going through. It also emboldened her to know that others have a need to be assertive and uncompromising in order to get the care they wanted and to be heard by providers. Conversely, Sandra noted that it was also instructive to hear from those who were *not* very assertive and who did *not* complain. This information made Sandra aware of the negative results that can happen when one is passive or when one does not know what to do or to whom to turn.

Indeed, Sandra, who has also done her own qualitative research, voiced concern for people who may lack the social support, inner resolve, and assertiveness needed to insist on high quality care:

> I just think that for the person who doesn't have the resources, and who can't ask the questions . . . I think for many Afro American people that I've come into contact with and talked to even in the hall, [they say] "Well, I don't like my doctor because my doctor just doesn't . . . answer anything for me. I can't get what I need. They don't tell me these things, or the nurse does it.". . . And people want the information, but there seems to be something, a perception that "I am, you know, the doctor, and this is what I've said, and this is what is going to be done and what should be done.". . . And even with my study, I'm seeing [African American women with diabetes] who are saying "I can't get the information" or their experiences with their doctors are not good experiences. You know, and they hang in there, O.K., although they are not happy, many of them do because they don't know any other direction to take. You know, and I think . . . I was headed back to the first doctor after my experience with the second doctor. If it had not been for my girlfriend talking to that [chiropractor], I would not have met [the third doctor] . . . So I think you could call it a fluke, or divine intervention, but something guided, you know, that path. And my gut instinct—I'm very intuitive.

Instead of submitting to care provision that made her ill at ease, Sandra followed her gut and intuition as she drew upon the advocacy and help of others. Not everyone is as able to ask all the questions or walk out the door of a bad situation. Sandra admits that, without the intervention of key people, even she, an educated nurse who knows her way around healthcare, may not have been able to do so.

Lucy, a nurse, also emphasized the role advocacy plays. I asked Lucy for a description of the cases in which the doctors are less apt to make decisions quickly and/or without full consultation of a patient. In other words, in contrast to the lack of consultation regarding placement of a feeding tube for the woman from the islands, when do they slow down and consult more? Lucy responded, "Well, the patients who they know have a voice, you know what I'm saying? The family members that more—are more visible, that's always there, that's always questioning them. You know, they'll make sure they don't make any decisions without—because they know these family members are more involved."

Listening to Lucy reinforces in my memory the active roles people assumed on their loved one's behalf: María's daughter tenaciously stood up for her when she finally received the second cancer diagnosis from the doctor who was uncaring and cold. She also helped María access care elsewhere, instead of signing on the dotted line right then and there. If it had not been for Luz's friend and the friend's sister-in-law, Luz may very well not been able to get into the cancer clinic she had been calling for two days on her own.[35] Wanda also had key people in her corner. Her sibling worked in a hospital and connected her with the first breast specialist; other friends and work relationships helped her find and consult with two others. Despite evident power imbalances, these women with the help of loved ones were creative and bold in advocating for themselves. Also, many of them have used breast cancer support groups to help them gain information and support, which, in turn, strengthened their voice and resolve.

The Impact of Bureaucratic Processes and Financial Bottom Lines

According to all of the people with whom I spoke, hospital patients trying to get well and providers trying to care for them encounter many systemic challenges that can impede their respective progress. Well apart from the individual, interpersonal level of provider sensibilities, interactions, and (un)awareness of patient-provider power dynamics, the larger context in which U.S. healthcare is given plays a huge role in determining how respected patients feel. Being mired in red tape hinders respect for personhood. The financial pressures of bottom lines constrict what providers feel able to provide, especially in terms of "unbillable" things such as compassion. "Being processed" by impersonal and bureaucratic ways of managing the flow of people can be disheartening and dehumanizing. Marcela described this way of relating to people as treating them like "a piece of furniture," rather than as a person. Unfortunately, a present lack of questioning of the social and corporate context in which U.S. healthcare is situated weakens much of biomedical ethics and the healthcare initiatives and curricula aimed at cross-cultural competence among providers.

Bureaucracies

It is important to underscore the fact that Luz left the first hospital and doctor not only because of her lack of trust and disappointment in him, but out of frustration with how she was treated within the hospital context itself. She complained that the staff did not know her name. She also experienced staff being unable to tell her where her blood and/or chart were. When she would try to get to the bottom of such things, staff would be unable to tell her who was responsible for the different tasks related to her question:

> When you call these persons and they say, "Well I don't know who is doing this . . . I don't know who is responsible for this." Or, [you ask] "Where is the person that drives the ambulette that is supposed to pick up Luz Hernandez?" "We don't know who that person is." You sit at my hospital where I am: "Luz"—you don't even say my last name sometimes, there are millions of "Luz" at that hospital . . . Or, "Who's in charge of your blood?"

In other words, there was scant accountability. The straw that broke the camel's back was when the ambulette never showed up. This transportation had been arranged for by her doctor so that she could have the "pre-ops" done. Follow-up calls made by Luz, her husband, and even her doctor were of no use. None of the staff at the other end of the line knew anything about it.

What is interesting is that Luz told me about these things when I asked her what makes a person feel like a human being while ill. She answered by showing me the *opposite*, by giving me examples of a bureaucratic management system that *did not* work well. What is critical to understand is that such grievances are not simply annoyances or inconveniences. They eat at a person's sense of self. They insult dignity. Bit by bit, each call to a computerized "automated attendant"[36] that ends in a dead end, each encounter with a rude, ineffective, or impersonal staff member gnaws away at one's humanity.

In short, a lack of accountability at the most mundane level of office and administrative practices impairs genuine respect for persons seeking healthcare. The importance of the basics—courtesies and pleasantries, follow-up with answers to questions—ought not be missed. In Slimfat's words, "Courtesies. And some doctors are pretty good . . . But, you know, just don't think of me as a paycheck. Now, well, I *am* a paycheck, but now can I say it? Money in the bank." (Emphasis hers.)

It was the warmth, time, quality of attention, and respect that these women felt that made them glow about their favorite care providers. In Hannah's words, "We were, like, my relation with my doctor, was more personal, you know, we got more personal with one another. It wasn't just—I wasn't just, you know, paying a bill at her clinic or whatever. It was more personal. I felt more like she was part of my family. . . . [S]he remembered everything that I told . . . her." Hannah was not the only one to overflow with such affection for her doctor. Sophia, Sandra, María, Luz, Wanda, and Slimfat Girl all did as well. In addition, Luz and Slimfat Girl both had nurses who stayed with them while they cried and actively comforted them. One of Hannah's nurses prayed with her. In summary, it took some of them a bit longer to find care providers they liked, but in the end each woman did. And each spoke with strong praise and gratitude for these caregivers.

Undeniably, Black and Latina women are not the only patients frustrated by the difficulty in finding such quality care and relationships with providers. A nationwide survey conducted by Harvard University, The Kaiser Family Foundation, and the federal Agency for Healthcare Research and Quality (AHRQ) questioned 2,000 adults in 2004. The researchers found that, "55% of those surveyed said they were dissatisfied with the quality of their care, up from 44% in 2000; and 40% said the quality of care had gotten worse in the last five years."[37] *The New York Times* article goes on to explain that the nursing shortage, tight budgets, and shorter hospital stays all mean that it is more difficult for patients and staff to build good rapport with one another. Recurring patient complaints include the loss of identity, the disrespect for their privacy, the lack of social niceties (e.g., names being introduced, patient requests being remembered), and unacceptable noise levels coming from televisions, staff chatting outside the door, et cetera.

Sandra's insight into various bureaucratic mechanisms that can frustrate quality care was keen. As mentioned earlier, she was often disturbed by the way desk clerks and nurses acted as gatekeepers or screeners to the point that relevant information was not conveyed accurately. Sandra does not appreciate it when others ask her a series of questions whose answers she has to repeat several times to her doctors. This practice takes place a couple of different ways. Sometimes, nurses ask questions in order to speed up the doctor's examination and consultation time. Other times, medical students ask questions as part of their training and also to lessen the workload of the doctor. Both are short-cuts. "It doesn't work for me." Sandra spoke of becoming impatient with having to repeat herself endlessly—to nurses, medical students, and, finally, to her doctors. She said it's "like . . . a test to see if you got it right or told the truth the first time."

Specifically in terms of medical students, Sandra observed that having a doctor come into the hospital or examination room with a troupe of students behind without first asking permission to do so can feel invasive. As a nurse herself, Sandra understands that students need to learn and gain experience. Yet she also thinks it is not too much to ask of doctors that they ask a patient's permission for such observation and participation, rather than assuming they have blanket consent for every kind of student involvement in teaching hospital settings.

In fact, student participation can be rather invasive. For example, during an ethics class with second-year medical students, I heard one female student object to the practice that she had encountered first-hand of having students conduct numerous vaginal examinations on a woman under anesthesia. She said she had been told to do an exam by an instructor for practice, but she felt incredibly uncomfortable doing so without the patients' prior knowledge and consent to these practice sessions. She was certain the patient had not been told before going under that these practice exams would be taking place.

It is important to emphasize that it is not that Sandra always objected to the presence or participation of medical students. What bothered her was that her doctors did not consider her feelings or extend the courtesy of asking her permission. Presumptions of authority can make a patient feel less than a full agent in the exchange, and perhaps even invisible as a person.

Moreover, sometimes it is difficult to get past the nurses and clerk gatekeepers to see the doctor at all. Sandra has had several experiences where she will call the doctor's office and the nurse or clerk has to know what is wrong before she/he will relay the information to the doctor. Sandra said that sometimes she just feels what she needs to say is too personal or private to want to share with the nurse or desk clerk. She also commented that in some cases, she has called the doctor's office and left a message, only to receive a call back a couple of days later or not at all. As I reflected on how much aggravation this assertive and educated nurse has had with these bureaucratic practices, I also wondered about what others, perhaps less agile in these respects, go through.

For example, recall that Marcela had three different doctors in less than two years—and no say in the matter. No one gave her an explanation of why they left, other than to say it was no longer their turn to be there—that they had to work elsewhere. This makes me think that they were interns or residents, but Marcela did not see them as young or inexperienced doctors. Regardless of the reasons for their departure, the fact remains that she was not given a choice in retaining any of them. She was insured by Medicaid and that fact also restricts her choices in providers. It is true that while Marcela found this fact amusing, she was not angry or annoyed by it. She expressed strong satisfaction with her doctors.

On another level of functioning, it is significant to note that none of the three doctors during this time spoke more than a smattering of Spanish. All were white; two were men. Even as she laughed about the number of changes in doctors and their feeble Spanish, it is true that Marcela did not complain or express any resentment. She was accepting of these realities and limitations. She told me that on those occasions when her husband or a friend could not translate for her, she would make do on her own and that she was able to understand enough of what they said. She expressed satisfaction with the medical care she has received. I found myself a bit less accepting of certain aspects of her care.

Others may not fare so well or be as content as Marcela. Lucy observed, "We have patients that come in, they speak no English. And I'm amazed because they'll get informed consent; and I didn't see a family member. I didn't see a translator. And I'm wondering, well, how did you get an informed consent from somebody that speaks no English? And you don't speak the language. . . ." Antonia also gave an example of a noncommunicative linguistic exchange: "I remember one situation where a doctor was talking Spanish so horribly that the patient decided to talk her English so horribly because she felt that his Spanish—they were not going to be able to talk in Spanish. . . . And he continued to talk in Spanish and she continued to talk in English. . . . And I'm standing there, and I'm saying, this is not—this is not working." She went on to add that when a provider speaks Spanish so poorly, it is not only unhelpful, but it is also disrespectful to the patient. In such cases, fluent translators ought to be utilized instead.

Translation is a complicated and important task. Antonia, herself a Spanish speaker, even acknowledged her own limitations: "Sometimes, even with me, I don't know certain words, medical words. But I have a little pocket medical . . . book. I don't pretend to act like I know every word." She noted that translators can help, but that most often the effort is not made to bring them in. "I think a lot of the times people either try to get one of the staff to try and translate, or the family member to translate. And then you're dealing with issues of confidentiality." It is significant that hospitals cannot bill insurance companies for translation services. Thus, few have resources to pay translators or to fund the infrastructure needed to coordinate sufficient numbers of highly skilled volunteer translators. Moreover, while patients may be comfortable with this ad hoc translation, it nonetheless raises important questions about patient rights to privacy and confidentiality. And similar to

Antonia, ad hoc translators may not know all the needed terminology—in one or the other of the languages.

Indeed, Antonia had many sharp insights into the complexities of cross-linguistic/cultural communication. She identified language as a significant barrier to healthcare quality for communities of color. Given her knowledge of Spanish, she is both attuned to these barriers and able to help do something about them. "Well, I guess because I am Hispanic, and I can speak Spanish, I do find a lot of the times there are communication barriers, not only just with Spanish-speaking people, but in other languages as well."

She added that often, the real problem is a combination of fear and language, which can occur when patients are of different cultural backgrounds than their providers. I asked her to explain more of what she meant by fear: "Fear of . . . that the person, the physician or whoever, not understanding their culture, not understanding their reasons for thinking or doing something." Antonia thinks that this fear can then inhibit patients from asking for clarification or admitting that they do not understand everything said to them:

> And then so [patients who do not speak English] communicate, and they're sort of nodding yes and no's, but there really isn't [understanding], because the patient's trying to please, or trying to, you know, do their best at communicating or accepting or understanding what the doctor's telling them. But in the long run, after they've left that office, I think that there are times where they leave there not really knowing what's going on. And I think they try so desperately to, I guess, get the medication or try to tell [the doctors/providers] how they feel in a way that they get something done.

Antonia perceives how vulnerable patients can be. These comments reinforce the notion of the power imbalances—how patients want to please their doctors or are desperate to get medical treatment. In the scheme of things, they accept truncated understandings in order to access the needed medical intervention, be it medicinal, surgical, or something else.

Antonia related one situation involving a Spanish-speaking woman in her late sixties or early seventies where a language barrier led to a grossly flawed assumption. She explained that during admission, a standardized form is used to record basic facts about the person. In this particular instance, "[O]n the form, she was labeled as low educational level. And when I spoke to her—I said, 'Let me speak to her for a little while,' and I spoke to her. And she was a professor, you know? So because she did not speak English very well . . . they put down she was of low educational level. . . . And that's a stereotype." Antonia's story illustrates both the inherent problems with a system that does not make language translation a fundamental part of any assessment protocol for non-English speakers as well as showing again how stereotypes have tangible consequences. Indeed, when providers assume patients are uneducated or unintelligent, they may then make less effort to communicate important information. Antonia thinks that such dismissive practices are fairly common:

> And just basically a lot of times I think a lot of people, also, because like I said, their level of understanding English, they're assumed to not under-stand medical terms, or medical problems, or what's going on with them. And so it decreases your level, or their level, of wanting to communicate further and explain what's going on because you think they're just not going to know what's going on. . . . So you don't try. I've seen that a lot. Or patients, you know, ask me questions about certain procedures, ques-tioning things that's going on because they really don't know why they're having the test done, they don't know, you know, what's going on. They don't know. And that's unfortunate. Because if they don't understand what's going on with them, if they don't understand their disease, they're less likely to take their medicines when they go home. They're less likely to do what's told—what's asked of them.

Antonia makes several important points regarding the chain reaction that assumptions can trigger. If providers assume a patient is unintelli-gent, they may then make less effort to explain procedures, treatments, and goals to the patient. The patient may then, in turn, be less likely to follow through with the prescribed treatment plan. The irony is that such events are used as evidence of a patient's lack of intelligence and/or noncompliance—when, in actuality, it is the assumption, which instills fear and confusion, that is the real problem. It is a tautological game of spin in which a bias is used to substantiate and reproduce itself.

Bottom Lines

As a nurse case manager, Beef Stew's main responsibility is to "facilitate the treatment and discharge plan" for oncology patients. This work entails making sure that patients stay only as long as they need an acute care setting. It also means making sure that the insurance company is paying for the services.[38] "In a nutshell, I protect the facility's bottom line, you know, make sure that we get approvals and authorizations for the patient stay and the patient services. And when we're not getting approvals, that's when I get on the doctors." Beef Stew acknowledged that the influence insurance can exert upon the treatment and discharge plan is not optimal,[39] but she also noted that without this pressure, some patients would stay longer than is in their best interest.[40]

Rebecca Williams, a white social worker on the oncology floor, was even more blunt.[41] She commented, "In a hospital, when there's a money constraint, the first people to go are the people who don't contribute to the profit of the hospital, right?" While Beef Stew facilitates discharge planning, Rebecca is the one to do it—to get the referrals, find placements, and make the transition happen.

Rebecca was quick to qualify the above remark by saying that she loves the hospital and thinks it is a great place. Her main frustration with her work is that she has to spend an inordinate amount of time on paperwork and coming up with discharge plans, instead of simply being present to patients. This frustration with documentation was strongly echoed by the oncologist Leonard Orlando and by another social worker Kathleen O'Brian. In addition to discharge planning, the other main responsibility of Rebecca's job is offering psychosocial support. This latter responsibility is her favorite, but it gets compressed by the demands of the former. She noted that the hospital sees discharge planning as a vital function, but not the other. The difference is that discharge planning has a tangible result and benefit to the hospital's finances; sitting and listening to patients do not. Adding to the time pressure, Rebecca noted that she has a high caseload that continues to rise. At the time of the interview, the hospital was having difficulty hiring and retaining enough social workers for every unit. Consequently, Rebecca had been covering another floor for a prolonged period of time.

Leonard Orlando is an oncologist.[42] He has been an oncologist since 1998 and is still building his practice. He defined his racial-ethnic identity as Italian American. With respect to the reality of financial pressures, Leonard noted that his salary

> is very much tied to my productivity . . . And the reality is, I don't think that anyone—I mean, I don't think that insurance companies really pay for an emotional investment, really. . . . [N]ot that one wants to, you know, bill for compassion . . . But the point is that there are constraints that are very much in place that force one to kind of keep moving forward and moving ahead.

The point is not that this doctor does not value or offer compassion. Indeed, when I asked Leonard what drew him to oncology, he replied that he likes the emotional intensity often involved. He values connecting with his patients and makes concerted efforts to do so. Rather, the issue is that his desire to do so is at odds with the bottom line pressures. In fact, Leonard does not take Medicaid patients because the reimbursement rates are so low that he loses money in doing so.

As I listen to the provider insights about bureaucratic pressures and bottom lines, Sandra's story comes back to my mind. This nurse and educator felt terrified by being ill and uninsured. She has experience as both a provider *and* a patient. She has analyzed the financial bottom lines as an administrator. She has compiled and collated more than her share of documentation and forms. She knows hospitals. And when she realized that she likely needed intensive treatment and had no insurance, she feared that she had been given a death sentence.

Hearing how trapped Sandra felt while temporarily uninsured acts like smelling salts to my consciousness. Akin to Sophia's experience during her recurrence, Sandra's voice gives embodied witness to the glaring, but often ignored, reality of how the vast majority of U.S. inhabitants are just a breath away from becoming uninsured. As is clear from the analysis in chapter 2, a lack of insurance is not simply a problem of the poor or uneducated. As constituted by present structures, health insurance is a precarious benefit for most people, ready to flee the scene right when you need it the most. And this risk, which threatens especially those under the age of 65, weighs heavy upon the minds and hearts of millions.

Of course, there are notable exceptions. Those exempt from these worries include those who are independently wealthy, those who can afford private insurance indefinitely, and who do not depend upon employment for their income or insurance. In addition, one largely exempt population from this danger, ironically, is comprised of the federal legislators who make healthcare policy into law. Out of curiosity, I called the Payroll Office of Member Services, which handles benefits and payroll for the elected members of both the U.S. House and Senate. I was informed by a staff person there that members of Congress are eligible (but not mandated) to enroll in the Federal Employee's Group Health Insurance Program. They have to pay for this coverage as all federal employees do. If they are not reelected, they cannot automatically retain this coverage. However, if they serve at least five years in office *and* are at least 62 years old and retire from the House or Senate, they *may* elect to continue this coverage indefinitely after their term of service has ended.[43]

Both Sophia and Sandra reveal with startling clarity what a vulnerable position it is to be critically ill and without insurance. It is an agonizing worry that can cause as much, if not more, distress as having cancer. Being uninsured adds the fear that the cancer will not be treated with all the resources available in this technologically and therapeutically advanced (and costly) healthcare system.

Concluding Reflections: What I Did Not Hear

One thing that intrigued me from my conversations with the three white care providers is that the presence of racial dynamics between providers and patients was not especially visible to them. Perhaps somehow related is the fact that of this very small sample of white providers, Rebecca was the only one who verbally self-identified as white. Leonard seemed a bit befuddled by conceptualizing his racial-ethnic and cultural identity. At one point, he asked rhetorically, "So, you know, am I a WASP? I mean, I certainly am very privileged. I work very, very hard. I've always worked very, very hard. But I've had it easy in the sense that I've always had what I needed at my disposal. So I don't know, really, what I am. But, you know, different; but then we're all different."[44] He identified as Italian American and the other social worker identified as Irish Catholic.

None of the three gave examples of how they see racial-ethnic stereotypes or assumptions coming into play on the part of providers. Instead, they acknowledged that it is important to attend to cultural and language differences. They acknowledged that language barriers can be an issue; none speak Spanish. Each stressed how important it is to build trust within each individual relationship.

These providers are not alone in this regard. A national survey of 2,608 physicians published by the Kaiser Foundation in 2002 found the following: "The majority of physicians believe disparities in how people are treated within the health care system 'rarely' or 'never' happen based on factors such as income, fluency in English, educational status, or racial or ethnic background."[45] In fact, doctors are less likely to identify that disparities happen than members of the general public. However, there are differences in perceptions among doctors of different colors: "African American physicians are more likely than White or Asian Physicians to believe that the health care system at least 'somewhat often' treats people unfairly based on various characteristics, with differences particularly striking with regard to race and ethnicity."[46] For example, 77 percent of Black doctors and 52 percent of Latino doctors think that the healthcare system treats people unfairly based on their race or ethnic background, while only 25 percent of white and 33 percent of Asian doctors share this perspective. The comments of the providers with whom I spoke reflected a commitment to treat everyone as a person and to respect each individual, but lacked reflection on how racial dynamics might impinge upon or obstruct such goals and values. In this sense, they revealed more by what they did *not* say or see than by what they did.

This comment is not meant as an attack on the character of any of these three providers. All three struck me as genuinely competent, empathetic, and sensitive people. I liked each of them very much; none of them were cold or abrupt. All of them were very generous with their time and expressed appreciation for my research topic. They are clearly dedicated to the values of compassion and service. In particular, all expressed love for working with cancer patients. They like the emotional dimensions of their work.

For example, Leonard commented that he tries to listen and "resist the temptation to talk a lot." He added that he understands that a connection with the patient is critical to accomplishing his work. However, the way he put it struck me as, even if well intentioned, a bit "stiff": "[A]ll physicians have our agenda, because we know what we need to accomplish for medical reasons . . . But then the patients have their goals. And they need to be blended. In fact, . . . for my goals to be accomplished, I need to understand where a patient's coming from, you know, and what my—what the barriers may be to allowing my goals to be accomplished." He is right in acknowledging that in order to progress in treating the patient's disease, he, along with other physicians as a whole, needs to understand the patient's needs and priorities. Yet the way he communicates this awareness—the emphasis on "agendas, goals and barriers"—seems to me a bit sterile and overly abstract in its tone.

I asked Leonard how he tries to connect with patients of differing racial-ethnic and socioeconomic class backgrounds. He mentioned eye contact and physical contact, emphasized talking with them and not only *at* them. Then he added,

> And I probably use all three [methods], if I can, and also try to interrupt or interject a medical agenda with just some personal interjection, even if it's silly or stupidity. I often talk about nonsense during my physical exam, you know, in other words, ask them—follow up on some aspect of their social history, either where they grew up, or you know, where

they live, etc., in part to break the silence of the exam, but again maybe break down their defenses a little bit and make them more comfortable. And connecting with my patient is really important, particularly, you know most of my patients, my cancer patients, at least, will bring a family member with them, or family members. And there's often—the patient is often not the dominant family member, either because of fear, because of their illness or because of culture. And so—I try to set the family aside and really focus on the patient.

Again, his comments certainly demonstrate a profoundly well-intentioned, compassionate physician. Yet, what concerns me was his reference to social history as nonsense. And, while I understand that sometimes families can interfere and make it hard for the patient to direct her or his own care and make decisions, in some cultures, it does not work well to sideline the family and focus only upon the patient. In some cultures, familial configurations and relationships do not mesh well with the western bias toward individual doctor-patient relationships and individualistic notions of autonomy and informed consent.[47]

In summary, none of these three providers are afraid of the hard emotions. They are well-intentioned and skilled caregivers. I have no doubt that they have built many wonderful relationships with patients and families and that they have provided vital services to many patients and families. The problem lies not at the level of intention, but rather at that of perception. I think that they may not fully perceive some of the cross racial-ethnic and/or cultural dynamics potentially at work in provider-patient relationships; at least, they did not elaborate upon them with me.

It is true that no one has complete vision; all human perception is partial. Indeed, that is why we need one another's eyesight so that we can catch our respective blind spots. In addition, the amplifying and corrective lenses that come from other sources of information (theology, medical sociology, social ethics) must also be part of the dialogue. Moreover, none of what any of the collaborators said amounts to all that needs to be explored on any of these topics. They have each told me part of their story, but certainly not the whole of any story—of their lives, of the care they received, or of the institution in which they work.

However, here it is important to hearken back to the analysis of the preceding chapter: Even if any human vision is partial, still white people seem to suffer in general from a particular astigmatism. Specifically, we tend to fail in our perceptions of current forms of racism and of our own white privilege. Simply put, the social and racial contextual pieces informing patient-provider relationships were not as clearly on the radar screens of the white providers as they were of the providers of color. Leonard reflected that he probably has better success in building trust in his relationships with patients of lower socioeconomic classes than with affluent patients:

> To be perfectly honest with you, in terms of trust, I would generalize and say that I have more success with patients of lower socioeconomic classes than I do with those of higher. In other words, patients with means shop for doctors. And patients who live within their means, or who don't, aren't or even just barely making it, they're more willing to reach out and be more accepting . . . But it's interesting because those who are more sophisticated, they actually doctor shop.

What fascinates me about this comment is that Leonard did not connect the fact that patients of lower socioeconomic classes may be less picky because they may have, or feel they have, fewer options than the affluent ones. They may be enculturated by a legacy of societal discrimination to be accepting of limitations. Or they may feel subtle pressure to accept what they are offered because they may have less information or feel less confident in their own knowledge. Or they may be immigrants who are simply grateful to have any care at all.

For example, I went to two breast cancer support group meetings in which the women were mainly first generation immigrants. It is important to mention that, by in large, all of them expressed great appreciation for their doctors and for the care they have received. Many contrasted it with the state of healthcare in their home countries and emphasized how much more comfortable they felt with the care here. Alternatively, they may feel constricted by their insurance plans. In short, if given more room to move and breathe, it is possible that patients of lower socioeconomic classes might shop around as much as wealthy patients. The ability to shop around speaks to financial/insurance resources. It may also relate to the fact that certain people (white, affluent) may often be socialized in a way that encourages them to feel entitled to such options. Leonard did not reflect on any of these possible contextual scenarios.

Rebecca mentioned that in school she learned about racial and socioeconomic realities and how they shape human relationships, but that she does not see that they really do matter very much in the concrete relationships she has cultivated. Overall, she tends to think that people are people, and that as a provider, she needs to get to know and treat each one as an individual. For her, the biggest obstacle to giving care to people is not making connections across race, culture, or socioeconomic class, but rather the lack of time. And certainly, as providers are able to treat everyone "as people," and get to know them individually, Rebecca is right. Race and class do not necessarily need to obstruct human relationships. I only wish to add that "treating people as people" is not a simple venture and that what will feel respectful to one person may feel like an affront to another—in part, due to racial realities and particular cultural sensibilities.

Kathleen O'Brian, another white oncology social worker, also reflects this general perspective:

> I think the most challenging part is, on an emotional level, being able to feel that you've helped somebody, to be able to really feel that you've spent some amount of time to be able to—I guess what I'm trying to say is that it's very difficult to feel that you're doing all that you can because of the pressures of time. And it's hard to devote enough time to each person.[48]

Kathleen later emphasized the heavy weight of "all of the rules and regulations of the hospital" that pull her away from spending time with people. The biggest thing in healthcare that Kathleen thinks needs to change structurally is its funding. She commented that Medicare reimbursements from the government are being cut to teaching hospitals. She explained that the funding "gets less and less" and that hospitals are stretched and have to "cut corners," adding: "And unfortunately, what gets cut are often ancillary staff or nurses or the patient direct contact people."

Kathleen expressed strong awareness of the need to be attentive to the cultural background and spiritual aspects of patients, especially when working cross culturally. She spoke of trying to see patients holistically. However, her description of holistic care did not attend specifically to racial or socioeconomic aspects related to an individual's personhood or community membership. She addressed the spiritual and cultural aspects of people in a general way.

In summary, in terms of race, the three white provider comments were much less incisive than the three providers of color. When I asked the providers of color how/if racial dynamics and assumptions might affect patient-provider encounters or the quality of care, they offered several examples. In contrast, the white providers focused more on the roles of economics, bureaucratic obstacles such as tedious and large volumes of paperwork and insurance status. While they saw socioeconomic realities structuring patient-provider relationships, they were less articulate on how racial dynamics might do the same. They tended to focus their responses more at the level of one-to-one interactions and trust-building. They discussed general strategies for building rapport (e.g., actively eliciting information, eye contact, touch, sitting down) but did not reflect upon how the power dynamics and social dimensions might already be informing the interaction as soon as they enter the room.

I contend that part of white privilege includes the option to not reflect on these matters very much. These providers are not unique in this regard. Overall, white people in U.S. society fail to see or talk about the larger social patterns and systems that shape and inform human relationships across races and cultures in particular ways. The hope is that by bringing these tendencies to light, more white people will engage in critical reflection about matters we have too often overlooked or taken for granted.

This chapter has told several stories and has shared insights from 14 people in order to see how racial and socioeconomic dynamics have filtered into their experiences of receiving and giving healthcare. Each has a unique voice and perspective. In one sense I have not told very many stories; yet in another, one story may have sufficed. All of the four themes surfaced in each of Sandra's, María's, and Sophia's lives. The fact that a woman is bleeding and is told to go away and get insurance already tells me there is something seriously problematic in our healthcare system. The fact that a woman with a history of cancer goes from one doctor appointment to another for nearly two years without having tests done to determine if she has breast cancer already tells me that there is an ethical problem in healthcare delivery. The fact that a woman carries the heavy burden to be a "good Black Puerto Rican" so that her caregivers will be invested in her life already tells me that we live in a very scary world.

What I now understand with greater acuity from listening to these collaborators is how entangled they all are in an impossible dance. *Both* the providers and women with breast cancer are caught in a very frustrating system. The women try hard to establish and advocate for themselves. The providers sincerely want to give the best care they can. Yet the constraints of the healthcare systems and cultures to which they are all so integrally connected often work against them in pivotal ways.

Ethics cannot stop with lament or denunciation. It must—out of gritty determination and dogged hopefulness—articulate another way of being and living. Chapter 5 takes up theological and constructive visions of how things could be different—in healthcare settings and in scholarship.

5

Resisting Death, Celebrating Life:
Christian Social Ethics for Healthcare

won't you celebrate with me

won't you celebrate with me
what i have shaped into
a kind of life? i had no model.
born in babylon
both nonwhite and woman
what did i see to be except myself?
i made it up
here on this bridge between
starshine and clay,
my one hand holding tight
my other hand; come celebrate
with me that everyday
something has tried to kill me
and has failed.

—Lucille Clifton, *Book of Light*, 25[1]

There are many kinds of death; the physical cessation of life is only one among them. It is quite possible to breathe and move and yet to feel dead inside. Sometimes people feel emotionally or spiritually deadened by strife. Human hearts wither without love and recognition. A kind of death swarms over a person when she loses hope and/or the sense of herself as intrinsically beloved. So when Lucille Clifton speaks of celebrating the fact that every day something has tried to kill her and has failed, I consider the full scope of death and rejoice with her that neither her body, spirit, or hope has perished.

This research is one attempt to resist the death-dealing ways in which human beings and the systems we fashion dehumanize one another. Even more, this book is about life—about straining to articulate ways in which the critically ill might feel cared for and alive in the presence of others. To foster this flourishing of life—in all its complexity and uniqueness—we human beings need every constructive resource at our disposal: Risk-taking, loving, (com)passionate hearts; our sharpest critical thinking and intellect; our bodies and senses; and gritty—take a beating and stand up again—faith.

Before arriving at any ethical conclusions, I want to come back to theology. Specifically, this final chapter lifts up theological insights of the women with breast cancer who make visceral connections between what they know of God and what they know about what human beings owe one another. By beginning here, I hope that the kind of contribution theology can make to healthcare and medicine will be evident. After this groundwork is laid, the analysis then turns to more specific areas of concern for medical ethics and healthcare quality. The starting point is a description of the qualities of a patient-provider relationship that the women who have had breast cancer most prize. Taking these theological and practical insights seriously, the next main section considers what has to be in place—structurally—for such wisdom to be heeded within U.S. healthcare. The chapter concludes by articulating the methodological significance this interdisciplinary research has for the doing of ethics.

"God Has To Live in Each One of Us": Theo-Ethical Insights of Women with Cancer

Beyond insight into healthcare practices and realities that I have gained from doing ethnographic research, I have also learned a bit about God and God's relationship to humanity.[2] I asked each of the participants if and how her faith in God informs what dignity and respect mean; how human beings ought to treat one another; and how they try to treat others. Seven of the women with cancer identified explicitly as Christians.[3]

Before articulating how faith in God informs their sense of what dignity and respect mean, I need to touch upon another term: Gratitude. Gratitude to God was voiced so often that it seems fundamental to understanding anything else the women said regarding the relationship between God and humanity. Even as several of them were/are contending with cancer and uncertain futures, these women effusively thanked God and emphasized that they felt accompanied by God throughout their lives. They expressed ardent confidence in God and acknowledged that God is ultimately in control—that they live in dependence upon God and God's goodness. Slimfat Girl expressed her faith this way: "It's like this—He's always been there. He has never left my side. I have been in some situations, and I always thank God, and I thank the Lord that they pulled me through. So I do believe. I do believe there's a higher power than myself."[4] And Marcela has this to say: "And I thank God that I feel, that I am feeling really, really well—thanks to God. I appreciate this God that is up above because I ask Him for this every day."[5] She then added this description of the divine: "I think that He is support, where we find refuge, that if one looks, if we look for God day after day, He will unconditionally support us always."[6]

This theme of gratitude and thankfulness came up in the four breast cancer support groups that I attended as well. In each of these cases, I heard many and varied women in challenging life circumstances unreservedly thank God and "give God all the praise and glory": Immigrant women; undocumented women; Black and Latina women born and raised in New York City; women with limited economic means; women who had lost all their hair; women who were feeling poorly (some who had just had chemotherapy); women with poor prognoses. Through their tears, whether shed out of happiness or out of fear and worry, still they thanked God.

This gratitude was not a form of denial of their illness, nor did it seem at all superficial or cliché. I saw fear and strength—doubt and hope—in many pairs of eyes. I understand their words of gratitude to God to serve as *both* expressions of their active hope and faith *as well as* reassurance that there are reasons to have faith—as a way to combat the fear that gnaws away at hope. As a white, educated, physically well woman who can sometimes feel paralyzed by surveying all that is wrong in this world, I am humbled by their ability to stay rooted in hope in the midst of concrete suffering and reasons for despair.

Their praise did not mean that they never got angry with God or struggled with faith. Sophia openly acknowledged that having faith can be really difficult, that sometimes she felt like she was "faking it." I am sure that these and other women with cancer struggle so much and can be so angry or sad that they go to the point of losing any scrap of hope or faith. Yet what struck me about the dozens of women I met or observed was that both their faith in God and their hope for their own lives had grit. These interconnected hopes gave them staying power to endure the suffering and the uncertainty—at least in the moments that I have known them.[7]

It can be hard to find words to describe the divine-human relationship. When I asked Slimfat Girl how God wants people to treat each other, she exclaimed, "He wants everything—oh, boy! That's why Adam and Eve *did not* stay in the garden, O.K.? Because they didn't listen to what He said. And if they hadda' listened, if they had of listened, you know, maybe the—our world would be a better place." (Emphasis hers.) The question of how faith in and knowledge of God informs how people are to treat one another can be daunting. The complexities and brokenness of this world can make it hard to imagine what human beings can and ought to do.

Despite the mammoth problems of this world, however, Marcela eloquently expressed her understanding of who God is and of what this means for human relationships:

> God says that He is love, right? And so, God has to live in each one of us. If one says that they love, one can assume it is because he/she knows God. Therefore, God says we are going to love one another. . . . Love is so important that it is, how to tell you, something that one cannot even define. So, we are going to love one another, respect one another, support one another so that this way God is reflected in each one of us.[8]

Her logic is compelling: God is love—something so important that it defies the boundaries of any definition. Human beings love. To the extent that we love, God lives in each one of us. In fact, we are only able to love *because* we know God who is love itself. This radical incarnational understanding of the divine means for Marcela that in our concrete activities and lives, human beings are able and supposed to image God—to reflect this love and to be a refuge and support to others. Wanda made a similar connection: "I want to always treat people the way that they're supposed to be treated, with respect and dignity and the love of Christ and having them see that Christ-like example within me."[9] Wanda wants others to see divine love alive within her.

Reflecting on Marcela's and Wanda's words, I realized that their emphasis is the reverse of what I usually articulate as my aim; namely, to see Christ (or the divine) in the other. While both ways of putting it are important, their vision is an important corrective for me because it inspires creative moral agency, in addition to respectful listening to and recognition of others. In an emphasis on seeing the divine in others, it is possible to forget or de-emphasize the crucial insight that *by my own* actions and decisions, I can reflect and embody (if only very partially) God's love for the others I encounter in any given day. What matters is not only *seeing* the divine in others, but *expressing* divine love and justice in relation to others.

When I asked a couple of the women to define dignity, I again heard an emphasis on self-agency. Marcela told me, "Dignity is something that lifts your self esteem . . . What you think of yourself is what helps you have dignity." I clarified, "So dignity is not something that others give a person, it is what one has inside oneself?" Marcela readily agreed. Indeed, while she agreed that others in society do not have the right to make a person feel bad, she was quick to add, "But it is not them who will resolve this problem for me, it is me." I commented that if one has dignity in oneself it will be a kind of protection—to protect one against these influences—that others cannot rob this dignity because it is one's own internal property. Marcela concurred: "[Dignity] doesn't depend on them; *it depends on you.* But above all, you have to maintain it always no matter what happens, you have to go on." (Her emphasis.)[10]

I was surprised by her words. They place a great deal of weight on an individual to guard and maintain one's own dignity. When I subsequently asked Marcela to elaborate more upon her perspective, she said, "If you think you're garbage, how will that animate you? If you think you are intelligent, this will animate you. . . . Even if they look at you negatively, you have to be strong, you can say no—and not let it offend you." I initially felt that she was letting social and structural inequalities off the hook too easily. As I continued to ponder her thoughts, however, I remembered Luz's perspective. Even as Luz recalled her mother's words, that she was born with "three strikes against her," she too placed great emphasis on individual agency—speaking of how important it is to "be feisty"—to learn English, to get an education, to be assertive, and to prove them wrong.

I now understand that Marcela and Luz's point was that people who experience discrimination and prejudice must not internalize either. For persons and communities who regularly face racism, one way to contend with it is to deny and resist its power to determine their future or sense of self. "Dignity is yours to protect. It is not dependent upon others." In these words, I heard a strong refusal to see themselves or be seen by others as victims—as persons utterly dependent upon systems and forces outside of their control. While I still maintain that it is essential to hold systems and individuals accountable for the ways in which they eat away at the dignity of certain identities and communities, their insight chastened any inclination on my part to deny their agency out of misplaced pity or sympathy.

I learned something else about dignity. Its flip side is respect for others. What makes dignity genuine and what keeps it from devolving into narcissism or egocentrism is holding self-respect in dynamic tension with love and concern for others—being attentive to others as persons who also have dignity. From these women with breast cancer, I heard in a powerful way that part of respecting others *and* one's self involves humility. María commented that an inner balance is needed among humility, respect, and consideration for others. "None weighs more than another, the three all weigh (count) the same." Her words caused me to reflect that if one has authentic self-respect, she will be more humble with regard to others. Humility *does not* mean an absence of self-respect, but, rather, having a grounded sense of one's importance—not having to inflate one's ego—because one knows she is truly loved and worthy of love. Therefore, she can be less egocentric and instead turned more outward to face and address the needs and personhoods of others. Here I sensed a resonance with that premodern man Luther.

María gave an example of how gratitude to God and humility within herself help her to notice and respond to the needs of others. She said that when she sees hungry people on the street and she has two or three dollars, she often goes and buys the person something to eat. She does this, she says, not so that God will appreciate her, but because she is grateful to God. "I am very grateful to God, first of all, and then to my family and to [the second hospital]." She added that she is also grateful to the cancer support organizations and to their volunteers and staff.[11] And because she is so grateful for all the information and support she has received and for her life, she wants to give back. "God's given me a second chance and if someone is in the shoes I was in, I will try to help." In terms of giving back to the organizations that have helped her, she tries to be present for the events, walk-a-thons, and the marches on Washington—"as long as God permits." Her cancer support volunteering and her feeding of hungry people are expressions of both her self-respect and humility.

In a similar vein, Sophia explained that cancer has made her acutely aware of human fragility—that life can be gone in the blink of an eye. She vividly sees what really matters in life. She said that cancer has changed things in a positive way in this sense because it helped her get her priorities in order and to see what is truly important. She reflected,

"Cancer made me stronger in a lot of ways. It made me more vulnerable in a lot of ways. I'm more open than I was before. . . . Now I kind of want to do more, help more. Not just with cancer, but with anything, anything I can do . . . I listen more to people, too. It's less about me, you know?"

Self-respect and respect for others go hand in hand. Wanda brought this fact into full light for me. I asked her to define dignity. After a long pause, she said,

> I think just treating others the way that you would want to be treated, just with respect, not looking down on people, not—because a person, for example, may have, like, HIV, and, you know, not treating them with disrespect, but treating them like a human being, like they're some-body. And I use that example because that was a population that I worked with. And I used to see how people would treat them and just wouldn't want to be bothered or touch them or anything like that. And, you know, once I became educated about the illness, you know, it didn't frighten me. You know, I was, like, they're a human being too, you know. . . . [T]hey have a disease; but they're a human being, you know, they need to be treated with respect and not looked down upon or thrown away.

What struck me about this comment is that when I asked Wanda to define dignity, she reflected on a concrete change she had experienced in herself as she worked with a stigmatized population. Said differently, she did not speak about how others ought to respect *her* dignity, but rather she focused on how in one instance she herself had become more attuned to the *dignity of others*. This insight conveyed a great deal of self-reflexivity.

Moreover, Wanda explained how confronting her own biases and assumptions has not only helped her to respect others more, but to also have a more grounded sense of dignity and self-respect for herself. Specifically, she said that working with people with HIV has helped her to speak up for herself: "And I just think having the job of working with the HIV population has really helped me, you know? Not only did it help me empower my clients, but it helped empower myself, and to speak up for myself." Working with a community of people who are vulnerable in their own way gave her a window into her own life. In getting to know people with HIV and seeing what they go through, Wanda learned how to look out for herself *and* how to be more genuinely compassionate to others.

In all, by articulating what dignity in oneself and respect for others mean, these women also saw how far human beings are from what God wants for us. Yet this knowledge did not stop them from offering a vision of what ought to be. Several emphasized that it is important to strive for what is possible in one's life. To recall again Marcela's insight, "God has to live in each of us." When we love, it is because God is in us. And because God's love and grace make it possible for God to dwell within humanity, we had better get busy. Because we are loved so intimately and profoundly—because God has searched and dwells within all human hearts, knew each of us in our mother's wombs, and cherishes every one beyond description—we too can and must do all that we can to cherish one another.

"I Didn't See [a] 'Doctor.' I Just Saw a Woman": Patient Expectations of Healthcare Providers

That's how Hannah sees her breast surgeon—as a woman first. And that is how Hannah feels seen *by* her as well. This quality of relationship seems so fundamental. Yet it is not so easy to achieve in actual patient-physician relations. In what follows, I want to explore what I have learned from these women with breast cancer about what ingredients form the basis for high quality patient-provider relationships. I will touch upon four.

Above all other remarks, when asked what they most want from their doctors and/or other primary care providers, all of the women repeatedly emphasized authentic listening, empathy, and understanding. I cite Sandra to illustrate the point. She explained that the most important thing care providers and systems need to do in terms of showing respect and honoring the person is hearing—*genuinely* hearing—without being compromised by an impatience to move on. "Listening is the biggest thing. I don't know if it's an acquired skill, but it certainly diminishes and affects the dignity and respect of the person when they don't listen." The basic yet crucial act of listening may be the most direct way of respecting another person. Sandra went on to comment, "Those who did not hear forced me to seek more information so that I could feel comfortable." Indeed, when doctors or nurses rush the listening, they may end up having to spend more time with the patient and being less efficient in the long run. Being in a hurry, or overly relying on impersonal protocols for processing people—especially in the initial stages of a professional relationship—can inhibit trust and delay relationship-building.

Antonia Morales also understood that listening well makes the work easier for the provider:

> And I see amazing doctors. And I see some that are not. . . . [T]hose that are amazing are the ones that drive me. Because they are so much better physicians in what they do. And it is obvious. If you want to do a better job . . . communicate better with your patients. They're going to tell you what's going on if they feel they can trust you. If not, you know, I think it's going to be harder for you. Your patients are going to come back . . . or they're going to have problems, and you're always going to see them sick . . . I'm following an amazing doctor now. And even though she runs around, and she has a lot of work, when she comes into a room, the patient, I mean, shines. Because all she needs to do is come next to their bed, you know, come down to their level, and hold their hand, and talk to them face to face, smile at them, let them know everything's going to be O.K., let them know what's going on. It doesn't take that much time. . . . Come down, sit down next to them by the bed, you know, apologize for anything that's going on, you know, because things happen, nurses you know, or whatever. Apologize. Doesn't hurt, you know, and it makes them feel like you care about what's going on with them while they're [in the hospital]. Apologize for it. "I'm sorry." And "We'll try our best to do better."

Antonia points out that adequate listening is not only a function of the ears and brain, but also of one's quality of presence. Sitting down next to a patient can indicate that a doctor is truly present to the condition of the person in the bed. Even more, Antonia signals the importance of empathy—even to the point of apologizing. The act of offering an apology—communicating that one is sorry that another is uncomfortable or that things have not gone smoothly—seems something so obvious and yet it may be the last thing a care provider thinks to say to a patient. Indeed, perhaps some might worry that apologizing exposes providers to legal (and financial) liability. It would be a sad commentary on the state of affairs between providers and those in their care if people do not apologize out of a fear of being sued.

Finally, genuine listening involves not being put off by questions. Again, Sandra noted the importance of this quality by pointing out its absence in her relationships with her first two physicians. Interestingly, she noted that in her case, being educated did not make a difference in terms of being listened to or treated with respect. In fact, she felt her education worked against her. She felt treated as a "dumb nurse" by the first physician because she did not already know all the medical information, asked a lot of questions, and had let her insurance lapse. The second doctor, while less abrasive, also seemed threatened by her educated questions.

A second quality of healthcare providers that I heard the women desire is honesty. Slimfat Girl implored, "And just be honest with me. *Be honest, just be honest.* You know?" (Emphasis hers.) Honesty was also of paramount importance to Luz who poignantly articulated this need by explaining that part of the problem with her first doctor was that he was not honest with respect to what he did not know. He assured her that she was fine (or would be fine) before having test results to support this claim. Luz adamantly stated,

> A doctor tells you the truth of your illness. A doctor is professional enough to tell you, "This is what I understand from my studies, from the books—not from my feelings. . . ."And not a doctor that would tell you, "Oh, you're O.K., that's nothing." A doctor should never tell a patient "That's nothing," or "This looks like"—no. A doctor should say, "Let's take whatever it is, send it to a lab, let's see what it is."

Rather than saying, "I don't know what you have," or "We have to wait and do all the tests before we will know," this doctor tried to reassure Luz. Attempts at reassurance that are not based in facts quickly diminish in their value to a patient. Even if the words sound good at first, their hopefulness is eventually unmasked for what they are: Empty attempts to keep the patient from being upset (at least in the provider's presence). In this way, Luz explained that such attempts to be caring actually do the opposite:

> [E]ven though he spoke the same language, he was not like caring because he didn't understand my feelings. For example, you know that what you are telling me is from you, it's not from medicine. It's not like you have tested this and know that this is a fact. You just see a worried person and you are going to tell me something to make me feel better, not something that is medically correct. When I sat down with the doctor [at the second care setting], he told me, "Your cancer is aggressive. It's a bad cancer." He told me. He told me the truth about my cancer. He did not tell me something I wanted to hear. . . . Coat it with honey, coat it with sugar, do something, *but tell me the truth*, not something that I want to hear. So I have to do what I have to do to take care of my body. . . . [S]o I can make my decisions. (Emphasis hers)

According to Luz, the most caring thing to do is to give the patient the most accurate information possible. To reassure someone without knowing all the facts undermines respect for the other person as well as one's own agency. Luz needed to know the truth so that she could make the best decisions of what to do next to take care of herself. "Coat it with honey . . . but tell me the truth."

While María agrees that honesty is important, she would emphasize the need for the honey. Genuine compassion is the third ingredient. María's story shows that it matters *how* the truth is shared. Just as compassion without information has serious deficiencies, so does being candid without having tact. She felt her doctors were incredibly brusque with her—"*frío*" (cold). Providers need to be honest and they need to convey information in a caring and compassionate manner. It is a delicate but crucial balance.

Compassion and honesty need to be joined in a provider's relating to patients. Most nursing and medical school textbooks would emphasize this point. The harder question is *how* to achieve such a balance. I asked Wanda how she knows when compassion is genuine—and providers are not simply going through the textbook motions. She responded,

> I look at body language, the way they're talking, how they're expressing themselves. Body language is really important to me. If someone is—if I'm asking a question, and they're like, you know, shrugging their shoulders, and as if they don't care or it's not important, or, you know, trying to brush me off, then I look at that. I also look at just the way they speak, their voice, how they talk to me, and not talking down to me.

Patients are able to read their providers as thoroughly as their providers read their charts and test results. Feigning interest or concern rarely works. Wanda also commented that her primary cancer physician (a white woman) "really loved her job. She loved working with people." Her love both for her work *and* for people showed through in her words and actions. In dramatic contrast to two of Sandra's doctors, Wanda's physician enthusiastically (and without defensiveness) encouraged her to get a second opinion and gave her all her records to take with her. They have had an ongoing relationship since Wanda's diagnosis; they have come to know and trust one another. This relationship has been built on consistently good (honest) communication and positive rapport (genuine compassion and sensitivity).

Wanda underscored the weight of such qualities for patient-provider relationships. They are not mere courtesies; they can affect the patient on a profound level:

> I think that that can help soothe a person or help the healing process, if you have a very compassionate doctor working with you, or staff working with you . . . Because if a patient has to come back, and they'd be worried about how you're treating them, their immune system is already weakened, so that's stress on them. I mean, that's just going to bring them down even more.

While a brusque exchange with a person in authority can irritate a healthy person or cause her stress, it may not as easily threaten her well-being. Wanda introduces an important possibility that might be overlooked. An absence of honesty, compassion, or listening may very well beat down an already compromised immune system. The critically ill are in a weakened position—physically, emotionally—with respect to their caregivers. They have more to lose than their care providers.

Finally, I heard the women emphasize their need for their providers to be skilled clinicians. They want thorough workups and tests. This point, while obvious, ought not be taken for granted. María's story is just one indication of what can happen when the workup is not done, but deferred over the course of several months and visits. In delaying the biopsy, her tumor grew significantly and was joined by a second.

Luz and Marcela also emphasized the importance of having comprehensive and prompt testing. Marcela grew impatient with how long her providers were taking at the first hospital and so took her files to a second in order to speed up the determination of a diagnosis and to get a second opinion in the process. For her part, Luz was pleased with how fast and thorough her providers were when she got into the second care setting. There, in just three days, they did additional tests and performed the mastectomy because they found her cancer to be so aggressive. They took her and her medical situation seriously.

While everyone wants a skilled doctor, some experience more ease in finding one. Although she expressed overall satisfaction with her cancer care, Marcela (a woman insured by Medicaid) had no choice in providers. In less than a year, she had three different primary cancer physicians and was given little explanation for the changes. Luz was only able to access the second care site because of a friend who is a nurse who happened to work for one of their prominent cancer physicians. Recall that Luz called ten times over two days before asking this nurse's help. During this time, she was told again and again that there were no available appointments and that they would not accept her insurance. Indeed, all of the women were well aware of the role that money and insurance play. They either open up doors or close them. Similarly, all expressed an awareness of how financial dynamics/ assumptions can get in the way of good patient-provider relationships.

In all, the most poignant thing I heard from these women regarding what they want from healthcare providers is this: To be seen as a person. They used different expressions to get at this request, from positive statements such as Slimfat Girl wanting to be treated "as you would somebody else" to negative statements regarding how they do *not* want to be treated, such as not being a "bill." While some of these statements explicitly used financial metaphors, all made references to not wanting to be objectified.

For example, Hannah is grateful that her doctor does not see her a check or as income. Slimfat Girl expressed a similar sentiment when she said that she does not want to be treated as a "a paycheck," "money in the bank," or as a "guinea pig." And Marcela commented that it is important that providers do not treat patients "like a piece of furniture." She described that the best scenario is when providers "forget it's a job":

> [I] think that at least, even though it is a place of employment, one must think, if one is going to relate to another person as a human being and that this human being is going through a difficult situation, in this moment, one ought to forget it's a job. Do you understand me? This person is going through a difficult moment and needs help, above all, support. One cannot think that this [work] is as it were—as if I were making, hum, furniture. "I am going to make furniture and I will throw the furniture there." That—no. It is as if you take a piece of furniture and put it there—to take a person and check them and go—no.

"Forget it's a job." That may seem like an odd or unrealistic request. While Marcela does not use the terminology, I hear in these comments a reference to the difference between a "job" and a "vocation." A job is something one does to survive financially—to bring in the paycheck. In contrast, a vocation is one's "calling" into which one puts one's heart, mind, talents, and energy because one senses in a profound way that this is what "I was put on the planet to do." Of course, while living out one's vocation, making a living is still a basic necessity. The key difference is that the work is done out of a sense of purpose and service, not only for one's own financial sustenance or enrichment. To build upon Marcela's illustration, if one is working in healthcare primarily out of a sense of vocation, and not employment, he or she will not think of it as a paycheck so much as a way of serving and being present to others. In the process, Marcela thinks, patients will be less likely to feel objectified, "treated like furniture."

Marcela added that doctors need at least a bit of psychology background to realize what all is going on in their patients. She explained,

> I think that the doctors have to co-penetrate [the situation] with the patient. In one way or another, many times the patient does not say exactly what [the problem] is, just what they feel. Sometimes [the patient] does not want to talk, is sometimes timid. For one or another reason, [the patient] does not want to say exactly what she/he is feeling.[12]

Marcela later explained that what she means by *"conpenetrar"* is that the doctor enters the experience of the person in order to understand both it and the person more fully. Womanist ethicist emilie townes defines empathy in a way that resonates with Marcela's use of *"conpenetrar"*: "As a moral virtue, empathy means that we put ourselves in the place of another. This means sharing and understanding the emotional and social experiences of others and coming to see the world as they see it. We move away from 'those people' and 'they' language and behavior to 'we' and 'us' and 'our' ways of living and believing."[13]

In sum, genuine listening, honesty, compassion, and technical skill all facilitate trust. And trust is perhaps the most essential foundation upon which quality patient-provider relationships are built. Yet there is another way of describing this quality. To conclude this section, I want to return to where it began. What patients most integrally need may be personhood. Hannah glowed when she told me that she sees her breast specialist "as one of the girls." Her experience is a wonderful illustration of what is possible for patient-doctor relationships when the baggage of racial and socioeconomic assumptions, bureaucracies, and financial bottom lines do not interfere. I do not think it is insignificant that Hannah had excellent health insurance and that she and this doctor shared a similar racial-ethnic background. I conclude this portion of the discussion with her words. They convey so much of what each of the women I spoke with would like from their primary caregivers:

> *HJ*: [My breast surgeon]'s so down to earth, too, you know. When I saw her, I didn't know she was a surgeon [laughs] . . . you

know . . . just the way she, you know, just my experience with others, you know, doctors.

AV: She didn't come in, total, all, "I'm the doctor."

HJ: No. She was just one of the girls. She just had that air about her
that, you know. . . . I didn't see her, I didn't see, you know, "I'm a
medical doc," you know. No, I didn't see "Doctor." I just saw a
woman, you know. She's a woman first, you know. Yes, she's a doctor, but she's also a woman.

AV: And maybe that's how she saw you first, not as patient.

HJ: Not as a patient, but just as a woman, you know, like you and I,
just sitting here talking . . . You know, she didn't see . . . "here's
another bill." [laughs]

AV: Right. "Here's another check."

HJ: Right . . .

AV: That shows a lot right there, you know.

HJ: Yes, it does.

AV: That you saw her as a woman, and she saw you as a woman, first.
And that's where you connected.

HJ: And that's where we connect.

In this relationship, Hannah and her doctor were first and foremost
women—persons—in one another's eyes. When I told the qualitative
methods writing group about this exchange, Mindy Fullilove
remarked, "It is saying the obvious, but it's the most profound thing
we need to keep learning over and over again."[14] In a society where
human interactions are often structured by and filtered through external
roles and internal expectations, it is no small matter to be seen simply
as a woman by one's doctor and to have the courage and self-confidence
to see one's doctor in the same way.

"Keeping it Real" While Staying Out of the "Loony Bin": Social Ethics for Healthcare Systems

These women who have survived or are living with breast cancer
shared a great deal of embodied wisdom with me. They know a lot
because they have been through a lot. They see and appreciate what is
good in some healthcare contexts and what is problematic in others,
and they offered up descriptions of what most matters to them as
particular persons. What I have learned from them has significant
implications for healthcare discussions. As discussed in the prior chapter,

four themes emerged as persistent obstacles to quality healthcare. So my questions now are: What has to be in place in healthcare institutions for these themes to be more adequately addressed within the cultures and practices of healthcare than they are now? How might healthcare organizations and providers heed the wisdom of these women? As a way to explore these questions, I will use the four themes of the previous chapter as guideposts in order to reflect upon what they mean for the doing of healthcare. In making connections between these themes and ethical implications, I will touch upon four constructive possibilities for healthcare and medical ethics.

Racial and Socioeconomic Assumptions and Power Imbalances

The combination of these assumptions with the imbalance of power dynamics inherent in patient-provider relationships is potent and potentially deeply alienating. Undeniably, all breast cancer patients are in a position of relative vulnerability to their oncologists given that the patients are physically compromised by cancer and depend on their doctor for care and help. However, it is clear that communities of color, along with those who are poor and/or who lack health insurance (or who have inadequate medical coverage), experience additional forms of vulnerability. Indeed, they are doubly or triply at risk because they may not be able to access care as easily and they may carry the burden of providers' assumptions related to race and/or socioeconomics.[15]

Race and class are distinct but interwoven realities within U.S. mindsets and social structures. While they cannot be conflated, their intersections need to be understood. The combination of racial-ethnic and class assumptions can make a huge difference both in terms of the degree of access and visibility that darker skinned women have when negotiating healthcare as compared with lighter skinned women. Having excellent insurance coverage does not magically dispel these assumptions from the minds of care providers.

Sophia's story testifies to this fact. Her sense that providers expect her to change their minds lingers in my consciousness. There is something seriously—systemically—wrong when patients such as Sophia feel the burden to change provider assumptions—to demonstrate that they are "different," "one of the good Black Puerto Ricans" so that providers will be deeply invested in doing the absolute best they can for them. It is an unjust burden for her and others to bear. Given the relative power differences, the burden ought to fall on the providers—to work harder to know, understand and care for the patients who are most different from them. For it is in these scenarios where misunderstandings, mistrust, and poor communication are most likely to fester and cripple patient-provider relationships, treatment plans, and cure rates. In considering the weight and prevalence of these assumptions within a context of unequal power dynamics, two specific suggestions for change surface.

Conclusion #1: Educating Providers to See Their Own Assumptions

Providers need to be attuned to the peril of compartmentalizing people. Seeing patients primarily though the lens of their physiological condition, insurance status, or through assumptions based on racial-ethnic and/or class background diminishes and limits the quality of their care. Such narrow vision can render the actual persons invisible.

Healthcare systems and practitioners need to understand that it is unjust to hoist the burden of changing provider assumptions onto patients. Instead, healthcare institutions and practices can and ought to support the seeing and understanding of the social contexts in which these lives are situated. Simply put, we—as providers, ethicists, healthcare practitioners and professionals, theologians—need to do our homework. For holistic care to be comprehensive, appreciation of the person as embedded within a network of socioeconomic, cultural, familial, and political relationships and structures is needed in addition to attending to her physical, spiritual, and intellectual dimensions.

Antonia spoke to these qualities when she described the kind of doctor she hopes to become:

> The kind of doctor that I want to be is a doctor who . . . truly, truly wants what's best for the patient, and is not just looking at the patient as an illness, but is learning about who that patient is, learning about their background, about the family home life, what's going on with them . . . You're constantly learning about diseases and illness [in medical school]. And a lot of times, you're not exposed to patients. And, but when you are, and you get that little piece of information about them which fascinates you—something you find out about them, and you're like, "Wow, this is a person who has a life, this is a person who has dreams." And you just learn so much more about them.

Rather than using such contextual information to stereotype a person, the provider can use it to be attentive to the complexity and richness of every human life. When doctors possess these skills, they stand out. Antonia observes, "But I personally have seen many, no, I've seen *a few* white doctors who are amazing to all their patients. . . . [T]hese physicians who are amazing were culturally competent. They were respectful. They were understanding. And it's interesting how that can cross over all cultures." (Emphasis hers.) I take heart in knowing that some of Antonia's white mentors have these sensibilities and skills.

Antonia mentions an important and increasingly discussed concept: Cultural competence.[16] There are many possible strategies for enculturating such understanding. I would like to highlight the need for *intensive* cultural competency training. By cultural competence education, I mean integrated attention to racial-ethnic, socioeconomic, linguistic, cultural, and religious particularities that shape patient needs, perceptions, experiences of health and illness, needs, and fears with which they contend. Such education must teach *both* appreciation of the complexity of others' lives as well as critical self-reflection. In other words, ethicists and providers alike need to analyze in-depth the socioeconomic contexts of healthcare provision and we need to articulate and attend to our own internal assumptions and biases.

The word integrated is important. One course or class segment devoted to "cultural diversity" will not suffice. Instead, a cultivation of these skills ought to be integrated throughout courses as well as be reflected in how clinical training is taught and modeled. Antonia worked for a not-for-profit organization before going to medical school and still volunteers with women of color cancer support programs. In light of these experiences, she suggested that immersion in a racial, socioeconomic, and cultural context that is different from the student's should be a part of one's professional development:

> I think that everybody, before they go to medical school, should really spend a year someplace where they wouldn't see themselves. Just someplace where they really have no clue about those people, or that group of people . . . Yeah, just to sort of, you know, go away, go somewhere, go to the Caribbean maybe, or go to Puerto Rico, or the Dominican Republic, go to Cuba, come up to Harlem. They'll go to East Harlem, spend time in a small HIV clinic. That's what I did. I was a—I went to an HIV clinic for about six months, and I volunteered there. It's putting yourself in the position to learn from others . . . And just seeing something from a different view, and being around people [who have a different view].

Antonia is right that such experiences are a wonderful way to prepare for medical school. However, given that all students may not seek out these experiences on their own before gaining entrance into a formal medical program, the schools need to provide them as well. Immersion experiences, mentoring programs, and clinical experience in socioeconomic and racial-ethnic contexts that differ significantly from the student's are all ways in which assumptions and beliefs might be questioned in ways that enrich understanding and care. Sophisticated methods for critical self-reflection must be a part of such curricular programs. Additionally, greater emphasis on speaking and understanding second languages is needed both at undergraduate and graduate curricular levels than is currently oftentimes present.

However, such suggestions may be hard to realize. The cultures of many medical programs are predominately focused on the important matters of learning the physiological and technical dimensions of healthcare. Antonia herself does not expect her formal education to teach her the skills of relating to patients:

> I wouldn't say there's an actual push for us to really bond with patients— you know, to really learn about the patient. But there are bits and pieces, sort of to remind us, you know, that you—you're going into this medical profession . . . You need to know how to communicate with your patients, and that's very important. But I think it's something within you. It's . . . very difficult to learn. It's not going to be part of your medical education. You've got to either develop it through experience or have it.

Antonia is right that such things are challenging to teach and instill in another. Yet it gives me pause that she does not expect such values to be part of her formal education. I wonder how many medical students have similar experiences and expectations of their curricula. I know that some medical and nursing programs do foreground an ethos of service to, and understanding of, our diverse society; however, I am not at all certain of how widespread this pattern is.

There are still ample opportunities to gain such skills after graduation. Many hospitals periodically offer diversity trainings to their staff. However, brief diversity trainings held for current healthcare professionals can fall short of what is needed. Staff sometimes view them as nothing more than a bureaucratic hoop for accreditation. Indeed, a couple of the care providers were clear that short diversity trainings do little to alter provider assumptions. Beef Stew was pointedly candid in her criticism of them:

> That's a bunch of bullshit. O.K. Because how it is conveyed is not from a person of color. It's from a person who says, "O.K., these people are

complaining about there's a problem. O.K., how do we be nice to them? O.K., this is how we're going to be nice to them.". . . That's putting a Band Aid on it. That's not, like, "O.K., well, let's try to understand the problem, O.K.? This is a problem. Why is this problem happening? . . . All right, now, how are we going to change this to improve the dialogue between us, to improve the communication so this doesn't happen again?" That's not the spirit that it's coming from. It's coming from, "Look, O.K., the Department of Labor says we have to do this."

The impetus behind the training matters. It also matters if the hospital and practitioners are open to rigorous self-critique, or if they want to apply "Band Aids" that give an appearance of serious attention to the issues. Indeed, interpersonal communication techniques cannot be employed as "tricks" to build trust with a patient. Attempts at understanding and compassion need to be sincere. If not, none of the strategies will help much because they are motivated by self-interest rather than concern for others.

Moreover, the narrow scope of these trainings and cultural sensitivity courses can limit the scope of the analysis as well. In chapter 2, I discussed how the culture of medicine and the medical gaze may make it difficult for communities of color and/or lower socioeconomic classes to be seen as persons. Researchers Good and Good add that such classes often focus on the culture of patients without incorporating social analysis:

> Until recently, when cultural analyses were proposed, the focus was largely on patient culture. Burdens of difference were on patient communities, and medicine and health professionals were expected to learn to be culturally competent in attending to the diverse populations that make up American society. When we are challenged to examine the culture of medicine and of our healthcare institutions, we are also challenged to bring a critical perspective that has largely been ignored by most research to date or that has circumscribed cultural inquiry to the differences between patients' and physicians' "beliefs." Disparities in medical treatment are not simply matters of differences in "beliefs." Clearly, political and economic factors that shape our medical commons and our larger society are implicated in the production of these disparities.[17]

Culturally competent care involves more than learning about different foods, beliefs, and religious practices of patients. It must also rigorously and self critically analyze the socioeconomic and political forces that structure healthcare institutions and practices themselves.

I asked Wanda who has been both a patient in and an employee of hospitals how hospitals can engender respect for persons:

> I think you have those culture sensitivity courses. And you stay on that. You—not just have the courses, and then, O.K., they've got the training, but see how the staff is treating the patients. Walk around, you know, be involved in something. Because what I think tends to happen is that people will go—some hospitals offer the culture sensitivity course. And then the staff will go. But then what happens after that? How do you follow up and how do you make sure that they're doing what they're supposed to do? Because, like I said, I worked in a hospital, and I've seen what happens. And even if you take culture sensitivity classes, people don't follow, follow those things. So I think having the higher-up staff oversee it, making sure that it's being done, instilling that in their staff. . . .

Wanda understands that periodic trainings will not change the culture of institutions. Real change must be consistently promoted and instilled at all levels within the organization. In particular, Wanda notes the importance of those in leadership positions. Akin to mentoring medical and nursing students, administrative managers, senior physicians, and nurse managers need to see the value and need for such efforts and change.[18]

While a simplistic "top-down" approach can alienate staff, so too will efforts flounder at the staff levels if change is not supported by the leadership of a hospital. Both levels need to be engaged for cultural competence to take hold within the practices and sensibilities of care settings. Instilling such awareness and sensitivity is a complex process of moral and professional formation to which both honest self-criticism and social analysis are integral.

Conclusion #2: Emphasizing Healthcare Leadership of Color

Apart from the ability to cross cultures to build trust and understanding, there is also the matter of increasing the number of providers of color. More leadership of darker skinned people within healthcare will transform the cultures of institutions in ways that no number of diversity trainings can. As noted in chapter 2, some quantitative studies have found that race concordance between patients and doctors aids patient satisfaction. Undeniably, many patients and doctors succeed in creating strong bonds regardless of race concordance or its absence. However, having more staff of various racial-ethnic backgrounds will affect medical cultures and assumptions in ways that are both broader and deeper than a singular focus on cross-cultural patient-provider relations. For example, care providers of color might propose changes for how various religious traditions are accommodated, for how language translation services are provided, and for how a hospital connects with its surrounding neighborhoods and communities through education and prevention programs.

Such diversity among healthcare providers is especially needed at leadership levels—senior physicians and medical school faculty. Beef Stew observes that there are numerous staff of color at her hospital, even doctors, but not in leadership roles: "[T]here's plenty of doctors of color. I'm talking managers. I'm talking head honchos. I'm talking calling the shots. I'm talking, you know, nurse managers, vice presidents, CEOs, board of trustees. That is what'll make an impact." For substantive changes to take hold, it is not sufficient to have a diverse staff at the level of technicians, nurses, nurse assistants, and clerical support.[19]

Presently, the racial-ethnic diversity represented within the general population is not reflected in the population of healthcare providers. Recall from chapter 2 that Latinos represent 14 percent of the total population and that Blacks represent 13 percent of the total population. Yet Latinos "make up 2% of registered nurses, 3.4% of psychologists, and 3.5% of physicians . . . and while one in 8 Americans is black, fewer than 1 in 20 physicians or dentists is black."[20] Similarly, the September 2004 Sullivan Commission Report found that even as they together account for over 25 percent of the U.S. population, Blacks, Native Americans, and Hispanics only comprise "nine percent of the nation's nurses, six percent of doctors and five percent of dentists . . . [M]inorities make up less than 10 percent of baccalaureate nursing faculties, 8.6 percent of dental school faculties, and only 4.2 percent of medical school faculties."[21] These latter statistics raise the concern of the need for more and varied role models and mentors among teachers of future care providers.

In a related vein, the Association of American Medical Colleges reports that as of 2000, 9 percent of all medical school graduates are members of one of these four communities: African American, Asian American, Latino, and Native American. One current estimate is that within this total percentage, Latino graduates comprise 2.25 percent of the total population of medical graduates.[22] Latinos now constitute the largest and fastest growing ethnic community (comprised of many differing racial-ethnic and cultural communities) in the United States.

Yet their numerical growth within the ranks of healthcare professionals continues to sputter.

Unfortunately, change in this reality does not look promising. *The New York Times* recently reported that the current administration's budget does not see leadership of color as a priority: "President Bush's budget would cut spending for the training of health professionals and eliminate a $34 million program that recruits blacks and Hispanics for careers as doctors, nurses and pharmacists."[23] It is disturbing that such cuts are being proposed even as the administration has been criticized for trying to downplay the realities of racial-ethnic disparities in healthcare.[24]

Having drawn this conclusion, it is also important to not see the problem only as one of numbers. Good and Good make the case that the medical gaze is potent in training students to focus in upon certain information relevant when listening to and giving care to patients. In short, students of whatever color are taught to "speak the language of medicine." They argue that this culture is strong and pervasive even though there has been "a sea change in the gender, and to a lesser extent, the racial and ethnic profile of medical students. In addition, extraordinary developments in medical technology, biomedical science, and the political economy and financing of medicine and the delivery of healthcare appear to be subsumed into this culture and way of learning medicine."[25] Having more providers of color is essential, but it is not a simple solution to the complex nest of problematic disparities. The very way in which medicine and healthcare are taught needs substantial revision as well.

The Imperative of Advocacy and the Impact of Bureaucracies and Bottom Lines

After surveying the extensive and growing medical sociological literature on healthcare disparities and interviewing a few patients and care providers, I have come to the conclusion that radical changes are needed in the structures of U.S. healthcare provision. Piecemeal approaches cannot sufficiently address systemic problems. A system where doctors are reimbursed different amounts for different patients—or even worse where they are compensated to attend to some but not others—already sets up structural care disparities in which some lives are more valued than others. Indeed, the political economy embedded within the financing, organization, and delivery of healthcare dehumanizes some by making available to others (those with the financial, political, and social resources) healthcare that is more comprehensive and better matched to their health needs and cultural backgrounds. Simply put, initiatives aimed at making individual providers more sensitive will falter miserably if they do not address the economic systems and institutional cultures in which the providers are supposed to learn and practice this sensitivity.

To make this case does not mean that no poor person or person of color receives good care. In fact, many, many do—the women with whom I spoke testify to this fact. Rather, the point is that regardless of the fact of whether or not some individuals encounter exceptional care, skill, and compassion, an intrinsically unjust system is in place that contradicts the egalitarian principles and ideals to which it aspires. Simply put, it is hard to defend the notion that all lives are respected equally when the costs of medical care are reimbursed at widely different rates, depending on one's insurance status. As Leonard Orlando, the white oncologist, put it to me in our conversation, "I'm very idealistic, and it's very important for me to be a human, humanistic. But I don't think the environment supports that. . . . [T]he system promotes—encourages us to be otherwise." Significant disparities in care due to combinations of access and quality issues mock and transgress the moral obligations of a democratic society. Therefore, the fact that some lives are more fully seen, valued, and respected than others represents a serious moral problem with which ethicists, healthcare policy makers, and theologians all must wrestle. In response to the failings of present structures, I offer two specific recommendations.

Conclusion #3: Funding and
Support of Community Networks
Several of the women told me stories of how they were only able to access acceptable care because of a friend or a contact in a healthcare network that helped them make a change: María's daughter sought out care at another hospital; Luz would not have been able to get into a site of care she preferred without the help of a friend and the friend's sister-in-law (a nurse). As a nurse case manager, Beef Stew acknowledged that while she does her job for every patient, she takes additional time to educate patients who do not have many resources at their disposal.[26]

In short, without advocating for themselves along with the advocacy of others, many would have remained in care settings with which they were neither satisfied nor comfortable. Quite literally, advocacy and connections help you be seen. Consequently, I find that community not-for-profit support and information networks provide vital services to women. They help them process everything they are going through and make informed decisions.

I shudder when I contemplate the traps in which those who are ill and who do not have these networks or connections—those who are timid or isolated—may find themselves. A 2004 investigative article by Katherine Boo recounts the story of Juana, an uninsured woman in Texas who died at the age of 36 of cervical cancer, two years following her diagnosis. Because she had no insurance, she was shut out of all of the for-profit hospitals near her in Cameron County, Texas. Boo reports,

> While federal law requires those hospitals to treat the uninsured in emergencies—gun shot wounds, heart attacks—the institutions usually decline to accept uninsured supplicants who need chemotherapy, radiation, or other longer-term treatments. Juana, like most uninsured patients with advanced cancer in Cameron County, had to travel back and forth to the state public hospital in Galveston. It is an eleven-hour bus trip each way.[27]

From reading the entire article, it was clear that Juana was *not* an undocumented inhabitant. Recall from chapter 2 that Texas has the highest rate of uninsured of any state in the union.

One of the breast cancer support group facilitators with whom I met coordinates a Latina group to which predominately new immigrants come. Many of the participants speak only Spanish and some are undocumented. Many have no benefits or health insurance and find it difficult to attend the support groups after they are well enough to work. They cannot afford to stay at home during their recovery because of their need of the income, however meager.

This facilitator explained to me that many of these immigrants are scared—because of the cancer, because of their immigration status, and because of their very limited income levels. She observed that many of them come from cultures in which it is expected that patients trust their doctors and do not ask questions. These insights gave me a sense of why I may not have heard more immigrants complain about the quality of their care when I spoke to them at the support meetings. Indeed, the facilitator said that many of the Latina immigrants she has worked with are so afraid of dying or being deported that they are simply grateful for whatever care they do receive—even if there are no translators or doctors are rude, inattentive, or hurried. Without groups such as The Witness Project of Harlem, Share, Cancer Care, and Gilda's Club, many women would not have a safe place to ask questions, learn about their disease and treatment options, and receive emotional support.

Moreover, these organizations intensively work to create deep connections in the communities they serve. Rather than using a white staff person coming to facilitate a group in Harlem or Queens, for example, all of the above organizations make it a priority to have group facilitators who share the cultural and racial backgrounds of the communities in which the groups take place. More ample funding and support of such community networks is essential.[28]

Unfortunately, these nonprofit organizations, which rely heavily upon volunteers and donations, are not prioritized in healthcare funding budgets. Community health programs—community-oriented prevention and educational services—tend not to be emphasized by either government or private healthcare institutions. Many of the organizational representatives spoke to me about how strained their budgets are and how precarious their futures can be from one year to the next.

Conclusion #4: The Value of Continuity and Choice

All patients benefit from the opportunity to work with the same provider over time so that trust and rapport can develop. On the other hand, they also benefit from being able to switch providers if they are uncomfortable with their care in a given setting. Given the social, economic, and structural power imbalances, patients of color and/or lower socioeconomic status need to be able to keep *or* change a given provider without fear of losing healthcare coverage. Hannah's story describes the experience of one woman who, because of the comprehensive and generous nature of her health plan, has felt free to interview prospective doctors as needed before settling on one. And once she has made her choice, she has not had to worry about a change in doctors being made without her involvement. (However, a few months after our interview, Hannah Jacobs lost her job after over 20 years of service due to corporate downsizing.)[29] What amazes me is that Sandra, temporarily without insurance, forged ahead and switched doctors until finding one to whom she could relate to as a person. And it is important to note that she was able to do this both because she is a strong woman who is also a well-educated nurse *and* because she had nurse friends and contacts helping her to navigate her way through this harrowing time.

Indeed, the current makeshift safety net of care for people who are either uninsured or underinsured and/or who have limited funds to pay for care has many gaping holes. Simply put, the combinations of Medicaid programs, Medicare programs, and charity care offered by hospitals and providers is not at all sufficient to meet current needs. Too many Americans delay seeking care for chronic conditions, fail to fill prescriptions or to have follow-up care and tests because of the severe limits of this safety net.[30]

In stark contrast, while having excellent health insurance is not a guarantee of receiving excellent care, what it *can* do (both literally and metaphorically) is buy more time. Not having to worry about what services and tests will be reimbursed or how many visits will be covered can create a context in which there are sufficient opportunities for women of color to break down provider assumptions and to build up relationships. Sophia's story represents one example of this transformation. She was clear that when her breast cancer was first diagnosed, she was able to get through to her doctors because she and they knew that they would be working together over time. There was continuity of care. She developed a strong relationship not only with her breast surgeon, but with her oncologist and the nurses and nurse practitioners as well. As a team of providers and as individuals, they crossed their cultural, racial, and socioeconomic differences to come to know Sophia as a unique and valuable person.

The point is that such transformations take time. When I asked Sophia how it is possible for providers of differing backgrounds from a patient to create genuine relationships and to see the patient as a person instead of as a stereotype, she remarked, "Unfortunately, it's not something that you can go in and change off the bat, like with people of the same race. Like if a white person goes in to see the doctor, there are no defenses. You know. Unfortunately, with me personally, it's something that comes in time." I then added, "So it's kind of like you have to work harder." Sophia responded,

> Yeah. It's something that you—that, in time, kind of works itself hopefully and just disappears. And there's always the little underlining of, "When are they going to show their true colors?" . . . Yeah, like, you know, I don't think now they think that there are any true colors. You know? I think they see this is her true color. But I, you know, that took—that takes a little longer.

Ultimately, this need for continuity and choice means that universal healthcare needs to get back on the table as a serious topic for healthcare policy reform. Since the 2000 and 2004 elections, the bulk of congressional healthcare debate has taken the form of prescription drug coverage for seniors and what to do with respect to the internet availability (and substantially lower prices) of Canadian prescription drugs. Prescription drug coverage is a topic worthy of public debate. By itself, however, it makes for anemic healthcare reform. Current political platforms are a far cry from the healthcare reform agenda on which Clinton and Gore ran in 1992. Now, 14 years later, a comprehensive approach to healthcare reform is sorely absent from the public scene. This reality is unacceptable.

A form of universal healthcare may help to make healthcare less of a private commodity purchased by some and more of a public service provided to all. Without universal coverage, providers are compensated differently for different patients. Leonard, the white oncologist, laments that he cannot take Medicaid patients because the rates do not adequately compensate his services. Even as he defended the free market economy, he cautiously noted: "[C]ancer care is so complicated and comprehensive that it's hard to do a lot of *pro bono* work. But it wouldn't matter, a patient's economic status, if [doctors] had full-time positions. You know? With just a set salary."[31]

Leonard also noted that there ought to be fewer administrative hassles in order to give more time and better care. He complained that his days are too occupied by the piles of paperwork—not done only as medical charting—but as formulaic, duplicative documentation for insurance companies. Rebecca Williams, a white oncology social worker, also commented that her main frustration is that she has to spend an inordinate amount of time on paperwork, instead of offering psychosocial support to patients. Discharge planning has a tangible benefit to the hospital's finances; sitting with and listening to patients do not.

A recent report, *Closing the Gap: Solutions to Race-Based Health Disparities*,[32] offers examples of actual programs and policies in various locations around the United States that address similar themes as those found in these four conclusions. In particular, the report highlights healthcare programs that have successfully integrated services, developed rigorous cultural competency components to their practices, prioritized meeting diverse language needs, and increased access to healthcare by dealing creatively with financial barriers. In addition, the report features community-based programs that seek to improve the health status of people living in low-income communities and that consciously address structural racism. The strength of this report is that through its field research and interviews with various providers across the nation, it offers a collection of in-depth case studies that concretely show how these kinds of recommendations can be effectively implemented. Change *is* possible.

To conclude this analysis of recommendations for change, I would like to come back to Sophia. Of all the 14 collaborators who shared enlightening insights and experiences, Sophia spoke with the most candor and critical reflection. She both powerfully named how current dynamics affect her life and care and had a clear vision of how health-care relationships and healthcare could be structured. I was deeply saddened to learn that Sophia died of cancer on October 18, 2004. I will always be grateful for her keen perception, sharp wit, and for her willingness to speak with this stranger.

Sophia had no trouble naming the fact that human beings arbitrarily create systems of meaning (such as those focused on wealth) and that in doing so, we have fashioned a world light-years away from what God wants for us. In not shying away from stark honesty, her words took on a prophetic quality for me. Akin to all genuine prophets, she knows that being real and speaking truth can put one in danger—they can "end up in the loony bin." I heard this prophetic voice most clearly at the end of our interview when Sophia described the ideological framework in which U.S. healthcare is conceived and given. Her incisive analysis needs no further introduction or commentary from me. Its wisdom speaks for itself. Indeed, without realizing its Greek meaning, Sophia chose her pseudonym well:

> *SA:* It's this world that we've created. And money is something that's created. And, you know, gold is in the ground, I mean, that's, like, free, really, when you think of it. You know, we've made this—we've given it so much importance. And when you think about the rest of the world, like the backwoods, and we think that they're really primitive, but places in Africa and places in Nicaragua and places all the way back in the hills, they have medicine men who cure people. And they would never think of taking a dime for doing what is the most natural thing to do in this world, which is make you well if you are sick. People will give them food and give them donations. And— but they would never think of taking money for something that, in their eyes, is a God-given gift. And, you know, I think, you know, there are a lot of healthcare providers and healthcare facilities that try, you know, to do things. But in the math, in the math of it, you know, medicine is a corporate business. It's not a business of sacrifice like that anymore. I'm not saying that everybody's like that.

And there's healthcare professionals out there who do. But I think self-sacrifice is, like, such a big thing. And I think that God would like that.

AV: But the context of the institution or the system isn't set up to facilitate that.

SA: No, no. And it all comes down to the almighty dollar that we ourselves have given all this importance to. Well, we still have to pay our bills and all that. I mean, there's got to be—I guess for people who don't have the same kind of faith, they have to have something to hold onto, and something that is important. So you can make up anything and make it important. I can make that picture important. I can make it the most important thing in this house, you know. But it really—that's what it is. It's not real.

AV: No.

SA: And I think that's what God wants. I think that's what God wants from all of us. You know?

AV: Yeah.

SA: It's really, really out there, though.

AV: No. But it's also just right here.

SA: Yeah. It's right here, which is why nobody's going to do anything about it.

AV: It's too close.

SA: It's too close. It's too real. And people that tend to be too real are the ones that end up in the loony bin.

Why These Stories Matter: Methodological Implications for the Doing of Ethics

Before drawing this work to a tentative close, I would like to discuss one last relevant area of analysis: Implications this research has for the doing of social ethics itself. The conclusion I draw is simply this: It matters who is at the table. This book does not presume to solve the various problems related to healthcare disparities. Neither my desk nor brain is big enough to bear such weight. In other words, no single person or group is able to arrive at such a resolution. Indeed, well apart from offering the above constructive points for changes in healthcare delivery, this book has sought to contribute to changing the way in which we as academics and professionals search out these answers. Not only does the content of ethical and policy decisions fundamentally matter, *but the process used to come to them* matters as well. It is my conviction that adequate and dynamic understandings of dignity, respect, or personhood only happen through the course of sustained and broad relationships and conversations in particular communities—and out of profound dialogue across difference. Moral deliberation and formation are neither onetime nor individual events. Even more, they are not the sole property of scientists, policy makers, or academics.

This insight is as true for theology, the social sciences, and health-care policy as it is for social ethics. Across disciplines, a shift is needed in how we think about and tackle the pressing problems and questions facing us. With respect to healthcare quality disparities, those who have most directly confronted healthcare quality disparities ought to be at the tables and involved in setting the terms of the conversations convened to eradicate them. We need to find the answers together. Ethicists, physicians, social scientists, healthcare policy analysts, and theologians all need the knowledge of those who may be laypersons with respect to our fields, but who know viscerally what it means to feel disrespected and disregarded in society.

Beyond this argument, I want to consider the methodological impli-cations by considering a few specific changes in how scholarship might be done. Then I want to turn to a brief discussion of what solidarity means and of how, given the complexity and need for so many partic-ipating voices, normative claims may still be made. In this section, then, you will hear me speaking first as white academic calling other white academics into new modes of research and then as a white the-ologian and ethicist speaking in particular to theology and social ethics. Throughout, my core commitments to listening, to decentering the "experts," and to calling all of us who occupy relative sites of privilege into accountability will be visible.

Ethnography and the Value of Acknowledged Ignorance

James Spradley begins *The Ethnographic Interview* with a basic but crucial distinction: "Rather than *studying people*, ethnography means *learning from people*."[33] (Emphasis his.) In order to learn from people, you need to assume that you do not already know what they are going to teach you. Spradley goes on to acknowledge; "Ethnography starts with a conscious attitude of almost complete ignorance."[34] The value of this insight is multifold and is not limited to those in academia. First and foremost, I—whether I am a white scholar, activist, teacher, social worker, doctor, friend, or church member—will learn more if "what

I think I know" does not get in the way of actual learning and listening. An even bigger payoff, especially in terms of the formation of a white scholar, is that when one is not overly focused on being an expert, but rather on being a person, there is great potential to cultivate humility both within one's vocational endeavors and inner spirit.

Moreover, there are ramifications here not only for individual scholars, but also for entire disciplines. To put it bluntly: White scholars may profit greatly if/when we spend significant, sustained time and energy *outside* of libraries/offices and *inside* a variety of relationships and activities. My time with the Reverend Dr. Powell and others indicates not only *why* I chose a particular research topic, but also *how* I learned about it in the first place. I came upon inequalities in healthcare not primarily by deducing the problems from books of social theory, ethics, and theology, but by listening—to patients, loved ones, and staff—and by working in relationship with them.

In a related vein, it would be helpful if more academics would push ourselves to speak and hear fluently second and third languages—not only to read or translate them. Even if English is a common language between a researcher and the people with whom she is working, meanings cannot be taken for granted. Semantic differences, even when the same language is being spoken, ought not be overlooked.

For example, especially when I, a white person, attempt qualitative research within communities of color, I do not want participants to translate meanings for me, to cease speaking their own language, and begin to speak in ways that are more familiar to the white and/or professional ear. If I want to hear people in their own voices, then they need not alter what they are saying to overly accommodate me. The burden is upon me, the white scholar, to understand (or to learn to understand) what others are saying—their experiences, culture, worldview—in the fullest sense possible.[35] Of course, the persons with whom I am working will always be accommodating me to a degree and every description is a translation. But the important point is that I must make every attempt possible to ensure that my descriptions flow as directly as possible from the concepts and meaning of the people with whom I am working or interviewing.[36]

For white academics to engage racism and white privilege adequately in our scholarship, we need to find avenues of contact and relationship with the people who most directly confront racial inequalities. Learning from scholars of color is vital and we need to ever expand our treatment of their texts. Yet we ought not stop here. The incorporation of works by scholars of color will be stronger and more credible if it bears out in relation to concrete movements, projects, and experiences. It not only matters whom I have read, but also with whom I worship, eat lunch, volunteer on weekends or evenings, lobby politicians, and canvass the neighborhood. It takes time and effort to cultivate the sensibilities and skills within white academics that will curb the presumptuous and self-righteous qualities often present in white identity.

While not all white scholars will do formal qualitative fieldwork in their research, more ought to consider it. Moreover, there are other avenues for similar involvement (volunteering with grassroots organizations that address housing, poverty, education, environmental racism, prison reform, healthcare, or migrant labor issues). I am well aware of the pressure to increase one's "scholarly" credentials—to publish books and articles, to give public lectures, to get grants. But perhaps an additional measure of an accomplished scholar ought to be given more weight: The hours one spends working with community programs dedicated to social, economic, and racial transformation. Perhaps seminaries, colleges, and universities might more intentionally promote and support the notion of a public scholar, whose task in whatever field is not only to advance knowledge, but also to contribute concretely to the shaping of people and communities in which the scholar lives and works.

In sum, there is a claim upon all scholars in whatever field (and of whatever racial-ethnic background) to envision and create even a small corner of the good society. Intrinsic to any such creation is a specific claim upon me, as a white person and scholar, to cultivate sustained, concrete relationships with communities of color in entirely different life situations and vocations from myself. These kinds of practical engagements and relationships are of paramount importance especially for white scholars and other scholars of privilege. For if we do not get it right in our day-to-day interactions and relationships, we will not get it right in our scholarship either.

Catching a Glimpse of the Reign of God: What Solidarity Means

The theological case made in this book is this: For any theological description of what it means to be a child of God, or made in the image of God (*imago dei*) to be adequate, it needs to be concrete—incarnate—and reflective of the needs and experiences of the most vulnerable—in a city, in a region, in the world. From this theological starting point, I have argued in the language of ethics that for any positive change in healthcare quality and access to take place and last in institutional and interpersonal ways of being, we need attuned and sustained listening to those who occupy vulnerable positions in both society and healthcare settings. I am trying to envision and articulate what justice and solidarity mean and how they might be realized more fully, even if imperfectly.

Sustained and self-critical attention to those marginalized by systems of injustice is the only basis upon which efforts at solidarity are possible. Those in relative privilege (white, middle and upper socioeconomic classes, the well-insured, the presently healthy, the educated, members of the First World) need to not only "care" or "feel badly" about the plight of those less privileged, but must also understand that we are both implicated and accountable for their life situations. In responding to economic globalization, white, Lutheran ethicist Cynthia Moe-Lobeda defines solidarity this way:

> Solidarity entails seeing, hearing, and heeding what is obscured by privilege: People and other parts of creation destroyed, degraded, or impoverished by five centuries of globalization, culminating in the contemporary form. Said differently, people of economic privilege will seek out and hear the stories of those who experience globalization as a threat to life and will respond to those voices.[37]

Whether the topic is globalization or healthcare disparities, Moe-Lobeda's emphasis upon *seeing, hearing, and responding* to the stories and peoples most threatened by present structures is crucial. Calls to solidarity ring hollow if they are not accompanied by profound efforts to listen, perceive, understand, and respond. As I argued in chapter 3, listening on the part of the relatively privileged ought to involve a cost to the hearers—and a fundamental change in their dispositions and practices.

Moreover, solidarity necessarily involves recognition of others in their particularity and uniqueness. Differences are honored not erased. No one is left unaccounted for or rendered voiceless. No one is superfluous. Everyone's unique heart, perspective, and abilities are needed. This is how I envision the reign of the divine. In contrast to an autonomous and individualist notion of the self, Womanist theologian M. Shawn Copeland understands personhood only within the context of complex and diverse peoples living and working together. Indeed, such efforts at solidarity offer a glimpse of the dominion of God in which everyone in bright and varied array is present and participating. Copeland casts solidarity in an explicitly theological light by contending that attempts at solidarity are a way to worship God.[38]

Copeland's conceptualization of the relationship between person hood and solidarity calls those of us in positions of privilege to radical accountability: "If personhood is now understood to flow from formative living in community rather than individualism, from the embrace of difference and interdependence rather than their exclusion, then we can realize our personhood only in solidarity with the exploited, despised, poor 'other.'"[39] The significance of solidarity is found not only in the possibility of social transformation or in an embodied respect for exterior differences, but also in its potential for inner transformation. As discussed in chapter 3, not only is the care of vulnerable communities at stake, but so is the moral formation of those less vulnerable—the affluent, the lighter skinned, the healthy, the well insured. If we do not push ourselves and our communities to live and act in ways that are in solidarity with those socioeconomically, politically, and physically at risk, we stand to lose our own humanity.[40] By putting ourselves above such struggles or denying that we are inherently implicated, the formation of white and privileged beings continues to be woefully misshapen. The consequences are both devastating to others and shame-producing for us.

Indeed, we can be downright ugly and nasty. Two of the care providers I interviewed, Beef Stew and Lucy Bristol, spoke of a personality characteristic that they would like to see disappear, which seems prevalent among both their white patients and colleagues. Lucy explained how she has noticed that white and/or affluent patients can be less appreciative of and feel more entitled to healthcare. She observed that they are less likely to say "please" and "thank you" whereas less fortunate patients "are so grateful for any little thing you do for them." She found that in the city hospital where she once worked, the patients (the vast majority of whom were impoverished and persons of color) were more respectful of the nurses than some of her white and affluent patients at the well-respected private hospital where she is currently employed.

More than Lucy, Beef Stew was sharp in her description of this trait:

> It's amazing how people believe that they have this white card, and they can do anything that they want . . . And I would really love . . . to find out how that has happened, so that we can knock that down. Because once someone gets taken down a peg, not to humiliate, but to understand

that, look, you are not privileged because your skin is white, you're a blonde, You're a human—take that off . . . you bleed the same way I do.[41]

I have started to refer to this pernicious disposition noted by Lucy and Beef Stew as a "white entitlement syndrome." Beef Stew makes a very important distinction: Calling white and other privileged people into accountability for our presumption is not done to humiliate us, but rather to stop allowing white persons and communities to be the center—the standard and the norm. "Taking us down a peg" is done so that we might be who we most truly are: Human beings intrinsically interrelated and accountable to other varied but equally beloved human beings.

Ultimately, combating white entitlement, privilege, discrimination, and bias involves not only education, but also conversion. People of privilege, perhaps especially the ones who espouse and cling to "good intentions," need vehicles for honest self-reflection. For example, I commented to Wanda that most likely healthcare providers do not want or intend to look down on anyone. Yet when there are differences between providers and patients—race, socioeconomic class, HIV status, culture, religion, language—it is complicated to meet the other as a person. I then asked her how care providers might learn to more fully understand and respect people within such particularity. She responded,

I think it takes a lot of soul searching within the individual self, you know, because I know people, they know that they're doing something wrong because I'm pretty sure they're getting complaints, you know, the way they may have treated a patient or something like that. They get complaints on that so they know . . . But I think you have to be willing to accept that you did that, and be willing to make that change. But a lot of people are not willing to do that because they think, "Oh, it's not me, I'm not like that."[42]

Both hearts and minds of the privileged must turn in new directions in order to see and appreciate the humanity of others. This work has tried to articulate methodological steps that may facilitate the soul-searching and intellectual analysis needed. A combination of different and sharp tools are needed to cut through the tough, encrusted layers of denial that keep peoples' eyes, intellects, and souls from seeing how our assumptions and sites of privilege wound the well-being of others.

The Possibility and Necessity of
Making Normative Claims

All human beings will always have to reevaluate the world that we are creating or want to create. We must always be on the lookout for who is not among us, who has not spoken, and who has been left out or put aside. Revision *does not* equal relativism in ethics. However, it *does* mean that all our expressions of justice, faith, right relationship, grace, and love are approximations—finite and imperfect and ever in need of critical reevaluation.

When we think we arrive at the last word or the final and complete sense of a value, virtue, principle, or theological concept, we have fallen into idolatry. This statement does not mean that there can be no norms. For me, to love one another as our self and to love God with everything we've got transcends time, space, and context. Yet its meaning must always be worked out in the particular and in concrete relationships. What loving the neighbor means in one context may not look or translate exactly the same in another. Appreciation of this reality helps to keep the norms vibrant within embodied relationships and structures, rather than eroding into "pretty" but abstracted concepts that fail to manifest in lived reality.

We cannot deny the impartiality of all knowledge or the particularity of social locations. Ironically, recognizing particularity may actually open the door to a kind of universality. In Carter Heyward's words, "Knowing our particular social locations and our limits . . . is intellectually empowering as a lens through which we may catch a glimpse of what is, paradoxically, universally true—that all people are limited by the particularities of their life experience."[43] The reality that all people are particular and limited in our knowledge and perspectives is something shared by all humanity. This fact shows again how deeply we need one another's stories, experiences, and wisdom in order to arrive at adequate social norms. The descriptions, philosophies, theologies, and perspectives of an individual or a relative few will not suffice. Human beings are forever and inescapably interdependent creatures.

Having said this, it is also imperative to recognize that some forms of relationality and interdependence are more desirable than others. Some structures and practices actively promote justice, health, and right relation. Others capriciously prey upon the needs of some while simultaneously profiting from the resources they possess. Undeniably, suffering, abuse, and exploitation occur across cultures, societies, and nations. In the case of this research, U.S. healthcare quality disparities are a problem for which lighter skinned and affluent communities (found at all levels of government, healthcare institutions, insurance companies, and lobbyists) are most pointedly accountable.

While the process of arriving at normative conclusions is arduous and fraught with thorny complexity, theological and social ethicists nonetheless have a responsibility to offer persuasive and compelling visions that carry normative weight and that hold privileged communities accountable. What is needed now, both in academic circles and also in the larger society, are thorough descriptions of present social realities along with constructive proposals for what ought to be and for how people ought to be regarded. Roman Catholic, white, feminist ethicist Margaret Farley understands that

> [a]n obligation to respect persons requires . . . that we attend to the concrete realities of our own and others' lives. . . . We can risk considering seriously the meaning the other gives to the world; building communities of support that have openness to the other at the center of their strength; surrendering our tendencies to omniscience without surrendering to despair; learning the particular content of just and fitting care.[44]

Respect for persons and difference does not negate the possibility of making normative claims. Human beings—as moral agents facing daunting and myriad injustices—dare not give up on creating pragmatic strategies and conceptual frameworks that foster right relationship among human communities living in a fragile and precious creation. Ventures into theological and social ethics are not sufficient if they stop at the place of description and deconstruction of present realities. We must also take the risk of offering constructive, bold, and hope-filled vision.

As Copeland asks questions about differences, commonalities, and solidarity, she articulates concrete measures by which to assess if the full humanity of persons is being respected or not. For insight into these questions, she turns to an understanding of the demands and obligations, which human beings (specifically Christians) must bear as fitting responses to the incarnation of the divine. In doing so, she offers the following description of human identity that is inextricably woven together with human responsibility:

> Our search for the *humanum* is oriented by the radical demands of the incarnation of God; . . . [T]o be a human person is to be (1) a creature

made by God; (2) a person-in-community, living in flexible, resilient, just relationships with others; (3) An incarnate spirit, i.e., embodied in race, sex, and sexuality; (4) capable of working out essential freedom through personal responsibility in time and space; (5) a social being; (6) unafraid of difference and interdependence; and (7) willing daily to struggle against "bad faith" and resentment for the survival, creation, and future of all life ... Taken together, the various theologies for human liberation push us, in self-giving love, to forward this realization in "the forgotten subject"—exploited, despised poor women of color. Only, in and through solidarity with them, the least of this world, shall humanity come to fruition.[45]

In this description, Copeland makes the connections between theology, anthropology, social analysis, and ethics explicit. The full meaning and implications of these points may only be spelled out in particular communities of dialogue and action. What is clear is who the normative anthropological subject is. The test, then, will be if social, theological, and medical ethics can remember this "forgotten subject" and if, in doing so, transformative practices, institutions, and communities are creatively fashioned by imperfect yet beloved human beings working together for the sake of those most in need of love and care.

Concluding Words for Beginning: (Re)Creating the World through Scholarship

There are three methodological insights I hope this book will contribute to the way in which scholarship is envisioned and created: First, qualitative methods such as those found in ethnography are helpful and needed tools for grounding and evaluating theological and ethical claims. How does a given theological construct relate to the lives and experiences of members of faith communities who are not professional theologians or ethicists? How do people embody, challenge, and practice—make actively real—the theological and/or normative claims put forward by scholarship or public policy? Stated more strongly, practical engagement is not only helpful, but it is also morally incumbent upon us as scholars. We need to test what we think not only against what others write but against what others live.

Qualitative research can expose problems in perception—whether our own or that of others. For example, it can reveal how assessments of healthcare issues may be impaired by socioeconomic class and racial assumptions. Perception matters. If we do not see rightly, we will not act rightly. Thus, qualitative research can be a vehicle for honoring the sacred within each person by checking perception and by learning about the intrinsic complexity within each and every person.

Second, healthcare and medical/bioethics ought to turn toward the social. Some of the most common topics and approaches of biomedical ethics (informed consent, genetic and stem cell research, a discussion of abstract principles and virtues, euthanasia, etc.) while important are not comprehensive enough to constitute the main points of an ethical agenda—especially if they are framed in a way which ignores socioeconomic and political structures and power dynamics. Issues such as universal healthcare, racial and ethnic disparities, poverty, inadequate nutrition, and education ought to have an important place on medical and bioethical agendas. I concur with Jewish ethicist Laurie Zoloth who has been frustrated with the absence of the social in bioethics. Here are a few excerpts of her lament and challenge:

> We tend to think about bioethics, even health care justice and access, as a problem of the highest tech medicine, the access to the scarcest commodity, rather than the access to what we could have much of: human touch, conversation, responsibility for attention. . . .
>
> We speak of food only when we get to discuss genetic alteration, not hunger and poverty and health. . . .
>
> The uninsured have all but disappeared except as a coda at the end of articles. . . .
>
> There is little debate over why it is that health care plans for the poor typically provide only older, less efficacious drugs for the side effects of chemotherapy, for example, or pain control. . . .
>
> There is no serious conversation about race and class in the debate about health care . . . little about how the enactment of class and racial inequalities frame much of the relationships n the clinic . . . or how the uninsured are disproportionately Hispanic or Black.[1]

Adequate analysis of healthcare and medicine must delve seriously into the socioeconomic, cultural, and political dimensions in which any topic (patient autonomy, patient-provider relationships, health status and healthcare quality disparities, cloning, reproductive technologies, etc.) is inherently situated. Without this context, these debates quickly devolve into abstracted dialogues in which only scientists, physicians, lobbyists, and a relatively narrow range of ethicists participate.

Third, theological insights and language also ought to have a place at the table. No theological position can be absolute or imposed. However, the truthful speaking out of one's own tradition may add to the moral imagination of the public debate on a variety of healthcare and biomedical topics. In chapter 3, I worked substantively with theological anthropology. I did so because how people conceive of what it means to be human and of what one human being owes to another in terms of respect and dignity affects how they will treat others— interpersonally and collectively. For example, such subjective assessments shape not only hospital protocols and mission statements, but also the amount of time staff persons spend with a patient and family and the kind of treatments presented as options. On structural levels, these same assumptions influence the degree and quality of a range of services and sensibilities, including cultural competencies, translation services, and the accommodation of diverse religious practices and spiritual needs.

For sustained social transformation, conversion of laws, practices, cultures, minds, *and* hearts is needed. Theology is a discipline and language especially gifted at expanding and critiquing moral imagination. Theo-ethical insights may make a unique and appropriate contribution when they engage their own traditions, scriptures, and communities of moral imagination in order to advocate for the equal care and regard of all persons.

Sophia's words show the kind of contribution theological language can make in shifting the terms and frameworks for healthcare discussions. Sophia spoke eloquently about what God wants from *and* for human beings. I asked her how she thinks God wants human beings to treat each other. She answered,

> What does God want human beings to do for each other? That's an easy one, although it's hard to practice sometimes. Everybody is supposed to be more Christ-like. . . . That means that we're supposed to . . . treat each other kind. We are each other's keeper. And everything that I feel I deserve, you deserve. I mean, that's what God wants us to do. We're supposed to treat each other with humility. We're supposed to treat each other with kindness, with sympathy, with affection. This is what we're *supposed* to do. . . . And we're here to take care of each other. And if, somebody—if we don't take care of each other, we're not taking care of ourselves. There's no way around it. We're all one people. There's no way around it. Anything that you do to me that isn't right, you're saying that it's O.K.—you're saying it's O.K. for it to be done to you. Right? I mean, O.K., we have all this medical profession, and it's all well and done. The world in itself was made perfect, and there's a natural remedy for everything anyway. So we made up all of these other things around it, and we're wrapped up around it. But let's just keep it real. And that's what God wants us to do. And all of our creation, and all of our manmade things, we still, at the end, as human beings, have to keep it real. (Emphasis hers.)

I asked, "And how do we keep it real?" Sophia answered,

> By not getting caught up in all of that, and remembering at the end what it is that matters, and that is life. That is human life. And how it is that we're treated, and how fragile it is, and how much we can just lose it. At a blink of an eye we can be gone. And it all revolves around love. And love is, you know, a big thing when you think of everything that's thrown in there. It's hard to have unconditional love for strangers. You know? In a perfect world, that's exactly what it should be, though. Because we are—we're all blue blood until it comes out of our body.

I mean, it's just—but that's in a perfect world. I mean, that's like, in this world right now, that's a fantasy. But that would be ideal, right? And I think that's what God would want. And He gave us the power of choice. . . .

While she clearly sees the harshness of this world, Sophia also stays grounded in what is most real and in what most matters. She has not allowed the language and structures of meaning within corporate healthcare to define ultimate meaning for her. Even if it means swimming upstream against strong financial, cultural, and ideological currents, human beings have a choice. Sophia reminds us that God has given us all a crucial choice regarding how we will live, what we will value, and how we will treat others. No singular entity—whether philosophical, scientific, bureaucratic, or biomedical—has the right to dominate the terms and frameworks for discussion of such critical matters.

The breadth and depth of healthcare quality disparities for darker skinned peoples and members of lower socioeconomic classes communicate something important about how we as a society value human life. These disparities affect people when they are not only generally vulnerable within the structures of society, but when they are acutely vulnerable—when they are seriously ill. Those of us who are Christians profess faith in a God who knows and loves each strand of hair on each human head. We are called to love God and to love one another as ourselves. Thus, such disparities in care represent both a moral and theological crisis. Simply put, we are not seeing or loving our neighbors as fully as we ought.

A distinctive and important kind of learning can happen when human beings faithfully and descriptively hear and retell stories— whether they are scriptural, their own, or from another's life experience. Such listening can facilitate a kind of transformation within both the intellect and the heart of the hearer. In short, what I have attempted to do in this interdisciplinary endeavor, imperfectly to be sure, is to help close what can be a cavernous gap between abstracted numerical realities and the concrete lives of people with respect to healthcare disparities.

To do so, I have listened to just a few stories from a very few people, from Latina and Black women with breast cancer and from select healthcare providers. My prayer is that my retelling of their stories and perspectives has been faithful and that it has neither idealized nor demonized any of them. The critical thing is that they are neither heroic exemplars nor utter failures, but human. The beauty is that they are unique *and* ordinary members of the human species. I hope that substantive reflection on these few individuals might help those who read this text to not lose particular peoples in the generalities and statistics of our times.

Indeed, I have seen professionals and academics pass over statistics without being moved by them. One of my questions has been, How do you get through to people? It is relatively easy to post a set of principles on the wall that lists every patient's bill of rights to respect and to being treated with dignity. It is not as easy to embody them consistently—on both interpersonal and structural levels. While policies and laws can regulate much (never all) external behavior, they cannot legislate the kinds of interactions, relationships, attitudes, and efforts that will make such respect and concern for dignity most deeply embodied and concrete. A genuine commitment to seeing people in a new light is a fundamental part of creating justice and social transformation.

While I have learned much from these collaborators, I cannot offer any perfect solutions for safeguarding human dignity across time and location. It is wise to recognize, as Ivone Gebara does that, "We have no consistent record of humanity's progressing in virtues and moral values. Instead we have the impression that at each moment of our history, we have to learn all over again the meaning of giving and receiving respect."[2] That is what this research and text are all about— trying to facilitate ways in which—in this particular historical moment and context—ethicists and healthcare providers may rethink and relearn what it means to give respect. My goal is not to create a universal ethical framework, but rather to add one additional way for individual and communal moral formation and discernment to happen that helps us to keep reevaluating our tentative embodiments of larger ethical norms. Again, in Gebara's poetic words, "We have to construct among different groups provisional agreements, always capable of revision, in order to allow the common good to be effective, not just a beautiful expression stated in a document, like the Universal Declaration of Human Rights, that lacks any force."[3] Time and time again, human beings—moral agents—have to translate and implement what it means to love truly and deeply our neighbor as ourselves. This is our common gift and task. While humbling, it seems most honest to stay grounded in the dust, joy, and particular dynamics of the times and places in which we find ourselves.

To discover anew what respect and love mean in the concrete is not simply an intellectual assent; rather, a conversion to love is required. And such conversions happen not so often when one is distanced from social and moral conundrums (or when one is in diversity and cultural competency training sessions held for hospital staff). Instead, they happen, sometimes unexpectedly, through a process—over time—of actual conversations, projects, struggles, and relationships pursued together by diverse peoples.

Through meaningful encounters with those who most directly confront healthcare disparities and inequalities, perhaps we—social, theological, and biomedical ethicists along with those who work in healthcare—might not only learn about the disparities, but might also turn anew to our neighbor and glimpse the sacred. Equally important, perhaps this kind of learning will contribute not only to the amelioration of human suffering, but also to our own moral and vocational re-formation. Perhaps we will discover more concretely what it means for us to be responsible, accountable, and present to another.

The Reverend Dr. Martin Luther King Jr. once observed, "Of all the forms of injustice, discrimination in health care is the most cruel."[4] Latina and Black women with breast cancer have much to teach the larger society about healthcare quality. This knowledge embedded within their particular experiences may contribute a vital measurement for assessing the adequacy of healthcare policies and practices. Knowing one counts among the living can mean the difference between life and death, between healing and alienation, between redemption and despair. My deep hope is that attentive listening to those most vulnerable might make U.S. healthcare more humane for all persons.

Appendices: The Recruitment Fliers

¿Es Usted una Mujer Latina o Afro-Americana Viviendo con Cáncer?

¿Qué Significa Recibir Tratamiento de Buena Calidad?

¿Cómo Le Gustaría A Usted Ser Tratada por Su Médico, Enfermera, Trabajadora Social, etc.?

¿Tiene Usted una Experiencia o algunos Conocimientos para Contar?

Una estudiante doctoral en Ética Social de *Union Theological Seminary* en Nueva York está haciendo entrevistas con mujeres latinas y afro-americanas con cáncer para aprender de sus experiencias y puntos de vista. ¿Qué signífica para usted ser tratada con respeto, dignidad, y como un ser humano?

Este estudio consiste de una entrevista de una hora de duración. Desafortunadamente, no hay compensación para este proyecto.

Usted es elegíble si es una mujer afro-americana o latina que tiene, o es una sobre viviente de, una forma seria de cáncer y tiene entre 18 a 75 años de edad.

Are You a Black or Latina Woman Living with Cancer?

What Does Good Quality Care Look and Feel Like to You?

How Do You Want to be Treated by Your Doctor, Nurse, Social worker, etc.?

Do You Have a Story to Tell?

What Suggestions or Wisdom Do You Have?

A student researcher in Social Ethics at Union Theological Seminary is interviewing Black and Latina women with cancer to hear your experiences and perspective. What does is it mean to you to be treated with respect, dignity, as a full human being?

This study consists of conversation-like interview of approximately one hour. There is no compensation for participation.

ELIGIBILITY: You must be either a Black or Latina woman who has, or is a recent survivor of, cancer and be between the ages of 18–75.

Notes

Preface

1. Evan Handler, a relatively affluent, Jewish, young actor recounts how he was disregarded and mistreated by some of his healthcare providers at Memorial Sloan Kettering in New York City during treatment for leukemia. See Evan Handler, *Time on Fire: My Comedy of Terrors* (New York: Little, Brown, and Co., 1996).
2. "Womanist" refers to Black feminist theology and/or ethics. This term was introduced into scholarship by Alice Walker. See Alice Walker, *In Search of Our Mothers' Gardens* (New York: Harvest/HBJ, 1983), xi–xii. Later, many Black feminist theologians began using the term to refer their scholarship. See, e.g., Delores S. Williams, *Sisters in the Wilderness: The Challenge of Womanist God-Talk* (New York: Orbis Books, 1993). (Citation abbreviated hereafter as Williams, *Sisters in the Wilderness.*) In a similar vein, some Latina feminist ethicists and theologians use the term "Mujerista." See Ada María Isasi-Díaz, *En La Lucha: Elaborating a Mujerista Theology* (Minneapolis: Fortress, 1993). (Citation abbreviated hereafter as Isasi-Díaz, *En La Lucha.*)
3. emilie m. townes, *Breaking the Fine Rain of Death: African American Health Issues and a Womanist Ethic of Care* (New York: Continuum, 1998), 42. (Citation abbreviated hereafter as townes, *Breaking the Fine Rain of Death.*)
4. Note to the reader: As a way to decenter whites and western frameworks from being the norm or standard, I do not capitalize these terms while I do capitalize "Latino" and "Black." In a related vein, sometimes I use "she" and "her" to suffice for "he/she" or "his/her." I will not alter the original language of quoted sources.
5. See townes, *Breaking the Fine Rain of Death*, 2, 111–112.
6. Most often, I use the terminology of "communities/persons of color" and "white persons/communities." However, the problem with this terminology is that it can make it sound like "white" is not a color or that racism does not involve everyone. I am grateful to emilie townes for encouraging me to keep searching for language that gets at the reality that we all—in all our colors—are implicated in racism. To this end, she suggested using the language of "lighter skinned" and "darker skinned."
7. Those invested in cryogenics dispute this fact. Yet until unfrozen people start reclaiming their place in society, I will work from the premise of human mortality.

8. As a part-time chaplain intern, I was the only non-Latino staff person who spoke Spanish with any degree of efficacy. When I was not on duty, the hospital called an AT&T operator or a family member translated. On other occasions, a member of the housekeeping or food service staff was called to translate. Such realities question claims and procedures regarding informed consent. This experience took place in 1995–1996. During this time, Proposition 187 was in effect. This CA state ballot initiative was passed by voters in 1994. Its purpose was to deny undocumented immigrants access to social services, healthcare, and public education. Proposition 187 was later found unconstitutional by a federal judge, but at this time it still had force. Consequently, many Latinos (regardless of their immigration status) felt viewed with suspicion and were uncomfortable in the hospital environment.

9. The terms "Black" and "Latina" are used because the book's scope is not limited to African Americans or to women related to a particular Spanish-speaking country. Some Black women prefer terms such as "African, Afro-Caribbean, Jamaican, Puerto Rican," etc. When speaking with women of color during the ethnographic portion of this research, I asked them how they define their identity and which term(s) they prefer that I use to describe them.

10. I first told this story in an earlier publication. Reprinted, with changes, from *Disrupting White Supremacy from Within: White People on What We Need to Do*, ed. Jennifer Harvey, Karin A. Case, and Robin Hawley Gorsline (Cleaveland: Pilgrim Press, 2004), 219–223, by permission of the author and the publisher.(Citation abbreviated hereafter as Harvey et al., *Disrupting White Supremacy from Within*.) © 2004 by Jennifer Harvey, Karin A. Case, and Robin Hawley Gorsline.

11. While not experienced uniformly, white people in the United States are often socialized in ways that encourage us to take charge, assume leadership, and make decisions. Socioeconomic class and gender are variables that certainly qualify this experience. However, I nonetheless contend that *relative to communities of color*, white people are enculturated by social systems to assume a right to supervision or authority over others and to recognition of special skills or expertise.

12. In the western dichotomy of mind/spirit/intellect/purity versus emotions/body/carnal/sin, women of whatever racial-ethnic background have been associated with the latter instead of the former. However, white women, through their association with white men, have accrued significant benefits over Native Americans, Blacks, Mexicans, among others. Kelly Brown Douglass offers an insightful analysis of this legacy and its significance for how the contemporary Black Church often views homosexuality. See her article, "The Black Church and Homosexuality: The Black and White of It," *Union Seminary Quarterly Review* 57, nos. 1–2 (2002).

13. Jennifer Harvey assisted me in clarifying my thoughts and arguments related to these insights.

14. W.E.B. Du Bois used this phrase in 1903. Since then, it has been theorized and expanded upon in different ways by numerous scholars. See W.E.B. Du Bois, *The Souls of Black Folk: Essays and Sketches* (New York: Blue Heron, 1953). However, the phrase had been used earlier by his teacher and mentor,

William James. And before James, Josiah Royce and Ralph Waldo Emerson had both used it. emilie townes alerted me to these earlier uses.
15. Nell Morton, *The Journey is Home* (Boston: Beacon, 1985).

I Introduction

1. Audre Lorde, *The Cancer Journals* (San Francisco: Aunt Lute Books, 1980), 54.
2. Reprinted with permission from Brian D. Smedley, Adrienne Y. Stith, and Alan R. Nelson, eds., *Unequal Treatment: Confronting Racial and Ethnic Disparities in Healthcare*, Institute of Medicine (Washington, DC: National Academy Press, 2003). (Citation abbreviated hereafter as Smedley et al., *Unequal Treatment.*)
3. Marsha Lillie-Blanton et al., *Key Facts: Race, Ethnicity & Medical Care*, published by the Henry J. Kaiser Family Foundation (June 2003):1–35, online: www.kff.org/minorityhealth/6069-index.cfm.
4. For a thorough review of literature on cardiac care, see Marsha Lillie-Blanton et al., *Racial/Ethnic Differences in Cardiac Care: The Weight of the Evidence*, a summary report published jointly by the Henry J. Kaiser Family Foundation and the American College of Cardiology Foundation (October 2002):1–24, online: www.kff.org/uninsured/20021009c-index.cfm.
5. "Study: Disparities in Care Kill 80,000 Blacks," published on CNN.com (March 10, 2005), online: www.cnn.com. Satcher made these statements in an article published in a special issue of the journal *Health Affairs:* See David Satcher et al., "What If We Were Equal? A Comparison of the Black-White Mortality Gap in 1960 and 2000," *Health Affairs*, March/April 2005, 24(2):459–464.
6. Ibid.
7. Shankar Vedantam, "Racial Disparities Found in Pinpointing Mental Illness," *The Washington Post*, June 28, 2005, A01.
8. Ibid.
9. Ibid.
10. Will Pitt et al., *Closing the Gap: Solutions to Race-Based Health Disparities*, jointly published by the Applied Research Center and the Northwest Federation of Community Organizations (June 2005):1–66, online: www.arc.org and www.nwfco.org. (Citation abbreviated hereafter as Pitt et al., *Closing the Gap.*)
11. Lawrence D. Bobo, "Racial Attitudes and Relations at the Close of the Twentieth Century," in *America Becoming: Racial Trends and Their Consequences*, vol. 1 (Washington, DC: National Academy Press, 2001), 273. Neil J. Smelser, William Julius Wilson, and Faith Mitchell (Citation abbreviated hereafter as Bobo, "Racial Attitudes and Relations at the Close of the Twentieth Century.")
12. Ibid., 278.
13. Ibid., 294.
14. J.Z. Ayanian et al., "Unmet Health Needs of Uninsured Adults in the United States," *Journal of the American Medical Association* 284, no. 16 (October 25, 2000): 2061–2069, online: jama.ama-assn.org. Copyright © (2000) *American*

Medical Association. All rights reserved. (Citation abbreviated hereafter as Ayanian et al., "Unmet Health Needs of Uninsured Adults in the United States.")

15. In this effort, my aim bears some resemblance to others such as Robert N. Bellah et al. and Patricia Hill Collins who engage their respective disciplines with the similar purposes—social transformation. In Collins' case, she does Black feminist social theory specifically for the sake of the empowerment of Black women. See, e.g., Robert N. Bellah et al., *Habits of the Heart: Individualism and Commitment in American Life* (Berkeley: University of California Press, 1985); Patricia Hill Collins, *Black Feminist Thought: Knowledge, Consciousness, and the Politics of Empowerment,* 2nd ed. (New York: Routledge, 2000).

16. "Vulnerable populations" is a specific term used in healthcare research and can have a few different meanings. One manual for protecting human subjects in research defines it in this way: "Group/individual that cannot give informed consent because of limited autonomy (e.g., children, mentally ill and prisoners). Also refers to subjects who may be unduly influenced to participate (e.g., students, subordinates and patients)." Cynthia McGuire Dunn and Gary Chadwick, *Protecting Study Volunteers in Research: A Manual for Investigative Sites* (Boston: Center Watch, Inc., 1999), 224. (Citation abbreviated hereafter as Dunn and Chadwick, *Protecting Study Volunteers in Research.*) Healthcare researcher Lu Ann Aday defines the term somewhat differently: "Vulnerable populations are defined as being at risk of poor physical, psychological, and/or health risk." She then identifies nine specific vulnerable populations and groups them within three types of needs: *"physical needs—* high risk mothers and infants, the chronically ill and disabled, persons with AIDs; *psychological needs*—the mentally ill and disabled, alcohol and substance abusers, the suicide- or homicide-prone; *social needs*—abusing families, homeless people, and immigrants and refugees" (italics is in the original). Lu Ann Aday, *At Risk in America: The Health and Health Care Needs of Vulnerable Populations in the United States* (San Francisco: Jossey-Bass, 1993), xviii. While Aday's definition is a bit broader than the first, both lack any mention of race, and socioeconomic class is only present by way of inference (homeless, refugees). In this project, I explicitly emphasize these vulnerable communities: Persons and communities of color, those in poverty, and/or the lower socioeconomic classes and those who do not speak or understand English.

17. The cancer support networks include SHARE, The Witness Project of Harlem, and Gilda's Club.

18. The terms "medical ethics," "healthcare ethics," and "bioethics" are closely related and are sometimes used interchangeably in certain contexts. I have noticed that often those who use "bioethics" focus more on upon topics related to biotechnologies and science (e.g., genetic research, cloning, artificial reproductive technologies, organ transplantation) than on other aspects of healthcare (e.g., informed consent, patient-provider relationships, end of life care). For the purposes of this work, I address all ethicists who take up the world of medicine in some fashion or other. I tend to use the terms "medical ethics" and "healthcare ethics" to describe my own work.

19. See John H. Evans, *Playing God: Human Genetic Engineering and the Rationalization of Public Bioethical Debate* (Chicago: University of Chicago Press, 2002); John H. Evans, "After the Fall: Attempts to Establish an Explicitly Theological Voice in Debates over Science and Medicine after 1960," in *The Secular Revolution,* ed. Christian Smith (San Diego: University of California Press, 2003).

20. See Tom L. Beauchamp and James F. Childress, *Principles of Biomedical Ethics,* 5th ed. (New York: Oxford University Press, 2001). (Citation abbreviated hereafter as Beauchamp and Childress, *Principles of Biomedical Ethics.*)

21. Allen Verhey, *Reading the Bible in the Strange World of Medicine* (Grand Rapids: Eerdmans, 2003), 18. (Citation abbreviated hereafter as Verhey, *Reading the Bible in the Strange World of Medicine.*)

22. Ibid., 15.

23. Lisa Sowle Cahill, "Can Theology Have a Role in 'Public' Bioethical Discourse?" in *On Moral Medicine: Theological Perspectives in Medical Ethics,* 2nd ed., ed. Stephen E. Lammers and Allen Verhey (Grand Rapids: Eerdmans, 1998), 57–62. (The anthology will be abbreviated hereafter as *On Moral Medicine.*)

24. See townes, *Breaking the Fine Rain of Death* (full citation appears in the preface chapter, note 3); Karen Lebacqz, "Bio-Ethics: Some Challenges from a Liberation Perspective," in *On Moral Medicine,* 83–89; Margaret Farley, "Feminist Theology and Bioethics," in *On Moral Medicine,* 90–103.

25. townes, *Breaking the Fine Rain of Death,* 2.

26. See Paul Tillich, *Systematic Theology,* 3 vols. (Chicago: University of Chicago Press, 1951); Paul Tillich, *Dynamics of Faith* (New York: Harper and Row, 1957).

27. Gregg Bloche laments,

> Notably missing from the national political agenda, though well-documented in the research literature, are the larger problems of population-wide racial gaps in health status and access to medical care . . .
>
> [T]here is no serious prospect of public action to ameliorate these disparities. . . . The more intractable problem of racial disparities in health status has attracted some of the research attention recently paid to social determinants of health, but our politics has not focused on these disparities as a problem in urgent need of a public policy response. ((M. Gregg Bloche, "Race and Discretion in American Medicine," *Yale Journal of Health Policy, Law, and Ethics* I (2001):97–98. [Citation abbreviated hereafter as Bloche, "Race and Discretion in American Medicine."]) Extracts appear with permission from *Yale Journal of Health Policy, Law, and Ethics.* All rights reserved.)

28. *Health, United States, 2005 With Chartbook on Trends in the Health of Americans with Special Feature on Adults 55–64 Years,* published by the U.S. Department of Health and Human Services, the Centers for Disease Control and Prevention and the National Center for Health Statistics, Publication No. 2005–1232:12, online: www.cdc.gov/nchs/hus.htm.

29. The Centers for Disease Control and Prevention, "Cancer Health Disparities Overview," downloaded November 17, 2005, online: www.cdc.gov/cancer/

minorityawareness/overview.htm. (Citation abbreviated hereafter as Centers for Disease Control, "Cancer Health Disparities Overview.")

30. Alina Salganicoff and Usha R. Ranji, *Women and Health Care: A National Profile, Key Findings from the Kaiser Women's Health Survey*, report published by the Henry J. Kaiser Family Foundation (July 2005):11, online: www.kff.org/womenshealth/whp070705pkg.cfm. (Citation abbreviated hereafter as Salganicoff and Ranji, *Women and Health Care.*)

31. Centers for Disease Control, "Cancer Health Disparities Overview."

32. Bloche, "Race and Discretion in American Medicine," 98.

33. In particular, emilie townes has done critical work that combines attention to both health status and healthcare in Black communities. See townes, *Breaking the Fine Rain of Death.*

34. Verhey, *Reading the Bible in the Strange World of Medicine*, 21–22.

35. I would like readers to know of an important book that specifically explores end of life care issues for inner-city poor and interviews several people in the end stages of disease. See David Wendell Moller, *Dancing with Broken Bones: Portraits of Death and Dying Among Inner-City Poor* (New York: Oxford University Press, 2004).

2   U.S. Healthcare 101: What Everyone Ought to Know about How U.S. Inhabitants are Treated (or Not)

1. Carmen DeNavas-Walt, Bernadette D. Proctor, and Cheryl Hill Lee, U.S. Census Bureau, Current Population Reports, P60–229, *Income, Poverty, and Health Insurance Coverage in the United States: 2004* (Washington, DC: U.S. Government Printing Office, 2005), 16, online: www.census.gov/prod/2005pubs/p60–229.pdf. (Citation abbreviated hereafter as DeNavas-Walt et al., *Income, Poverty, and Health Insurance Coverage in the United States: 2004.*)

2. In 2002, whereas 15.2 percent of the general U.S. population was uninsured for the entire year, 30.4 percent of all people living in poverty were uninsured. See Robert J. Mills and Shailesh Bhandari, U.S. Census Bureau, Current Population Reports, P60–223, *Health Insurance Coverage in the United States: 2002* (Washington, DC: U.S. Government Printing Office, 2003), 6, online: www.census.gov/prod/2003pubs/p60–223.pdf.

3. DeNavas-Walt et al., *Income, Poverty, and Health Insurance Coverage in the United States: 2004*, 18.

4. In 2003, there were 1.4 million more people uninsured than in 2002. See Carmen DeNavas-Walt, Bernadette D. Proctor, and Robert J. Mills, U.S. Census Bureau, Current Population Reports, P60–226, *Income, Poverty, and Health Insurance Coverage in the United States: 2003* (Washington, DC: U.S. Government Printing Office, 2004), 1, online: www.census.gov/prod/2004pubs/p60–226.pdf. In addition, 2002 saw the biggest increase in ten years when 2.4 million more people were reported to be uninsured than in 2001. In

2001, 14.6 percent were uninsured—an increase of 1.4 million people from 2000. See Robert Pear, "Big Increase Seen in People Lacking Health Insurance," *The New York Times*, September 30, 2003, online: www.nytimes.com.

5. DeNavas-Walt et al., *Income, Poverty, and Health Insurance Coverage in the United States: 2004*, 27. These percentages are based upon three year averages.

6. Stephanie Strom, "For Middle Class, Health Insurance Becomes a Luxury," *The New York Times*, November 16, 2003, online: www.nytimes.com. (Citation abbreviated hereafter as Strom, "For Middle Class, Health Insurance Becomes a Luxury.")

7. DeNavas-Walt et al., *Income, Poverty, and Health Insurance Coverage in the United States: 2004*, 27.

8. Ibid., 16.

9. Families USA, "Census Bureau's Uninsured Number Indicates Fourth Increase in a Row," Press Release (August 30, 2005), available online: www.familiesusa. org/resources/newsroom/statements/census-bureau-uninsured-number-indicates-fourth-increase-in-a-row.html. On the website, the organization identifies itself in this way: "Families USA is the national organization for health care consumers. It is nonprofit and nonpartisan and advocates for high-quality, affordable health care for all Americans."

10. In Spanish *botánica* literally means botany. It is often used in everyday Spanish to designate stores that specialize in herbal and/or spiritual remedies that are well-known in Latino cultures.

11. Salganicoff and Ranji, *Women and Health Care*, 16 (full citation appears in chapter 1, note 30).

12. Ayanian et al., "Unmet Health Needs of Uninsured Adults in the United States" (full citation appears in chapter 1, note 14). They used a random telephone survey in all 50 states and surveyed a total of 105,764 adults (ages 18–64) in 1997 and 117,364 in 1998. Of these totals, 9.7 percent were uninsured for a year or longer, 4.3 percent were uninsured for less than a year, and 86 percent were insured. The authors summarize their findings:

> Our study provides recent, nationally representative estimates of unmet health needs experienced by uninsured adults—two thirds of whom had been uninsured for one year or longer. Nearly half of uninsured adults with annual incomes below $15,000 reported they could not see a physician when needed in the past year due to the cost of care. Uninsured adults with clinically important chronic conditions and health risks were much more likely than insured adults to report this problem, even after adjusting for income and other potential confounders.

13. This study footnotes several studies done in the mid-1990s that show that lacking health insurance has significant clinical consequences. Commenting on this prior research, "[U]ninsured adults encounter greater barriers to preventive services and treatment for chronic illnesses than to acute care. They are more likely than insured adults to report poor health status, delay seeking medical care, and forgo necessary care. . . . Uninsured adults receive few screening services for cancer and cardiovascular risk factors, present with

later-stage diagnoses of cancer, and experience more avoidable hospitalizations. They also face an increased risk of death . . ." Ibid.

14. Ibid.

15. Ibid.

16. Starting with the 2000 Census, respondents were permitted to identify themselves with more than one race. Thus, the Census records those who identify in the following ways: "White alone," "White alone or in combination," "White alone, not Hispanic," "Black Alone," and "Black alone or in combination." With respect to Latinos, the Census Bureau uses the term "Hispanic" and specifies that they may be of any race. Those who identify as Asian may respond as "Asian alone," as "Native Hawaiian and/or other Pacific Islander," or as Asian in combination with one or both of these designations. For an explanation of these categories, see DeNavas-Walt et al., *Income, Poverty, and Health Insurance Coverage in the United States: 2004*, 1.

17. U.S. Census Bureau, "The Face of Our Population," online: http://factfinder.census.gov/jsp/saff/SAFFInfo.jsp?_pageId = tp9_race_ethnicity. See also ibid., 46–50.

18. DeNavas-Walt et al., *Income, Poverty, and Health Insurance Coverage in the United States: 2004*, 17.

19. Ibid., 9.

20. David Leonhardt, "More Americans Were Uninsured and Poor in 2003, Census Finds," *The New York Times*, August 27, 2004, online: www.nytimes.com.

21. DeNavas-Walt et al., *Income, Poverty, and Health Insurance Coverage in the United States: 2004*, 9. For information on poverty rates in 2002, see Lynette Clemetson, "More Americans in Poverty in 2002, Census Says," *The New York Times*, September 27, 2003, A1 and A10. (Citation abbreviated hereafter as Clemetson, "More Americans in Poverty in 2002, Census Says.")

22. DeNavas-Walt et al., *Income, Poverty, and Health Insurance Coverage in the United States: 2004*, 9.

23. Ibid., 45.

24. See Strom, "For Middle Class, Health Insurance Becomes a Luxury."

25. Cathy Schoen, Michelle M. Doty, Sara R. Collins, and Alyssa L. Holmgren, "Insured But Not Protected: How Many Adults Are Underinsured?" Health Affairs Web Exclusive, June 14, 2005 W5-289-W5-302, abstract available online: http://www.cmwf.org/publications/ publications_show. htm?doc_id = 280812. The entire article can be accessed online: http:// www.healthaffairs.org.

26. DeNavas-Walt et al., *Income, Poverty, and Health Insurance Coverage in the United States: 2004*, 16–17, 19, and 60.

27. Ibid., 18.

28. See, e.g., Carl Hulse, "Congress Rushes to Tie Up Loose Ends Before Break," *The New York Times*, November 19, 2005, online: www.nytimes.com; Editorial, "Congress's Threadbare Budget Politics," *The New York Times*, November 15, 2005, online: www.nytimes.com.

29. See Robert Pear, "U.S. Gives Florida a Sweeping Right to Curb Medicaid," *The New York Times*, October 20, 2005, online: www.nytimes.com.

30. Strom, "For Middle Class, Health Insurance Becomes a Luxury."

31. *Parade* recently featured three such working and middle-class families who cannot afford health insurance. See Dotson Rader and Isadore Rosenfeld, "Can You Pay for Your Health Care?" Cover Story of *Parade, The Chicago Tribune*'s Sunday Magazine August 15, 2004, 4–6.

32. John Leland, "When Health Insurance Is Not a Safeguard," *The New York Times*, October 23, 2005, online: www.nytimes.com.

33. DeNavas-Walt et al., *Income, Poverty, and Health Insurance Coverage in the United States: 2004*, 19.

34. Medicaid coverage in many places in the Unites States is often not as generous or comprehensive as private insurance. For example, the oncologist that I interviewed explained to me that he does not take Medicaid patients because the reimbursement rates for physician services are so low. However, he noted that Medicaid does cover other procedures and medications during hospitalization. Also, the social workers and nurse case manager with whom I spoke commented that Medicaid will often not cover many out-patient or in-home services (e.g., physical therapy) upon discharge.

35. María de Lourdes Maldonado, interview by author, New York, NY, August 23, 2003. Her name has been changed.

36. See R.S. Morrison et al., " 'We Don't Carry That'—Failure of Pharmacies in Predominantly Nonwhite Neighborhoods to Stock Opioid Analgesic," *The New England Journal of Medicine* 342, no. 14(2000):1023–1026.

37. Robert Moses was responsible for the monumental transportation and infrastructure projects throughout New York City in the mid-twentieth century. In particular, he orchestrated the construction of the Cross Bronx Expressway and determined where it would go such that it cut off the South Bronx from the rest of the Bronx. Furthermore, this roadway went over the South Bronx instead of through it, which meant that it did not serve any of the inhabitants of this neighborhood. The Reverend Heidi Neumark discusses some of the implications of Moses' work. See Heidi B. Neumark, *Breathing Space: A Spiritual Journey in the South Bronx* (Boston: Beacon, 2003).

38. Ibid.

39. Robert Pear, "Emergency Rooms Get Eased Rules on Patient Care," *The New York Times*, September 3, 2003, A1.

40. Some doctors and hospitals, along with the administrator of the federal Centers for Medicare and Medicaid Services, Thomas Scully, praise the change. They express the view that it will reduce the costs of hospital compliance, reduce the risk of lawsuits and fines, and lift bureaucratic regulations without affecting patient care. Ibid.

41. Lynette Clemetson, "Census Shows Ranks of Poor Rose in 2002 by 1.3 Million," *The New York Times*, September 3, 2003, A16. Also according to this article, this increase adds up to a depressing total of 34.8 million individuals, 7 million families, and 12.2 million children who live in poverty. (Citation abbreviated hereafter as Clemetson, "Census Shows Ranks of Poor Rose in 2002 by 1.3 Million.")

42. U.S. Census Bureau, "Poverty: 2002 Highlights," uploaded September 26, 2003, online: www.census.gov/hhes/poverty/poverty02/pov02hi.html. This webpage explains, "The data presented here are from the Current Population

Survey (CPS), 2003 Annual Social & Economic Supplement (ASEC), the source of official poverty estimates. The CPS ASEC is a sample survey of approximately 78,000 households nationwide. These data reflect conditions in calendar year 2002." In a follow-up article, Clemetson reported the revised Census poverty figures to reflect those of this report. While poverty increased, the article notes that the median household income decreased by 1.1 percent. See Clemetson, "More Americans in Poverty in 2002, Census Says."

43. Clemetson, "Census Shows Ranks of Poor Rose in 2002 by 1.3 Million."
44. Robert Pear, "Rising Costs Prompt States to Reduce Medicaid Further," *The New York Times*, September 23, 2003, online: www.nytimes.com. (Citation abbreviated hereafter as Pear, "Rising Costs Prompt States to Reduce Medicaid Further.")
45. Bob Herbert, "Curing Health Costs: Let the Sick Suffer," *The New York Times*, September 1, 2005, online: www.nytimes.com. However, at this writing, a federal judge has currently stopped these cuts from taking effect on the basis that ending coverage for up to 323,000 would violate their constitutional rights. See Anita Wadwhani, "Judge Bars TennCare Cuts Again," *The Tennessean*, April 29, 2005, online: http:www.tennessean.com/government/tencare/archives/05/03/68866139.shtml?Element_ID = 68866139.
46. Robert Pear, "U.S. Gives Florida Sweeping Right to Curb Medicaid," *The New York Times*, October 20, 2005, online: www.nytimes.com.
47. Ibid.
48. Pear, "Rising Costs Prompt States to Reduce Medicaid Further."
49. See Elisabeth Bumiller, "Bush Seeks $87 Billion and U.N. Aid for War Effort," *The New York Times*, September 8, 2003, A1.
50. COBRA is a federal law enacted in 1985 under which employer group health plans with 20 or more employees must offer continuation of coverage for up to 18 months to employees (and their dependents) who leave their jobs. The catch is that the former employee must pay the entire premium during this period of extended coverage.
51. See Strom, "For Middle Class, Health Insurance Becomes a Luxury." The *Village Voice* made similar comparisons. See James Ridgeway with Phoebe St. John, "A Post-9-11 Reality Check: The Soaring Cost of Iraq 'Peace,' the Soaring Cost of Life in America," *Village Voice*, September 10–16, 2003, 26.
52. Donald G. McNeil, Jr., "Africans Outdo U.S. Patients in Following AIDS Therapy," *The New York Times*, September 3, 2003, A1.
53. Ibid.
54. Ibid.
55. Take the example of South Africa, the country with the largest HIV positive population. Richard Morin reports that "[o]ne out of nine South Africans—about 5 million people—are infected with HIV, the virus that causes AIDS . . . By 2010, AIDS is expected to cut life expectancy in South Africa almost in half, from 68 years to 36." In an interview with Morin, Sister Pricilla Dlamini who works Holy Cross AIDS Hospice told him, "For a whole generation, it is too late. The deaths are increasing every month. The dying is just beginning." Richard Morin, "A Wave of Death, Surging Higher; Government Faulted as AIDS Claims Much of a Generation," *Washington Post*, April 1, 2004, A1.

56. Smedley et al., *Unequal Treatment*, 1 (full citation appears in chapter 1, note 2).

57. Here is a sampling of research that are among those cited by the IOM bibliography: J.Z. Ayanian et al., "Racial Differences in the Use of Revascularization Procedures after Coronary Angiography," *Journal of the American Medical Association* 284(2000):1670–1676; L.C. Einbinder and K.A. Schulman, "The Effect of Race on the Referral process for Invasive Cardiac Procedures," *Medical Care Research and Review* 57, supplement 1(2000):162–180; J. Etchason et al., "Racial and Ethnic Disparities in Health Care," *Journal of the American Medical Association* 285(2001):883; K. Fiscella et al., "Inequality in Quality: Addressing Socioeconomic, Racial, and Ethnic Disparities in Health Care," *Journal of the American Medical Association* 284(2000): 2579–2584; R.M. Mayberry et al., "Racial and Ethnic Differences in Access to Medical Care," *Medical Care Research and Review* 57, supplement 1(2000):108–145; S.L. Furth et al., "Racial Differences in Access to the Kidney Transplant Waiting List for Children and Adolescents with End-Stage Renal Disease," *Pediatrics* 106(2000): 756–761; M.P. DelBello et al., "Effects of Race on Psychiatric Diagnosis of Hospitalized Adolescents: A Retrospective Chart Review," *Journal of Child Adolescent Psychopharmacology* 11(2001):95–103; A.L. Whaley, "Racism in the Provision of Mental Health Services: A Social-Cognitive Analysis," *American Journal of Orthopsychiatry* 68(1998):47–57; K.L. Kahn et al., "Healthcare for Black and Poor Hospitalized Medicare Patients," *Journal of the American Medical Association* 271(1994):1169–1174; J.Z. Ayanian et al., "Quality of Care by Race and Gender for Congestive Heart Failure and Pneumonia," *Medical Care* 37(1999):1260–1269. See ibid.

58. Eric C. Schneider, Alan M. Zaslavsky, and Arnold M. Epstein, "Racial Disparities in the Quality of Care for Enrollees in Medicare Managed Care," *Journal of the American Medical Association* 287, no. 10(2002):1290. They gathered this data by analyzing the 1998 Health Plan Employer Data and Information Set (HEDIS) which annually tracks these four quality of care measures. (Citation abbreviated hereafter as Schneider et al., "Racial Disparities in the Quality of Care for Enrollees in Medicare Managed Care.")

59. Ibid., 1292. The authors found the greatest degree of disparity in the area of mental health follow-up.

60. See Anne Fadiman, *The Spirit Catches You and You Fall Down: A Hmong Child, Her American Doctors, and the Collision of Two Cultures* (New York: Farrar, Straus, and Giroux, 1997).

61. For example, in its review, the IOM found "no studies where the quality of care for American Indian, Alaska Native, or Pacific Islander populations were explicitly studied, or where the sample size of these groups permitted analysis." Smedley et al., *Unequal Treatment*, 78.

62. It is critical to understand that Latinos are not a homogenous population. This diversity is often not recognized or documented in either research or on hospital admission forms. Too often, they are lumped under the ethnic umbrella of "Hispanic." For example, Guatemalans, Ecuadorians, and Hondurans are often misidentified as Mexicans. Some Dominicans and Puerto Ricans are assumed to be African Americans.

63. See, e.g., S.C. Collins et al., *U.S. Minority Health: A Chartbook* (New York: Commonwealth Fund, 1999).

64. The film *A Day Without a Mexican* (2004) directed by Sergio Arau offers viewers an interesting vision of what it would be like if Latinos, specifically in this case all Mexicans, went on strike or suddenly disappeared from U.S. society.

65. According to the IOM, "Hispanic Americans face greater barriers to health insurance than all other U.S. racial and ethnic groups. The probability of being uninsured among Hispanic Americans is 35%, compared with 17.5% of the general population. This disparity . . . largely results from the lack of job-based insurance provided to Hispanic Americans, who disproportionately work in blue-collar and service-oriented jobs. The vast majority (87%) of uninsured Hispanics are in working families, yet only 43% of Hispanics receive health insurance through work." Smedley et al., *Unequal Treatment,* 87. The numbers the IOM is using reflect Census data that predates the 2004 Health Insurance Coverage in the United States cited above.

66. J. Emilio Carrillo, Fernando M. Treviño, Joseph R. Betancourt, and Alberto Coustasse, "Latino Access to Health Care: The Role of Insurance, Managed Care, and Institutional Barriers," in *Health Issues in the Latino Community,* ed. Marilyn Aguirre-Molina, Carlos W. Molina, and Ruth Enid Zambrana (San Francisco: Jossey-Bass, 2001), 67. (Citation abbreviated hereafter as Carrillo et al., "Latino Access to Health Care.")

67. R.A. David and M. Rhee, "The Impact of Language as a Barrier to Effective Health Care in an Underserved Urban Latino Community," *Mount Sinai Journal of Medicine* 65, nos. 5–6(October/November 1998):393–397. (Citation is abbreviated hereafter as David and Rhee, "The Impact of Language as a Barrier to Effective Health Care in an Underserved Urban Latino Community.")

68. See E.A. Jacobs et al., "Impact of Interpreter Services on Delivery of Health Care to Limited-English-Proficient Patients," *Journal of General Internal Medicine* 16(2001):468–474; K.P. Derose and D.W. Baker, "Limited English Proficiency and Latinos' Use of Physician Services," *Medical Care Research and Review* 57(2000):76–91.

69. Kevin Fiscella et al., "Disparities in Health Care by Race, Ethnicity, and Language Among the Insured: Finding from a National Sample," *Medical Care* 40, no.1(2002):52–59. The researchers gathered a national sample through the use of a telephone survey tool.

70. Carrillo et al., "Latino Access to Health Care," 67.

71. D.W. Baker, C.D. Stevens, and R.H. Brook, "Determinants of Emergency Department Use: Are Race and Ethnicity Important?" *Annals of Emergency Medicine* 28, no.6(1996):677–682, cited in Smedley et al., *Unequal Treatment,* 142.

72. To my knowledge, there have not been specific studies exploring the quality and satisfaction of telephone translators. It would be interesting to compare the experiences of patients who have had a professional translator present in the room with those who have had a translator on the telephone.

73. Two studies raise this point: David and Rhee, "The Impact of Language as a Barrier to Effective Health Care in an Underserved Urban Latino Community," 393–397; L.S. Morales et al., "Are Latinos Less Satisfied with Communication by Health Care Providers?" *Journal of General Internal Medicine* 14(1999):409–411. Both cited in Carrillo et al., "Latino Access to Health Care," 68.

74. P. Ebden, O.J. Carey, A. Bhatt, and B. Harrison, "The Bilingual Consultation," *Lancet* 1, no. 8581(1988):347, cited in Smedley et al., *Unequal Treatment*, 143.

75. Cross-cultural nursing curricula often make this point. See, e.g., Larry D. Purnell and Betty J. Paulanka, *Transcultural Health Care: A Culturally Competent Approach*, 2nd ed. (Philadelphia: F.A. Davis Co., 2003). (Citation abbreviated hereafter as Purnell and Paulanka, *Transcultural Health Care*); Bette Bonder, Laura Martin, and Andy Miracle, *Culture in Clinical Care* (New Jersey: Slack Inc., 2002). (Citation abbreviated hereafter as Bonder et al., *Culture in Clinical Care*.)

76. J. Cho and B.M. Solis, *Healthy Families Culture and Linguistics Resources Survey: A Physician Perspective on their Diverse Member Population* (Los Angeles: LA Care Health Plan, 2001), cited in Smedley et al., *Unequal Treatment*, 90.

77. Carrillo et al., "Latino Access to Health Care," 68.

78. S. Woloshin, N.A. Bickell, L.M. Schwartz, T. Gany, and H.G. Welch, "Language Barriers in Medicine in the United States," *Journal of the American Medical Association* 273, no. 9(1995):724–728, cited in Smedley et al., *Unequal Treatment*, 141.

79. Certainly the experience of not getting all the information one would like from a physician is not unique to patients who do not speak English well. For example, in one study of Black and white patients who had had cardiac stress testing that yielded positive results, the researchers found that both Black and white patients expressed that the information they had received from their doctors was "incomplete, vague, ambiguous, and unclear." Both groups of patients also reported that they needed further convincing "of the need for additional, invasive tests and procedures." Interestingly, however, the Black patients in particular consistently emphasized "a preference for building a relationship with physicians (meaning trust) before agreeing to an invasive cardiac procedure *and* just as consistently complained that such trust was lacking." Both white and Black patients agreed that they wanted more and clearer information from their doctors. Yet it is important to note that the Black patients were the ones in particular to express how important trust was as a precondition for further treatments and that this trust was lacking. See Tracie C. Collins et al., "Racial Differences in How Patients Perceive Physician Communication Regarding Cardiac Testing," *Medical Care* 40, no.1(January Supplement 2002):I-27-I-34.

80. Smedley et al., *Unequal Treatment*, 114.

81. Carrillo et al., "Latino Access to Health Care," 66. See also ibid., 114; *Associated Press*, "Report Urges Diversity in Health Jobs," February 5, 2004. They cite from the 2004 Institute of Medicine Report, Brian Smedley, Adrienne Stith, and Lonnie R. Bristow, eds., *In the Nation's Compelling Interest: Ensuring*

Diversity in the Health Care Workforce (Washington, DC: National Academies Press, 2004), online: www.iom.edu.

82. The Sullivan Commission on Diversity in the Healthcare Workforce, *Missing Persons: Minorities in the Health Professions*, published September 2004, 2, online: www.sullivancomission.org.

83. See V.L. Bonham, "Race, Ethnicity, and Pain Treatment: Striving to Understand the Causes and Solutions to the Disparities in Pain Treatment," *Journal of Law Medicine, and Ethics* 29(2001):52–68, cited in Smedley et al., *Unequal Treatment*, 168.

84. Michelle van Ryn and Jane Burke, "The Effect of Patient Race and Socio-Economic Status on Physicians' Perceptions of Patients," *Social Science and Medicine* 50(2000):814. (Citation abbreviated hereafter as Van Ryn and Burke, "The Effect of Patient Race and Socio-Economic Status on Physicians' Perceptions of Patients.") Reprinted from Michelle van Ryn and Jane Burke, "The Effect of Patient Race and Socio-Economic Status on Physicians' Perceptions of Patients," *Social Science and Medicine* 50(2000):814. Copyright © (2000) with permission from *Elsevier*.

85. Certain instances when such information is relevant to a medical diagnosis, e.g., the connection between sickle-cell anemia and some African Americans, represent an exception to this rule.

86. Kevin Schulman et al. drew national attention when they published their study in 1999, which found significant differences in how doctors responded to identical heart disease symptoms as presented by white and Black actors playing the role of patients. This study has been critiqued and responded to by others who found catheterization mistakes that exaggerated Schulman's findings. However, other studies on referrals for cardiac confirm Schulman's analysis as noted in chapter 1. Moreover, even with more modest appraisals, Schulman's study was nonetheless an important impetus in the congressional rationale for the commissioning of the IOM study.

87. For the IOM's caution, see Smedley et al., *Unequal Treatment*, 10–11.

88. A.I. Balsa and T.G. McGuire, "Prejudice, Clinical Uncertainty and Stereotyping as Sources of Health Disparities," *Journal of Health Economics* 22, no. 1(2003):89–116. (Citation abbreviated hereafter as Balsa and McGuire, "Prejudice, Clinical Uncertainty and Stereotyping as Sources of Health Disparities.")

89. See Smedley et al., *Unequal Treatment*, 162.

90. Van Ryn and Burke, "The Effect of Race and Socio-Economic Status on Physicians' Perceptions of Patients," 815. Of the nonwhite physicians, 11 percent were Asian doctors, 1 percent were African American doctors, 3 percent were Hispanic doctors, and 1 percent classified themselves as some other race/ethnicity.

91. Ibid., 821. CAD refers to coronary artery disease. SES refers to socioeconomic status, as already mentioned earlier.

92. Ibid.

93. Ibid., 822. Van Ryn and Burke later note, "In considering the problem of group differences and stereotyping, it is important to distinguish the difference between content accuracy (the accuracy of a generalized belief about

a group of people) and application accuracy. This refers to the fact that the inappropriate use of stereotypic beliefs as a basis for responding to others, even if these beliefs are entirely accurate, is potentially damaging to the stereotyped individual." Ibid., 823.

94. "Among the patients in the lowest 33% of the SES distribution, physicians perceive Blacks to be less pleasant and rational than Whites. Blacks are only one-third as likely as Whites to be rated 'very' pleasant. As with all the analyses discussed, this difference persists even when patient depressive symptoms, social assertiveness, and feelings of mastery are controlled for in addition to the standard covariates. In addition, low SES Blacks are less than half as likely as their low SES White counterparts to be considered 'very' rational by physicians." Ibid., 821.

95. It is also important to note that it is possible that many Black patients come into clinical encounters with more negative feelings than their white counterparts due to the legacy of the Tuskegee Syphilis study as well as their own experiences with racism in other contexts.

96. Van Ryn and Burke, "The Effect of Race and Socio-Economic Status on Physicians' Perceptions of Patients," 823.

97. See their extensive citations of recent studies. Ibid., 825–828.

98. Ibid., 823.

99. See Bobo, "Racial Attitudes and Relations at the Close of the Twentieth Century." (First full citation appears in chapter 1, note 11.)

100. Saif Rathore et al., "The Effects of Patient Sex and Race on Medical Students' Ratings of Quality of Life," *American Journal of Medicine* 108(2000):561–566. Reprinted from *American Journal of Medicine* 108(1), Rahore et al., "The Effects of Patient Sex and Race on Medical Students' Ratings of Quality of Life," 561–566. Copyright© 2000, with permission from Excerpta Medica, Inc. All of the student participants had already received adequate theoretical instruction to identify angina and to understand its relationship to coronary artery disease. However, they were recruited specifically because they had not yet had much clinical experience and would thus "have limited knowledge of the incidence of coronary artery disease by race and sex." Ibid., 561–562.

101. Ibid., 564.

102. Ibid.

103. Ibid. Also, the male students "tended to rate the health state of the black female patient actor lower than the white male actor, whereas female students tended to rate both patient actors' health states comparably, although this difference by students' sex was not statistically significant." Ibid.

104. Ibid.

105. Michelle van Ryn, "Research on the Provider Contribution to Race/Ethnicity Disparities in Medical Care," *Medical Care* 40, no.1(2002): I-140-I-151. (Citation abbreviated hereafter as Van Ryn, "Research on the Provider Contribution to Race/Ethnicity Disparities in Medical Care.")

106. In addition to this kind of research, van Ryn also cites numerous studies that document that a patient's sex, age, diagnosis, sexual orientation, sickness, and, more recently, race and ethnicity, influence provider beliefs about, degree of affinity toward, and expectations of patients. Ibid.

107. Ibid., I–142. With respect to the other three medical issues: Kidney transplants: Significant studies have documented racial-ethnic disparities in the amount that the possibility of transplantation is discussed or recommended and in the likelihood of being put on a waiting list—for patients with clinically similar medical conditions, symptoms, states of health. Cardiac: Research demonstrates race and ethnicity differences exist in terms of how often revascularization procedures and cardiac surgery are recommended and performed—again, in clinically similar cases. Pain Management: A series of studies show that nonwhites are at a greater risk for inadequate pain management and assessment—even with identical patient complaints of pain. These disparities have happened in the management of cancer-related pain as well as in that related to broken bones and chest pain. Ibid, 141–142.

108. Van Ryn discusses six distinct, but interrelated explanations for such behaviors and treatment outcomes that result in racial-ethnic quality of care disparities. She explores six hypotheses and uses relevant findings from both social cognition and provider behavior literatures to support each. These hypotheses are as follows:

1: [T]he primary cognitive mediator of the effect of patient race/ethnicity on provider behavior is providers' conscious or unconscious beliefs about the patient.

2: [P]roviders' beliefs about patients influence their interpretation of patient symptoms.

3: [P]roviders' beliefs about patient social and behavioral character directly influence their clinical decision-making. [This means, a patient's character makes them more or less deserving of, and/or more or less appropriate for, a given treatment in the provider's eyes.]

4: [P]roviders' unconscious beliefs and unconscious stereotypes about patients influence interpersonal behaviors.

5 and 6: [P]roviders' interpersonal behavior influences, respectively, patient cognitive factors such as attitudes, self-efficacy, trust, and behavioral intentions and patient satisfaction, which, in turn, also influences patient attitudes.

Ibid., I-143-I-147.

109. For example, in their bibliography, the IOM cites the following: J.F. Dovidio, "Stereotyping," in R.A. Wilson and F.C. Keil, eds., *The MIT Encyclopedia of the Cognitive Sciences* (Cambridge: MIT Press, 1999); J.F. Dovidio et al., "Stereotyping, Prejudice, and Discrimination: Another Look," in N. Macrae, C. Stangor, and M. Hewstone, eds., *Stereotypes and Stereotyping* (New York: Guilford, 1996), 276–319; J.F. Dovidio and S.L. Gaertner, "On the Nature of Contemporary Prejudice: The Causes, Consequences, and Challenges of Aversive Racism," in J.L. Eberhardt and S.T. Fiske, eds., *Confronting Racism: The Problem and the Response* (Thousand Oaks: Sage, 1998), 3–32; and J.F. Dovidio et al., "Implicit and Explicit Prejudice and Interracial Interaction," *Journal of Personality & Social Psychology* 82, no. 1 (2002):62–68; S.T. Fiske, "Stereotyping, Prejudice, and Discrimination," in D.T. Gilbert et al., eds., *The Handbook of Social Psychology*, 4th ed.,

2 vols. (New York: McGraw-Hill, 1998), vol. 2, 357–411. See Smedley et al., *Unequal Treatment.*

110. Smedley et al., *Unequal Treatment,* 169.

111. Social cognition literature is helpful in understanding the functioning of stereotypes. See, e.g., these sources cited in Van Ryn, "Research on the Provider Contribution to Race/Ethnicity Disparities in Medical Care," I-147-151; C.N. Macrae and G.V. Bodenhausen, "Social Cognition: Categorical Person Perception," *British Journal of Social Psychology* 92(2001):239–255; Z. Kunda, *Social Cognition: Making Sense of People* (Cambridge: MIT Press, 1999); C.N. Macrae et al., "Stereotypes as Energy-Saving Devices: A Peek Inside the Cognitive Toolbox," *Journal of Pers Soc Psychol* 66(1994):33–47; C. Stangor, ed., *Stereotypes and Prejudice* (Philadelphia: Psychology Press, 2001).

112. See Van Ryn and Burke, "The Effect of Race and Socio-Economic Status on Physicians' Perceptions of Patients."

113. Ibid., 814.

114. See Balsa and McGuire, "Prejudice, Clinical Uncertainty and Stereotyping as Sources of Health Disparities."

115. See Bloche, "Race and Discretion in American Medicine" (full citation appears in chapter 1, note 27).

116. For example, one study found that in a study of nearly 300 cancer patients receiving radiation, doctors were less able to identify high levels of distress among low-income patients. In another study, cancer providers underestimated the amount of pain patients of color were having as compared with their white counterparts. See Van Ryn, "Research on the Provider Contribution to Race/Ethnicity Disparities in Medical Care," I–145.

117. Robert Pear, "Health Spending Rises to Record 15% of Economy," *The New York Times,* January 9, 2004, online: www.nytimes.com.

118. Donald L. Barlett and James B. Steele, *Critical Condition: How Health Care in America Became Big Business and Bad Medicine* (New York: Doubleday, 2004), 13. (Citation abbreviated hereafter as Barlett and Steele, *Critical Condition.*)

119. Uwe Reinhardt et al., "U.S. Health Care Spending in an International Context," *Health Affairs* (May/June 2004):12. (Citation abbreviated hereafter as Reinhardt et al., "U.S. Health Care Spending in an International Context.")

120. Barlett and Steele, *Critical Condition,* 13.

121. Carrillo et al., "Latino Access to Health Care," 55. As evidence for this claim, the authors cite G. F. Anderson, *Multinational Comparisons of Health Care: Expenditures, Coverage and Outcomes* (New York: Commonwealth Fund, 1998); and S. Woolhandler and D.U. Himmelstein, "The Deteriorating Administrative Efficiency of the U.S. Health Care System," *New England Journal of Medicine* 324, no.18(1991):1253–1258.

122. "WHO Press Release 2000: World Health Organization Assesses the World's Health Systems," Press Release WHO, June 21, 2000, online: www.who. int/whr/2000/media_centre/press_release/en/index.html. (Citation abbreviated hereafter as "WHO Press Release 2000.") See also the full WHO report: *The*

World Health Report 2000 Health Systems: Improving Performance
(Geneva, 2000), 1–207, online: www.who.int/whr/2000/en/index.html.
123. "WHO Press Release 2000."
124. Reinhardt et al., "U.S. Health Care Spending in an International Context," 13.
125. Nicholas D. Kristof, "Health Care? Ask Cuba," *The New York Times*, January 12, 2005, online: www.nytimes.com.
126. Carrillo et al., "Latino Access to Health Care," 55.
127. *The New York Times* printed a lengthy series of articles, entitled "Being a Patient," which explored various aspects of being hospitalized in U.S. healthcare in 2005. One of the featured articles in particular focused on the bureaucracy of bill paying, See Katie Hafner, "Treated for Illness, Then Lost in Labyrinth of Bills," *The New York Times* October 13, 2005, online: www.nytimes.com.
128. Smedley et al., *Unequal Treatment*, 144.
129. One group of researchers, upon their literature review, summarize these barriers:

These organizational, intrinsic, and systemic barriers oftentimes prevent minority, socioeconomically disadvantaged, and limited-English-proficient patients with insurance from having true access to health care. Some examples of barriers include those within health care systems that (1) lack interpreter services and language-appropriate health education materials and signage; (2) have bureaucratic, complicated intake processes, long waiting times for appointments, and limited operating hours (including after-hours availability); and (3) are located outside the community, making them difficult to reach via public transportation. (National Hispanic/Latino Health Initiative, *Public Health Reports* 108[1993]:534–558, cited in Carrillo et al., "Latino Access to Health Care," 67.)

130. Schneider et al., "Racial Disparities in the Quality of Care for Enrollees in Medicare Managed Care."
131. J.L. Hargraves, J.J. Stoddard, and S. Trude, "Minority Physicians' Experiences Obtaining Referrals to Specialists and Hospital Admissions," *Medscape General Medicine* 3, no. 4(2001):10, cited in Smedley et al., *Unequal Treatment*, 146.
132. An aside with respect to the culture of medicine is as follows: I interviewed a white oncologist, "Leonard Orlando." When asked, he identified his racial-ethnic identity as Italian American. However, he later added that if he has to identify most particularly with a culture, it would be the culture of doctors: "Now, if I had to identify myself culturally, I suppose, maybe the right answer is for me to identify myself as a physician. . . ." When I asked him to describe the culture of physicians, he responded,

[P]hysicians are trained to be decisive, to be comfortable with suffering, to actually put up with a lot and not necessarily tend to our own personal needs or comforts. . . . And so I think our culture is really one of—it's very puritanical. It's one of being uncomfortable, of being in pain, and also being—making a decision without necessarily—being forced to make a decision and not always having all the information. . . . I guess, you know, kind of covering up our ignorance or uncertainty.

I found his comment that part of the culture of medicine is to hide one's ignorance particularly interesting. He later added that, in his view, physicians tend to be competitive rather than mutually supportive or collegial.

133. Mary-Jo DelVecchio Good and Byron J. Good et al., "The Culture of Medicine and Racial, Ethnic, and Class Disparities in Healthcare," in Smedley et al., *Unequal Treatment*, 595. (Citation is abbreviated hereafter as Good and Good et al., "The Culture of Medicine and Racial, Ethnic, and Class Disparities in Healthcare.")

134. Ibid., 596. However, the researchers note that up to now, they have not identified how the medical hierarchy of healthcare institutions and the indoctrination into specific ideologies and virtues that comes with medical school may affect communities of color and/or low socioeconomic class backgrounds in particular.

135. Ibid., 597.

136. Ibid. They initially answer this question by arguing that "multidimensional processes are at the root of different types of ethnic and racial disparities in health status and medical treatment. These processes are structural, economic, environmental, political and attitudinal." Ibid., 597–598.

137. H. Jack Geiger, "Why is the HHS Obscuring a Health Care Gap?" *Washington Post,* January 27, 2004, A17. (Citation abbreviated hereafter as Geiger, "Why is the HHS Obscuring a Health Care Gap?") Geiger is the Arthur C. Logan Professor Emeritus of community medicine at the City University of New York Medical School and a past president of Physicians for Human Rights. In the first paragraph of this article, Geiger notes that he along with others have "read and reviewed more than a thousand careful, peer-reviewed studies documenting systematic deficiencies and inequities in the health care provided for African Americans, Hispanics, Native Americans and members of some Asian subgroups."

138. Ibid.

139. Robert Pear, "Taking the Spin Out of Report that Made Bad into Good Health," *The New York Times,* February 22, 2004, online: www.nytimes.com. (Citation is abbreviated hereafter as Pear, "Taking the Spin Out of Report that Made Bad into Good Health.") Pear also mentions the fact that on February 18, 2004, over 60 "influential scientists, including 20 Nobel laureates, issued a statement criticizing what they described as the misuse of science by the administration to bolster its policies on the environment, arms control and public health." This article gives several startling examples of text in the original AHRQ report that had been deleted by the HHS.

140. Van Ryn and Burke, "The Effect of Race and Socio-Economic Status on Physicians' Perceptions of Patients," 823–824.

141. "Although patchwork programs can fill gaps in specific services such as cancer screening for uninsured adults, national health goals represented in Healthy People 2010 objectives are unlikely to be unmet . . . without more

vigorous efforts to extend affordable health insurance to the uninsured for a wide [range of] basic medical services." Ayanian et al., "Unmet Health Needs of Uninsured Adults in the United States."

142. See J.J. Escarse et al., "Health Care Reform and Minorities: Why Universal Insurance Won't Equalize Access," *Leonard Davis Institute Health Policy Research Quality Review* 3(1993):1–2.

143. See Beauchamp and Childress, *Principles of Biomedical Ethics* (full citation appears in chapter 1, note 20).

144. "If anything distinguished the health field, it is the abundance of carefully crafted technical reports, studies, and policy recommendations. The last fifteen to twenty years have seen a constant stream of special national initiatives, reports, summits, and task forces to address the health needs of Latinos. Yet the goal of many of these endeavors have yet to be fully actualized." Marilyn Aguirre-Molina, Angelo Falcón, and Carlos W. Molina, "Latino Health Policy: A Look to the Future," in *Health Issues in the Latino Community*, ed. Marilyn Aguirre-Molina, Carlos W. Molina, and Ruth Enid Zambrana (San Francisco: Jossey-Bass, 2001), 461. (Citation abbreviated hereafter as Aguirre-Molina et al., "Latino Health Policy: A Look to the Future.")

145. See www.healthypeople.gov.

146. Aguirre-Molina et al., "Latino Health Policy: A Look to the Future," 462.

3   A Call to the Particular: Contributions from Theology and Qualitative Research

1. Portions of this chapter that treat theological anthropology, qualitative research, and the particular method used in this research first appeared in an earlier publication. Reprinted, with numerous changes and editions, from Harvey et al., *Disrupting White Supremacy from Within* (full citation appears in chapter 1, note 10).

2. As mentioned in chapter 1, John Evans and Alan Verhey have shown that theological language has largely been removed from deliberations regarding human genetic engineering and other bioethical topics, a development they see as contributing to the thinning of the public debate.

3. See Harvey et al., *Disrupting White Supremacy from Within*.

4. One can glimpse the evolution of the modern hospital in Philippe Ariès, *Western Attitudes Toward Death: From the Middle Ages to the Present*, trans. Patricia M. Ranum (Baltimore: John Hopkins University Press, 1974).

5. Larry L. Rasmussen makes this point eloquently and cogently in his work. See, e.g., Larry L. Rasmussen, *Earth Community Earth Ethics* (New York: Orbis, 1996).

6. Ivone Gebara, *Out of the Depths: Women's Experience of Evil and Salvation* (Minneapolis: Fortress, 2002), 130. (Citation abbreviated hereafter as Gebara, *Out of the Depths*.)

7. Grace Jantzen contends, "Those who have seen themselves and the world about them as embodiment and self-manifestation of God are unlikely to continue to treat it in a vulgar way or feel it utterly alien or devoid of intrinsic significance and worth." Cited by Cynthia Moe-Lobeda, *Healing a Broken World: Globalization and God* (Minneapolis: Fortress, 2002), 113. (Citation abbreviated hereafter as Moe-Lobeda, *Healing a Broken World*.)

8. Up until relatively recently in the history of feminist theology, most white feminist theologians have not explicitly identified themselves as white when doing their work. Some may note it in a footnote or in the preface to a book, but when they do their theology, they tend to simply call it feminist and/or liberation theology (or eco-theology or gay theology). Race, however, is hidden. In contrast, feminists of color have been more intentional and self-aware in their identification. Black feminists tend to identify themselves as Womanist or Black feminist theologians and Latina feminists tend to identify themselves as Mujeristas, Latina Feminists, or Chicana Feminists, etc. Many white feminists are not as forthright in locating themselves racially and socioeconomically as their colleagues of color.

9. Cynthia Moe-Lobeda has shown how Luther's theo-ethical vision constitutes a vibrant resource for Earth ethics. She emphasizes how Luther's panentheism and deep appreciation for sensuality and the body help to make a case for a conversion to the earth—to the needs and requirements of all life on the planet as an expression of "neighborSlove" in Luther. Moe-Lobeda, *Healing a Broken World*, 112–113.

10. I want to thank my father for first igniting a love within me for Luther. He did so long ago as we drove on the back roads of rural, northern Minnesota.

11. I am indebted to eco-theologians such as Sallie McFague who point out that there is a danger inherent in this anthropological claim because it has been used to prioritize human life over and against all other life. See, e.g., Salle McFague, *The Body of God: An Ecological Theology* (Minneapolis: Fortress, 1993).

12. I also turn to Luther because as a white, middle-class, educated Lutheran in North America, I feel it is my calling to recover the social dimensions of Luther's theology and ethics. His writings, at times polemical, offended those in high positions precisely because he boldly challenged their ecclesial and civil authority. Yet predominant strains within Lutheran traditions in both western Europe and North America have often sidelined the social in Luther. I seek to draw out the social significance of his theological work and the way in Luther challenged not only religious structures and practices but societal ones as well.

13. See Luther's explication of Genesis 1:26–27. Martin Luther, *Lectures on Genesis*, vol. 1, *Luther's Works*, ed. Jaroslav Pelikan and trans. George V. Schick (St. Louis, MO: Concordia Publishing House, 1965), 60. (Citation abbreviated hereafter as *LW* 1.)

14. See, e.g., Ibid., 164–165.

15. Though not developed here, it is important to note that the paradox of seeing human beings as always "saint and sinner" plays a central role in Luther's anthropology. For Luther, the crucial dimension to the Fall revolves not around eating a fruit, sensuality or the body, or even in disobeying God. Rather, sin signals the human will turning away from God. All sin, all evil,

stems from the loss of trust in God. Moreover, it is by far the most devastating because it means that human beings stop putting their lives in God's hands and instead begin to fashion devices of self-salvation. Luther sees all around him confidence in human reason and abilities run amuck (evidenced by greed, arrogance, and corruption) especially in the ranks of ecclesial and civil authority. Given the importance Luther places on the pervasiveness of sin, it is important to note that he also continually emphasizes all that God does, through grace, to reach humanity. For examples of Luther's explication of sin, see *LW* 1, 114, 141–148, 162, 177–179.

16. Moe-Lobeda expresses this relationship well: "Ceasing to strive for godlike-ness and instead receiving the transformation inherent in justification, we are saved unto what we were intended to be: Fully *human* and finite beings on Earth, humans in communion through union with Christ, humans as Earth creatures assuming the form of Christ, servant of all." Moe-Lobeda, *Healing a Broken World*, 78. Emphasis hers.

17. For example,

> But now the Gospel has brought about the restoration of that image. Intellect and will indeed have remained, but both very much impaired. And so the Gospel brings it about that we are formed once more according to that familiar and indeed better image, because we are born again into eternal life or rather into the hope of eternal life by faith, that we may live in God and with God and be one with Him, as Christ says (John 17:21). (*LW* 1, 64)

18. See, e.g., Luther's 1519 essay, "The Blessed Sacrament of the Holy and True Body of Christ, and the Brotherhoods" in *Luther's Works, Word and Sacrament* I, vol. 35, ed. E. Theodore Bachman (Philadelphia: Muhlenberg, 1960), 58–61 and ff. See also "Heidleberg Disputation," "The Sacrament of the Body and Blood of Christ—Against the Fanatics," "Two Kinds of Righteousness," and "The Freedom of the Christian," all found in *Martin Luther's Basic Theological Writings*, ed. Timothy F. Lull (Minneapolis: Fortress, 1989). It is important to note that Luther discusses this reality in terms of Christians being Christ for their neighbor. To avoid sounding as if the aim is conversion of others, I have chosen to emphasize how human beings may be vehicles of grace, love, and right relationship, but not to impose Christology onto those who are not Christian.

19. His words are as follows:

> Many a person thinks he has a God and everything he needs when he has money and property; in them he trusts and of them he boasts so stubbornly and securely that he cares for no one. Surely such a man has a god—mammon by name, that is, money and possessions—on which he fixes his whole heart. It is the most common idol on earth . . .
>
> [This first commandment] requires that a man's whole heart and confi-dence be placed in God alone, and in no one else. To have God, you see, does not mean to lay hands upon him, or put him in a purse, or shut him up in a chest. We lay hold of him when our heart embraces him and clings to him. To cling to him with all our heart is nothing else than to entrust

ourselves to him completely. (Martin Luther, "Large Catechism," in *The Book of Concord: The Confessions of the Evangelical Lutheran Church*, ed. and trans. Theodore G. Tappert [Philadelphia, PA: Fortress, 1959], 365–366. [Citation abbreviated hereafter as Luther, "Large Catechism."])

20. Luther writes,

> This word, "You shall have no other gods," means simply, "You shall fear, love, and trust me as your one true God. Wherever a man's heart has such an attitude toward God, he has fulfilled this commandment and all the others . . . . [T]he First Commandment is the chief source and fountainhead from which all the others proceed; again, to it they all return and upon it they depend, so that end and beginning are linked and bound together. (Ibid., 409–410)

21. Ibid., 390–391.

22. See Luther's exposition of the seventh commandment, "You shall not steal":

> [A] person steals not only when he robs a man's strongbox or his pocket, but also when he takes advantage of his neighbor at the market, in a grocery shop, butcher stall, wine- and beer-cellar, work-shop, and, in short, wherever business is transacted and money is exchanged for goods or labor . . . .
>
> In short, thievery is the most common craft and the largest guild on earth . . .
>
> These men are called gentleman swindlers or big operators. Far from being picklocks and sneak-thieves who loot a cash box, they sit in office chairs and are called great lords and honorable, good citizens, and yet with a great show of legality they rob and steal. . . .
>
> Daily the poor are defrauded. New burdens and high prices are imposed. Everyone misuses the market in his own willful, conceited, arrogant way, as if it were his right and privilege to sell his goods as dearly as he pleases without a word of criticism. Luther, "Large Catechism," 395–397.

A full discussion of Luther's economic and social ethics is beyond the scope of this chapter. Suffice it to say that Luther's economic ethics were not only concerned with individual transactions. His ethical vision extended to the social structures of his day—inclusive of agricultural, religious, financial, mercantile, and political institutions. For example, he vigorously denounced the banking and international commerce systems emerging around him. See Carter Lindberg, *Beyond Charity: Reformation Initiatives for the Poor* (Minneapolis: Fortress, 1993); Moe-Lobeda, *Healing a Broken World*.

23. Moe-Lobeda, *Healing a Broken World*, 85. Emphasis hers.

24. These are the words of "Sophia Andre" and this insight will be discussed in more depth in chapter 5.

25. It can be challenging to argue for Luther's definitive stance regarding the nature and status of women. At points, he does no more than reiterate the androcentric views of his time, inherited from earlier male theologians and philosophers. What is remarkable is that he deviates at times from this tradition to make some rather fresh statements, which indict the patriarchal attitudes of

his day that "despise" women. For example, with regard to the story of Eve and Adam and those who have used it to justify the subjugation and inferiority of women, Luther writes the following: "This tale fits Aristotle's designation of woman as a 'maimed man,' others declare that she is a monster. But let them themselves be monsters and sons of monsters—these men who make malicious statements and ridicule a creature of God. . . ." *LW* 1, 70. Another example is with respect to Eve: "Then there is also something absurd in making Eve the lower part of reason, although it is sure that in no part, that is, neither in body nor in soul, was Eve inferior to her husband Adam." *LW* 1, 185. In several places, Luther affirms that Eve bears God's image equal to Adam and that she was given dominion over all the earth, with Adam, as a full partner. Even after the Fall, Luther claims, "Whatever the husband has, this the wife has and possesses in its entirety. Their partnership involves not only their means but children, food, bed, and dwelling; their purposes, too, are the same. The result is that the husband differs from the wife in no other respect than in sex; otherwise the woman is altogether a man." *LW* 1, 137.

26. To his credit, Luther never intended to construct theological formations for all times and places. He was a contextual and occasional writer—deliberately addressing concrete peoples, societies, and religious questions that were all embedded in a specific historical moment.

27. Moe-Lobeda explores these resonances. See Moe-Lobeda, *Healing a Broken World*, 107–114.

28. To call a given anthropology "androcentric" means that it was developed from a male point of view and uses male persons as the implicit or explicit frame of reference for understanding what it means to be human. Kari Elisabeth Børreson explains androcentrism as meaning "that a doctrine is developed from a male point of view: Woman is referred to as man, who is regarded as the exemplary sex; *vir* (man) and *homo* (human being) are considered identical." Kari Elisabeth Børreson, *Subordination and Equivalence: The Nature and Role of Women in Augustine and Thomas Aquinas*, trans. Charles H. Talbot (Washington, DC: University Press of America, 1981), xvi.

29. Beverly Harrison, *Making the Connections: Essays in Feminist Social Ethics*, ed. Carol S. Robb (Boston: Beacon, 1985), 17. (Citation abbreviated hereafter as Harrison, *Making the Connections*.)

30. See, e.g., Elizabeth Johnson, *She Who Is: The Mystery of God in Feminist Theological Discourse* (New York: Crossroad, 1992); Catherine Mowery LaCugna, *God for Us: The Trinity and Christian Life* (San Francisco: Harper Collins, 1991).

31. Carter Heyward, *Touching Our Strength: The Erotic as Power and the Love of God* (San Francisco: Harper and Row, 1989), 93–94. (Citation abbreviated hereafter as Heyward, *Touching Our Strength*.)

32. Beverly Harrison claims that even abstract reflection depends upon the sensual: "[W]e recognize that all our knowledge, including our moral knowledge, is body-mediated knowledge. All knowledge is rooted in our sensuality. We know and value the world . . . through our ability to touch, to hear, to see.

Perception is fundamental to conception. Ideas are dependent on our sensuality."
Harrison, *Making the Connections*, 13.

33. Heyward maintains that a key place to see the intersection of knowing and the body is with regard to sexuality. She maintains that sensuality and sexuality are sacred because they are ways in which we know and experience God. To make this claim, Heyward draws upon the groundbreaking work of Audre Lorde to argue that "[t]he erotic is our most fully embodied experience of the love of God. As such, it is the source of our capacity for transcendence, the 'crossing over' among ourselves, making connections between ourselves in relation. The erotic is the divine Spirit's yearning, through our bodyselves, toward mutually empowering relation." Heyward, *Touching Our Strength*, 99. See also Carter Heyward, *Our Passion for Justice: Images of Power, Sexuality, and Liberation* (Cleveland, OH: Pilgrim, 1984), 139–141. Human beings know and experience God within erotic power. The erotic can serve as a profound vehicle for human experiences of loving communion with one another and with God. See also Audre Lorde, "The Uses of the Erotic," in *Sister Outsider* (Freedom: Crossing Press, 1984).

34. See Mary John Mananzan, ed., *Women Resisting Violence: Spirituality for Life* (Maryknoll: Orbis, 1996).

35. Harrison, *Making the Connections*, 16.

36. Isabel Carter Heyward, *The Redemption of God: A Theology of Mutual Relation* (New York: University Press of America, 1982), 1. Heyward draws on the insights of Martin Buber here. (Citation abbreviated hereafter as Heyward, *Redemption of God*.)

37. "We work with our bodies, in our bodies, as bodies, sensual bodyselves working, playing, making love, making justice . . . [O]ur sensuality provides our relational grounding. It keeps us in touch with one another and with who we are." Heyward, *Touching Our Strength*, 193.

38. Ibid., 104.

39. "Our shared experience of relational power, our sacred experience of sensual power, our erotic experience of the power of God, is the root of our theological epistemology. It is the basis of our knowledge and love of God." Ibid., 99.

40. Heyward defines God as "our power in relation to each other, all humanity, and creation itself. God is creative power, that which effects justice—right relation—in history." Heyward, *Redemption of God*, 6. See also her definition of God in ibid., 188–190.

41. I am indebted to the works of scholars such as Williams, *Sisters in the Wilderness* (full citation appears in the preface chapter, note 2); emilie m. townes, *In a Blaze of Glory: Womanist Spirituality as Social Witness* (Nashville: Abingdon, 1995); Isasi-Díaz, *En La Lucha*. (Full citation appears in the preface chapter, note 2.)

42. Mary McClintock Fulkerson, *Changing the Subject: Women's Discourses and Feminist Theology* (Minneapolis: Fortress, 1994), 381. (Citation abbreviated hereafter as Fulkerson, *Changing the Subject*.)

43. Ibid., 382–383.

44. Ibid.,12.

45. One demarcation in white feminist theology stands between those influenced more by post-structuralism and critical theories (Catherine Keller, Serene Jones, Rebecca Chopp) and those who gravitate more toward making claims about essence of human identity and formulating norms that they claim have moral weight across differences (Elizabeth Johnson, Catherine LaCugna, Carter Heyward). White Catholic feminist ethicists such as Margaret Farley and Lisa Cahill argue for a kind of foundational sense of *imago dei* while others, such as Fulkerson, immersed in critical and/or poststructural theories contest such a stance. At their respective bests, these perspectives serve as correctives to each other. Serene Jones has made an insightful assessment of this debate. She finds that some feminist theologians are "on a rock" while others choose a "hard place":

> For those theologians who build their projects on universal, foundational rocks, their constructive work in the area of Christian doctrine is refreshingly solid, strong, accessible, and steadily visionary . . . For theologians who stand in the hard place, their work remains restless and, as yet, lacking in constructive solidity, marking a place of healthy instability. Looking behind truths, testing the strength of good, and pulling back edges in search of ever-retreating margins, these texts offer hope in the form of rupturing voices and more particularized graces.
>
> For those who stand on universalizing rocks, the challenge of women's experiences which do not "fit" into the generalized categories of phenomenology, process metaphysics, psychoanalysis, or literary narrative will no doubt continue to make these foundationalists uneasy. Likewise, the pragmatic demand for sturdy visions and faith-filled truths will not doubt continue to keep those who stand in the hard places of cultural anthropology and poststructuralism wanting more substance than their methods seem able to deliver. (Serene Jones, "Women's Experience Between a Rock and a Hard Place: Feminist, Womanist, and Mujerista Theologies in North America," in *Horizons in Feminist Theology: Identity, Tradition, and Norms*, ed. Rebecca Chopp and Sheila Greeve Davaney [Minneapolis: Fortress, 1997], 53. [Citation abbreviated hereafter as: *Horizons in Feminist Theology*.])

46. "I propose a feminist theology of affinity rather than identity or solidarity with the other. Affinity acknowledges love's inability to know the other, to resist domination of the other. Affinities rather than shared identities are the best we can hope for in developing feminist theology toward the respect for all subjects now defined as women and support for the end of dominations that texture their lives." Fulkerson, *Changing the Subject*, 384.

47. Fulkerson writes,

> What distinguishes any situation of Christian communally shaped practice . . . is not that Christians have beliefs that are true because they are not-human (i.e., authorized by God and therefore not subject to scrutiny), or because their claims to truth are confirmed by a second-order level of reflection. The distinction is found in the recognition that the truthfulness

of these reasons, rules, and values is tied to the visions of the good (however temporary) that come from communities, their traditions, and the practices they produce. Ibid., 374.

48. "What I propose for feminist theological use of the *imago Dei* is development of its strength—stories, rather than explanations." Mary McClintock Fulkerson, "Contesting the Gendered Subject: A Feminist Account of the *Imago Dei*," in *Horizons in Feminist Theology*, 114.

49. Moe-Lobeda, *Healing a Broken World*, 124. Earlier, Moe-Lobeda observes that "where moral agency is missing, the community has not properly maintained certain practices" Moe-Lobeda, *Healing a Broken World*, 94.

50. Fulkerson, *Changing the Subject*, 391.

51. M. Shawn Copeland, "Critical Theologies for the Liberation of Women," in *The Power of Naming: A Concilium Reader in Feminist Liberation*, ed. Elisabeth Schüssler Fiorenza (Maryknoll: Orbis, 1996), 72. (Citation abbreviated hereafter as Copeland, "Critical Theologies for the Liberation of Women.")

52. For Copeland, the term "feminist" must function in a way that serves to "pluralize, to destabilize, to dismantle, to problematize any propensity to asphyxiate or suppress difference in critical theologies committed to the radical liberation of women." Ibid., 71.

53. Ibid. She adds, "[C]ritical theologies affirm black, brown, red, yellow, white women in all their diversities, histories and cultures, even as they problematize those diversities. . . . As the exercise of rationality in theology, such interrogation, engagement and problematization is extended through the notion of *difference*, which has increasingly displaced the notion of *sisterhood* as a key theoretical tool in critical feminist theologies." Ibid.

54. Ibid., 73.

55. M. Shawn Copeland, "The New Anthropological Subject at the Heart of the Mystical Body of Christ," *CTSA PROCEEDINGS* 53(1998):30. (Citation abbreviated hereafter as Copeland, "The New Anthropological Subject.")

56. Ibid., 37.

57. Gebara, *Out of the Depths*, 142.

58. Notes taken from our conversation, November 21, 1999.

59. Several feminist theologians have called for ethnographic study in theology. See especially Isasi Díaz, *En La Lucha* (full citation appears in the preface, note 2); María Pilar Aquino, "Latina Feminist Theology," in *A Reader in Latina Feminist Theology: Religion and Justice*, ed. María Pilar Aquino, Daisy L. Machado, and Jeanette Rodriguez (Austin: University of Texas Press, 2002), 133–160; and Kelly Brown Douglas, *The Black Christ* (New York: Orbis, 1994).

60. Bent Flyvbjerg argues that the antagonistic debates and relations between natural and social scientists stem from a fundamental misunderstanding about what each contributes to knowledge and from judging one by the other's standards. See Bent Flyvbjerg, *Making Social Science Matter: How Social Inquiry Fails and How It Can Succeed Again* (New York: Cambridge University Press, 2001).

61. The pharmaceutical company, Merck, sold this painkiller even as it was aware of the drug's heart risks. It was found liable for the death of a man who had been

taking the drug. Carol Ernst, his widow, was awarded "$24.5 million for mental anguish and economic losses. . . . [and] an additional $229 million in punitive damages after finding that Merck acted recklessly in selling Vioxx despite having knowledge of the drug's heart risks." *The New York Times* article added that in Texas, punitive damages are automatically capped at $1.6 million, "meaning the overall award would not exceed $26.1 million and could be reduced by Texas appellate courts." See Alex Berenson, "Jury Calls Merck Liable in Death of Man on Vioxx," *The New York Times*, August 20, 2005, online at www.nytimes.com.

62. See Robert Yin, *Case Study Research: Design and Methods* (Thousand Oaks: Sage, 1994); Michael Burawoy et al., *Ethnography Unbound: Power and Resistance in the Modern Metropolis* (Berkeley: University of California Press, 1991); and Michael Burawoy, "The Extended Case Method," *Sociological Theory* 16(March 1988):4–33.

63. James P. Spradley, *The Ethnographic Interview* (New York: Holt, Rinehart, and Winston, 1979), 10–11. (Citation abbreviated hereafter as Spradley, *The Ethnographic Interview*.) From *The Ethnographic Interview*, 1st edition, by Spradley 1979. Reprinted with permission of Wadsworth, a division of Thomson Learning: www.thomsonrights.com.

64. Mindy Fullilove, unpublished handbook for qualitative research for classroom use, 9. *The Little Handbook*, ed. Thompson Fullilove, created for use of the QRM 101 class, Mailman School of Public Health, Columbia University, New York, NY © 2001.

65. Akin to the significance of theological anthropology already discussed, a similar corrective in the conceptualizations in secular philosophy and the natural sciences is crucial because these generalizations and assumptions have concrete and devastating effects upon real lives as well. For example, missionary, colonialist, and anthropologist descriptions of Africans and Indigenous Americans routinely justified slavery, imprisonment, or displacement based on anthropological arguments. In dividing up the revenues of taxes and the right to representation by the new government, the framers of the Constitution designated African slaves as three-fifths of a person. In sum, for over 200 years, the majority of "scholars," "men of the cloth," "statesmen," "doctors," and "scientists" persuasively argued, to the benefit of the new world order/church/ new republic/white landowner/settler, that Africans, descendents of Africans and Indigenous peoples were not fully or equally human. Even as slavery and segregation are legally abolished in this country, white ethnocentric and paternalistic assessments of African, Middle Eastern, Eastern, and Latino cultures/peoples still deny their full humanity, either implicitly or explicitly. For example, they help to enable and justify the prolonged detention of persons from the Middle East in both U.S. jails and Guantánamo Bay along with the immigration policies and practices that police the Mexican-U.S. border. For further reading, see Harvey et al., *Disrupting White Supremacy from Within*.

66. In New York City, in February 1999, Amadou Diallo was killed by an "elite" police force designed to aggressively patrol "high-risk" drug areas. Mistaking his wallet for a gun, the officers shot at Diallo 41 times in rapid succession when he attempted to show them his identification; 18 bullets struck him.

67. Spradley, *The Ethnographic Interview*, 29. Emphasis mine.

68. Comments to the qualitative research methods writing group, February 4, 2004, New York NY; taken from field notes.

69. "By word and action, in subtle ways and direct statements, [ethnographers] say 'I want to understand the world from your point of view. I want to know what you know in the way you know it. I want to understand the meaning of your experience, to walk in your shoes, to feel things as you feel them, to explain things as you explain them. Will you become my teacher and help me understand?' " Spradley, *The Ethnographic Interview*, 34.

70. Indeed, many weeks in the streets of New York and Chicago, I witness white people becoming quickly indignant (and sometimes outraged) when we are not. Embedded within white identity is a sense of entitlement. For further reading, see Harvey et al., *Disrupting White Supremacy from Within*.

71. Loic Wacquant distinguishes Bourdieu's notion of reflexivity from others in this manner:

> Bourdieu's brand of reflexivity, which may be cursorily defined as the inclusion of a theory of intellectual practice as an integral component and necessary condition of a critical theory of society, differs from others in three crucial ways: First, its primary target is not the individual analyst but the *social and intellectual unconscious* embedded in analytic tools and operations; second, it must be a *collective enterprise* rather than the burden of the lone academic; and third, it seeks not to assault but to *buttress the epistemological security of sociology.* Far from trying to undermine objectivity, Bourdieu's reflexivity aims at increasing the scope and solidity of social scientific knowledge, a goal which puts it at loggerheads with phenomenological, textual, and other "postmodern" forms of reflexivity. (Pierre Bourdieu and Loic J.D. Wacquant, *Invitation to Reflexive Sociology* [Chicago: University of Chicago Press, 1992], 36–37. Emphasis Wacquant's.)

72. Ibid., 236.

73. Ibid., 39.

74. Wacquant summarizes the meaning of Bourdieu's reflexivity in this way: It entails . . . the systematic exploration of the "unthought categories of thought which delimit the thinkable and predetermine the thought" (Bourdieu, 1982a: 10), as well as guide the practical carrying out of social inquiry. The "return" it calls for extends beyond the experiencing subject [meaning the researcher] to encompass the organizational and cognitive structure of the discipline. What has to be constantly scrutinized and *neutralized, in the very act of construction of the object,* is the collective scientific unconscious embedded in theories, problems, and (especially national) categories of scholarly judgment (Bourdieu, 1990j). Ibid., 40. Emphasis Waquant's.

75. Spradley, *The Ethnographic Interview*, 14.

76. In 1976, in his discussion on strategies for revitalizing American culture, Spradley suggested several priorities for strategic research. Priority number one was "A healthcare system that provides adequate care for all members of the society." Ibid., 15.

77. These included one oncologist, one oncology nurse, one nurse case manager, two social workers, and one third-year medical student.

78. I transcribed the Spanish interviews myself. A professional transcriptionist transcribed the interviews in English, which I then went through line by line while listening to the recording and making corrections.

79. I am profoundly grateful to Dr. Mindy Fullilove and to the qualitative methods writing group she began for sharing so graciously their expertise in the collection and analysis of qualitative data. In addition, in a sense they were advocates for me with respect to the IRB process.

80. I also want to acknowledge that Dr. Linda Barnes was very helping in reviewing my IRB protocol and in making constructive suggestions for its improvement. Her advice was also key in addressing IRB concerns.

81. Comment made in the qualitative methods writing group, personal notes taken December 10, 2003. She later added, "I'm just a simple practitioner, not a grand practitioner. But, listening respectfully has great value for health studies and academia. People will tell you a lot." Along these lines, she referred me to a helpful article by Ruth Behar that powerfully tells the story of one Latina after having a hysterectomy. See Ruth Behar, "My Mexican Friend Marta Who Lost Her Womb on This Side of the Border," *Journal of Women's Health* 2, no. 1 (1993): 85–89.

82. See Dunn and Chadwick, *Protecting Study Volunteers in Research*, 23–24, 48–50 (full citation appears in chapter 1, note 16). For example, they stipulate that "[w]ithin the limitations imposed by the population of the study site(s), research should include sufficient enrollment of persons of diverse racial/ethnic backgrounds in order to ensure that the benefits and burdens of research participation are distributed in an equitable manner." Ibid.

83. Of the MDs, 1 also has a PhD in Neurology, 4 are Attending Physicians, 4 are Assistant Attending Physicians, and 9 are Associate Attending Physicians. Of the PhDs, 1 is in Psychiatry, 1 is in Psychology in Pediatrics and Psychiatry, and 1 is in Physics in Clinical Radiology. The Ad Hoc member is reported as having a MSc, PhD, Dipl in Mental Health.

84. I am not alone in having such an encounter with an IRB. See Elizabeth Herdman, "Pearls, Pith, and Provocation: Reflections on 'Making Somebody Angry,' " *Qualitative Health Research* 10, no. 5(September 2000):691–702.

85. IRB rejection letter, March 19, 2003.

86. In a related vein, the IRB did not like the wording of the recruitment flyer I had submitted because they felt it was negatively biased. They objected to two of the four questions on it: "What does good quality care look and feel like to you?" and "How do you want to be treated by your doctor, nurse, social worker, etc.?" Later, in their second letter asking for further clarification on the protocol (which I received after I had met in person with the committee), they noted that the flyer "may still be considered as somewhat 'inflammatory' and suggesting that Black and Latina women, in particular, may have some complaints about their medical care." IRB written response to the protocol, May 5, 2003. The appendix contains a copy of the flyer used in the recruitment of study participants.

87. Some scholarship has emphasized the importance of people telling their stories as part of recovering from illness. For example, see Arthur Kleinman, *The Illness Narratives: Suffering, Healing and the Human Condition* (San Francisco: Basic Books, 1988).

88. Several months before my meeting with the IRB, I had met individually with this particular IRB member on the recommendation of the chaplain. At that time, she did not raise objections to my topic, but it was clear that she had a very different idea of the approach I should use. For example, she recommended the use of set questionnaires and standardized research tools to ascertain whether any participant was depressed.

89. Field notes following our conversation, April 28, 2003. He emphasized again that it was a "clash of worlds, power, and self interest." Also, he noted that it takes time to "come to grips with new understanding . . . As an outsider, you're being taken with more seriousness and time than any other protocol." He stressed that some members were trying hard to understand. According to him, at one point one of the senior members of the committee said, "We need to have lectures on qualitative research. I don't know that much about it."

90. I should credit Clifford Geertz with the term "thick description." See Clifford Geertz, *The Interpretation of Cultures* (New York: Harper, 1973).

91. In reflecting on the IRB rejection letter, Mindy Fullilove remarked, "They're teaching you how they treat vulnerable populations. Silencing—that's what this letter is all about. They're teaching you about their hospital. So who's there to stand up for the Black and Latina women? This interaction reveals the workings of the system." She makes the connection more strongly than me, but her thoughts have been provocative for my own self-reflection. Field notes from qualitative methods writing group, March 26, 2003.

92. Indeed, if there are ways in which to utilize a sense of *imago dei* or neighbor-love within non-western and non-Christian contexts for the purpose of creating better quality healthcare, it is absolutely critical that nonacademic, non-western, non-Christian people—particularly members of subjugated races, classes, and sexual identities—be integral participants and agents in the dialogue and formulation.

4   Listening

1. The oncologist is a white male who identifies as Italian American; the oncology nurse is a Black woman originally from Jamaica, the nurse case manager identifies as an African American woman; the two social workers are both white women. One identified her racial-ethnic background as Irish Catholic and the other first commented that she is "white middle class, unfortunately," but then added that she is actually part Spanish—part Basque; the medical student identifies as a Puerto Rican woman.

2. To be even more precise, one of the two Dominican women sees herself as most intimately African Caribbean.

3. Hannah Jacobs, interview by author, New York, NY, June 18, 2003. Hannah has the distinction of being the first person I interviewed.

4. A lumpectomy is the removal of a portion of the breast that contains cancerous tissue. A mastectomy is the complete removal of the breast. Chemotherapy is a nonsurgical treatment involving chemicals given intravenously which kill cancer cells (along with healthy cells).

5. Wanda Kelly, interview by author, New York, NY, August 12, 2003.

6. Her husband is in the military and is often stationed away from home for long periods at a time. Wanda commented that his absence can be stressful—both logistically and emotionally for her and her son.

7. María de Lourdes Maldonado, interview by author, New York, NY, August 23, 2003.

8. Luz Hernandez, interview by author, New York, NY, August 24, 2003.

9. One of the things that initially impressed me about Luz is that she offered to show her mastectomy scar to a newly diagnosed woman in a cancer support group. She conveyed pride and a total lack of shame regarding this symbol of survival and life. She adamantly proclaimed that she does not miss that breast, that she does not need it any longer.

10. From Luz's description, I take "clean-up" to mean a cleaning of the area—taking out any visible cancer tissues. I am not sure if this procedure would be considered a lumpectomy or if it is less extensive than that.

11. Luz is determined but not hardened or cynical by the various challenges she has encountered in her life. She advocates for herself by staying grounded in love—for herself, for God, for her family. She gives herself credit for her initiative and hard work. Being feisty is a part of her survival strategy, and it has served her well.

12. Marcela Rodriguez, interview by author, New York, NY, September 5, 2003.

13. From her description, that they "put in a needle to take out [liquid]," I am not sure if the name of the procedure was aspiration or biopsy. In talking about it, she used the term "*biopsia*."

14. Slimfat Girl, interview by author, New York, NY, August 25, 2003.

15. I did not specifically ask her age, so this is a guess.

16. Sandra Gavin, interview by author, New York, NY, August 4, 2003.

17. Sophia Andre, interview by author, New York, NY, August 27, 2003.

18. Sophia's grandmother raised her and her siblings because her mother died when she was six years old. Sophia described growing up in her grandmother's care with much affection. Her grandmother subsequently died at home on December 8, 2003.

19. This diagnosis means that the cancer appeared again in the same breast and is in the lymph nodes, but has not appeared in any other regions or organs of the body. Breast cancer is diagnosed between stages one and four.

20. Several of the women had interesting insights into what dignity and respect look and feel like and how these concepts are related to their faith in God. This thinking represents more of a meta-reflection than a telling of their concrete experiences. I will discuss these perspectives in chapter 5.

21. COBRA, a federal law makes it possible for an employee (and/or their spouse/dependents) of a company with more than 20 employees to continue their health insurance coverage for 18 months (36 months for the dependent) after their employment is lost (if they are fired, laid off, or if the business closes) or after mandatorily losing health coverage for another reason (e.g., divorce, marriage of a dependent, a dependent turning 23 years old). The catch is that the person/family member must pay all the costs (premiums, deductibles, copayments) for this coverage each month.

22. Initially, Sandra did not tell the doctors at this clinic that she is a nurse and holds an advanced degree. She explained, "I wanted to be just an ordinary person, you know, at that point, because I really wasn't asking for any special treatment. And I think, too, I felt sort of ashamed because here I am, a nurse, an educator, an administrator, and I do something like this, you know, I let my insurance go, you know."

23. Within two months, Sandra went from being uninsured to being enrolled in her school's insurance. If only all U.S. inhabitants were not permitted to be uninsured the way some graduate students are.

24. Translation: Racism, brutality, and a lack of consideration—of each a bit.

25. Lucy Bristol, interview by author, New York, NY, August 20, 2003.

26. Lucy gave this example as well:

> Well, I remember recently we had this African American woman, and she was very angry because, like, nobody would talk to her, the doctors. You know, they would be—she was very sick. And she was an intelligent woman, which they didn't take the time to find out. You know, they just felt that, I don't know, maybe looking at her—I don't know . . . And they would order tests and procedures, and nobody would talk to her. You know, nobody was telling her what was going on. You know, and she was in a lot of pain, and she would get frustrated . . . so people saw her as being demanding. But she was more or less just frustrated.

27. Lucy and Beef Stew (an African American nurse case manager) both noted the fact that they, as healthcare providers of color, also contend with others' racial assumptions. For example, some new patients assume Lucy is a nurse's aide. Some have gone so far as to refer to her as "the girl." Both Lucy and Beef Stew acknowledged that they sometimes experience a distinctive "attitude" from some white patients—condescending, not trusting, rude—that they try to break through in order to care for them. Also, both noted examples of discrimination and prejudice that can still happen among the hospital employees/ management. They cited, e.g., more staff of color working night shifts, having to work harder to be promoted or to be entrusted with additional responsibilities. In short, they think that racism is alive and well but that it is better hidden—that people are less likely to verbalize things. When I asked Lucy to tell me what it looks like, she said: "It's not being promoted. Not being recognized for really what you're worth. Having to work harder. Having to prove yourself consistently. It's still there. . . . [I]t's just not exposed the way it used to be years ago."

28. A PEG tube is an intravenous feeding and hydration tube used with patients who are not getting adequate nutrition by mouth.

29. Antonia Morales, interview by author, New York, NY, November 5, 2003. I should note that Antonia does not specialize in care for cancer patients, although she has encountered cancer care on her rotations through different departments. Consequently, the encounters to which she refers do not pertain specifically to cancer patients. In addition to classes, much of her time is spent in clinical settings. She relates to patients directly, e.g., by taking medical histories and she observes physicians' interactions with patients. Over the course

of her rigorous training and long hours, she has taken note of how hospitals work. Her general observation about the state of healthcare was this:

> I was expecting so much more. And in reality there are a lot of areas that it's a completely open field, and that patients get really whatever they need and whatever they want. But there are some—sometimes it's very difficult for patients to get what they really need. And I'm noticing that sometimes—there are sometimes priorities. For whatever reason, whether it be health insurance, whether it be language barriers, there are a lot of barriers. And they're barriers that, you know, come from one side, that come from just basically communication, or just come from actually administrative or bureaucratic barriers.

30. In reflecting on this interaction, Antonia remarked, "So I don't know, I think that sometimes, you know, would it have been different if it was somebody else who had come in, you know, from a different educational level, you know, or a different—some assumed educational level? I think that [making assumptions based on stereotypes] happens. But it has no place. It just is a lack of respect."

31. Beef Stew, interview by author, New York, NY, August 13, 2003.

32. Beef Stew has also witnessed patients of color ringing the call bell several times and staff at the desk responding, "She can wait. She doesn't really need it," whereas a "VIP" will only have to ring once. She expressed her great frustration with such occurrences:

> It puts my panties in a bunch when I see patients that are . . . not getting treated the same way as a Caucasian person who has great insurance, who is endowing the facility with money so that they get that private room . . . that really pisses me off. . . . But I'm just saying, how dare you? You are supposed to be giving care and treating people equally, and you're in a position to give something that is so precious and so needed. But because this patient shares your ethnicity and, oh by the way, is paying this amount of money and has great insurance and what have you, you're going to treat them so much better, versus the patient who really needs it.

33. Her words were as follows: "I've seen simple things like they want to get a room ready. That patient might be going home. And they have an admission coming in. And I've seen them, they will take the patient and put the patient to sit in the solarium. Where there are other people who say, 'No, I'm not leaving 'til my family members come.' And they will still need that bed for an admission, and that patient stays in the room. . . . It's usually people of color that they put in the solarium."

34. Another explanation could be that the doctor was not comfortable in facing her emotions. One of the white social workers, Rebecca Williams, observed that in her experience, doctors "are not trained enough to deal with death—with their own view of death. And if you don't have your own acceptance of death, you're not going to be able to relate to these people. You're not going to want to. There's a lot of avoidance that goes on, a lot of detachment that goes on." Rebecca Williams, interview by author, New York, NY, August 13, 2003.

35. Luz credited the nurse as being another "feisty woman," originally from Cuba who, like Luz, had been determined to "beat the strikes against her" and get an education.

36. "Automated attendant" is the term used for the computerized telephone trees commonly utilized by businesses and large institutions to route incoming telephone calls.

37. Benedict Carey, "In the Hospital, a Degrading Shift from Person to Patient," *The New York Times,* August, 16, 2005, online: www.nytimes.com.

38. She explained, "For instance, let's say we have a patient in an acute care setting like this facility. And they really don't need the services. Yes, they're sick enough; but these services can be rendered at another level of care, for instance, a skilled nursing facility, or a hospice, or at home with home care. Basically, I, and with the team, determine what the level of care is, and basically how soon we can facilitate the transition from an acute care setting to an alternative level of care. I basically am the eyes of the facility. . . ."

39. "[T]he bottom line is a necessary evil that we have to deal with, O.K.? Now, what I do is manipulate the benefit package or the insurance package to get the patient everything that they need within it."

40. She explained that the hospital in which she works is not equipped for hospice care, e.g., and that patients who are dying benefit much more from being either in a home or institutional hospice setting than on the unit.

41. Rebecca Williams, interview by author, New York, NY, August 13, 2003.

42. Leonard Orlando, interview by author, New York, NY, September 3, 2003.

43. For further information, call (202)-224–3121 and ask to be transferred to "Member Services." The staff person explained that these policies and regulations are spelled out in the Public Law, specifically in the U.S. Code, Title 5, chapters 83–84.

44. Leonard later came back to this topic to say that if he had to identify with a particular culture, it would be the culture of physicians. When asked, he described this culture to me in detail (see the endnote in chapter 2 for this quotation). In a related vein, he also commented that, for him, the hardest type of patient is another doctor because you cannot fake what you do not know. This situation has the tendency to make him more self-conscious. I found this comment to be revealing as well.

45. Kaiser Family Foundation, *National Survey of Physicians*, March 2002, online: www.kff.org/minorityhealth/20020321a-index.cfm.

46. Ibid.

47. For example, see Anne Faidman, *The Spirit Catches You and You Fall Down: A Hmong Child, her American Doctors, and the Collision of Two Cultures* (New York: Farrar, Straus, and Giroux, 1997).

48. Kathleen O'Brian, interview by author, New York, NY, August 13, 2003.

5 Resisting Death, Celebrating Life: Christian Social Ethics for Healthcare

1. Lucille Clifton, *The Book of Light* (Port Townsend, WA: Copper Canyon, 1993), 25. Lucille Clifton's "won't you celebrate with me" from *The Book of Light.* Coperight © 1993 by Lucille Clifton. Reprinted with permission of Copper Canyon Press, P.O. Box 271, Port Townsend, WA 98368-0271.

2. In a future project, I hope to explore theological understandings of what it means to be human and of the human relationship to God of other religions, particularly in Islam, Judaism, and Hinduism.

3. Sandra Gavin explained that she was raised in the Black Church, but is no longer an active member. She did not specifically identify herself as Christian, although she played Christian music the one time I was in her car. Sandra said that she believes in a higher power, but that she has a lot of issues with the church, particularly the Black Church. She explained that she has problems with how many ministers are male while most of the active members are women and how ministers use women—she emphasized that she "uses the term 'use' loosely"—to serve a variety of functions in the church. She shared with me that her form of prayer is to ask her mother, as if she were still alive, to pray for her.

4. Given that the women are speaking of their personal faith and out of respect for it, I will not alter their language for God. When I refer to the divine, I will use gender-neutral terminology.

5. In Spanish, Marcela said, "Y gracias a Él me siento, me estoy sintiendo bien de bien, gracias a Dios. Yo agradezco este Dios que está arriba porque a eso todos los días le pido." The Spanish used when speaking about God and faith is more beautiful than my translation renders. So I have decided to include original phrasings in places so that Spanish speakers may compare it with my translation.

6. Her words in Spanish: "Pienso que Él es el apoyo, donde nosotros nos refugiamos, que si uno lo busco, si nosotros lo buscamos día tras día, Él nos va a apoyar siempre—incondicionalmente."

7. This quality seems important given that so many in the United States, as evidenced by the surge in sales and the size of spirituality books and products, are searching for meaning in their lives, even (or perhaps especially) the healthy, educated, and affluent in society. It is ironic that some who suffer so much are able to draw upon faith and hope that help to sustain them while others who may have less threatening life circumstances experience malaise.

8. Her words in Spanish are as follows:

   Siempre o sea Dios dice que Él es amor, ¿verdad? Y por lo tanto tiene que vivir en cada uno de nosotros. Si uno dice que uno ama supone es porque conoce a Dios. Entonces, Dios dice vamos a amarnos uno a otro, querernos. El amor es tanto significado que es, como te digo, algo no se puede ni siquiera definir. Entonces, vamos a amarnos, respetarnos, apoyarnos uno a otro para que así Dios se refleje en cada uno de nosotros.

9. Wanda credited being raised in the church for grounding her in an ability to love and respect others. She articulates the connection this way:

   I've always had a strong background in the church and been raised in the church since I was a little girl, and have always been raised to try to do, you know, the right thing, and treat other people with dignity and with the love of God. And so I think that that plays an important part for me because I want to always treat people the way that they're supposed to be treated, with respect and dignity and the love of Christ and having them see that Christ-like example within me. And that helps me to just be able to really work with people and to deal with people and to relate to people, just having a spiritual upbringing.

10. In Spanish, the dialogue went like this:

MR: Bueno, por lo menos la dignidad de uno es yo digo como algo . . . que levanta a tu auto estima . . . Pero por lo menos tú tienes este auto estima alto, eso te levanta todo—lo que tú piensas de ti misma es lo que ayuda tener buena dignidad.

AV: Entonces dignidad no es de otra persona, que ellos le dan. Es lo que tiene dentro de si misma.

MR: Claro, porque yo pienso que por lo menos tú . . . tienes que seguir en como ellos te van a tratar. Por eso, yo no sé, no me quiero definir como una persona diferente a todo los demás. Pero, si yo, por lo menos, trato de cuando tengo mi derecho—saber como voy a seguir para que esa persona no tenga el derecho de ofenderme de hacerme sentir mal. . . .

AV: Pero ellos no tienen el derecho de hacerlo tampoco.

MR: No, no tienen el derecho de hacerlo, hacer sentir mal. Pero no son ellos que me van a solucionar ese problema, soy yo.

AV: Y usted tiene que tener la dignidad dentro de si misma que no—que es una forma de protección—para protegerse contra estas influencias y es—no pueden robar esta dignidad porque es propiedad de usted.

MR: Sí exactamente.

AV: Y pueden enseñar respeto o no, pero la dignidad es su cosa—parte de su identidad—no depende de ellos.

MR: Sí, exactamente. No depende de ellos. *Depende de tí.* La dignidad depende de tí. Pero sobre todo, tienes que mantenerla siempre aunque pase lo que pase, ir para allá.

11. Specifically, María named Share and Cancer Care as two organizations that have been very important to her.

12. This and the previous quotation in Spanish is given below:

Sí, pero pienso que por lo menos áun sea un sitio de empleo hay que pensar si va a relacionar con la otra persona, como ser humano y que este ser humano está pasando por una situación difícil, en este momento deber olividarse que es un empleo. ¿Me entiendes? Esta persona está pasando por un momento difícil y necesita ayuda, sobre de todo apoyo. No se puede pensar que eso es como si fuera—que estoy haciendo eh—mueble. "Voy a hacer mueble, voy a tirar mueble allí." Eso no, es como cuando usted coge un mueble y ponerlo allí—coger a una persona checquerla y vete—no. Yo creo que los doctores tienen que conpenetrarse con el paciente. Por de una u otra manera, muchas veces el paciente no dice exactamente lo que es, simplemente lo que se siente. A veces no quiere hablar, a veces es timido. Por una u otra razón, no quiere decir exactamente lo que está sintiendo. . . . Y tiene [el doctor] por lo menos un poco de psycologia—se puede dar cuenta de algo pero si no, si se ve simplemente como un mueble que está fabricando—pues, tira el mueble para allí y coger otro mueble. . . .

13. townes, *Breaking the Fine Rain of Death*, 175 (full citation appears in the preface chapter, note 3).

14. Field notes, qualitative methods writing group, June 18, 2003.

15. Since I began this research, it has been pointed out to me a few times (interestingly always by white academics or professionals) that white working class,

the white poor, and whites living in rural areas also suffer a lack of healthcare due to socioeconomic assumptions and barriers. Undeniably, these lighter skinned populations are at risk and merit attention. However, the fact that they too are vulnerable ought not be used to deny or obscure the particular vulnerabilities of darker skinned communities.

16. For examples of this curriculum, see Purnell and Paulanka, *Transcultural Health Care* (full citation appears in chapter 2, note 75); Bonder et al., *Culture in Clinical Care* (full citation appears in chapter 2, note 75).

17. Good and Good et al., "The Culture of Medicine and Racial, Ethnic, and Class Disparities in Healthcare," 620 (full citation appears in chapter 2, note 133).

18. Wanda emphasized that hospital leadership needs to a lead in making the changes part of the institutional culture:

> [W]hen I worked in a hospital, we used to speak with the interns. And the first thing the social workers would do was, you know, give them a speech. And then, you know, they would leave and go to their—through their own same old stuff. But then they had doctors who were over them, teaching them, who didn't have bedside manners. So, I mean, you would need to get to the root of it, you know, the top doctors who are doing the teaching.

19. Beef Stew later commented,

> When you put money, and when you put power behind that change? . . . When you make the price high enough that when you don't do it, you're going to feel it, guess what, change is going to come. And that change will happen when you get a black head nurse, when you get a Hispanic CEO, when you an Asian board of trustees. . . . O.K., when you start reflecting diversity that way, on a high level, then guess what, that's when the change is going to come. Until then, you can put all the black staff nurses and all the Asian doctors and Hispanic whatever, anywhere you want.

20. *Associated Press*, "Report Urges Diversity in Health Jobs," February 5, 2004. They cite from newly published Institute of Medicine Report, *In the Nation's Compelling Interest: Ensuring Diversity in the Health Care Workforce*, online: http://www.iom.edu.

21. The Sullivan Commission on Diversity in the Healthcare Workforce, *Missing Persons: Minorities in the Health Professions*, published September 2004, 2, online: www.sullivancomission.org.

22. Smedley et al., *Unequal Treatment*, 114 (full citation occurs in chapter 1, note 2).

23. Robert Pear, "Taking the Spin Out of Report that Made Bad into Good Health" (full citation appears in chapter 2, note 139).

24. Recall the following article: Geiger, "Why is HHS Obscuring a Health Care Gap?" (full citation appears in chapter 2, note 137).

25. Good and Good et al., "The Culture of Medicine and Racial, Ethnic, and Class Disparities in Healthcare," 599.

26. Beef Stew confided,

> I will say—and maybe this is a bias—but I will say that, when I see a person of color, and it doesn't have to be a African American, can be Hispanic,

Asian, you know, Middle Eastern person, anyone, a person of color who is especially disadvantaged, like may have Medicaid, no insurance, worker's comp, no fault, I tell you, I do go out of my way and work a little harder in regards to making sure that they understand the process. Because usually people that may be disadvantaged or indigent, poverty-stricken, maybe not educated and affluent, they don't know the process. And sometimes they're lost in it. Versus people who have really good insurance, you know, and who are rich and everything, and are affluent, well, they know the system.

27. Katherine Boo, "Letter from South Texas: The Churn," *The New Yorker*, March 29, 2004, 72.
28. emilie townes explores models of care that developed within and are particularly attuned to African American communities. Her analysis offers important alternatives to western cultural productions of health and also includes several constructive examples of African American community programs and education strategies. See townes, *Breaking the Fine Rain of Death*, 147–167.
29. While I do not know the specifics of her prior company's situation or firing, it is reasonable to entertain the possibility that the high costs of health insurance for full-time employees figured into, at least in part, the company's decision to cut back on staff numbers. If this were the case, it highlights the fact that in present healthcare and business climates, even those who are presently insured are not exempt from the threat of losing such coverage at any time.
30. For a thorough analysis of this reality, see Catherine Hoffman and Susan Starr Sered, *Threadbare: Holes in America's Health Care Safety Net*, published by the Henry J. Kaiser Family Foundation, The Kaiser Commission on Medicaid, and the Uninsured (November 2005), 1–30, online: http://www.kff.org/uninsured/7245.cfm.
31. Leonard's internal conflict on the matter of universal health coverage was apparent:

> [I]f everyone is flatly salaried, then regardless of what you do, either in quantity or quality, then the forces are in place to do as little as possible . . . However, having said that, I think that we really all should be salaried, that there should be some kind of universal infrastructure, so that as physicians we are adequately compensated, and then have a little bit less or fewer administrative hassles. So, I do think that we need some type of national, you know if not, you know, national health insurance, some type of national healthcare system where we are adequately and appropriately compensated. . . .

32. Pitt et al., *Closing the Gap*, 1–66 (full citation appears in chapter 1, note 10).
33. Spradley, *The Ethnographic Interview*, 3 (full citation appears in chapter 3, note 63).
34. Ibid., 4.
35. Ibid., 18–22.
36. Ibid., 24.
37. Moe-Lobeda, *Healing a Broken World*, 121 (full citation appears in chapter 3, note 7).

38. She writes, "In this solidarity, the Creator is worshipped, the *humanum* honored, particularity engaged, difference appreciated. Solidarity affirms the interconnectedness of human be-ing in common creatureliness . . . Humanity is one intelligible reality—multiple, diverse, varied and concrete, yet one." Copeland, "The New Anthropological Subject," 42 (full citation appears in chapter 3, note 55).

39. Ibid., 31–32.

40. See Jennifer Harvey, PhD dissertation, *The Moral Crisis of "Being White" and the Imperative of Reparations*, Union Theological Seminary in New York, New York, NY (Submitted and Defended April 2004).

41. On this point, Beef Stew encouraged me to see the film, *A Day in Black and White*, which treats the differences in perception between Black and white people.

42. Wanda continued,

> And I think that's what helps me, that I can look at myself and say I don't want to be like that; or if I did something, I can just, you know, pray about it, and ask God to forgive me for that, and change, you know, work towards the changing, you know, because I am not perfect. And I pray every day that when I walk out of my house, that I could, you know, I would treat people with respect, that I will not look down upon people, you know, wherever—wherever I'm working and wherever I'm going . . . Or, if I did something to someone, you know, that may have offended them, I can go to them and just, you know apologize or something like that.

43. Heyward, *Touching Our Strength*, 9–10. (First full citation appears in chapter 3.)

44. Margaret Farley, "A Feminist Version of Respect for Persons," in *Feminist Ethics and the Catholic Moral Tradition*, Readings in Moral Theology, no. 9, ed. Charles Curran and Margaret Farley (New York: Paulist, 1996), 179.

45. Copeland, "The New Anthropological Subject," 34–35.

Concluding Words for Beginning: (Re)Creating the World through Scholarship

1. Laurie Zoloth, "Heroic Measures: Just Bioethics in an Unjust World," *Hastings Center Report*, 31, no. 6 (November–December 2001):34–40.

2. Gebara, *Out of the Depths*, 96 (full citation appears in chapter 3, note 6).

3. Ibid., 142.

4. Quoted by Geiger, "Why is HHS Obscuring a Health Care Gap?"(full citation appears in chapter 2, note 137).

Index

access to healthcare, 28–35
  "axis of (in)access" and, 34–5
  defining, 28
  healthcare quality and, 28–35
  language barriers and, 37–43
  news stories concerning, 29–35
  provider bias and, 33–4
  research findings concerning,
    35–7
accountability
  collaborators first and, 96
  commitment to follow-up and
    feedback, 95
  nuance of description and, 95–6
  positive transformation of society
    and, 96–8
  in qualitative research, 92–8
  of reflexive mode of study, 92–4
  of white feminists, 81
  of white people, xxii, 81
advocacy, see patient advocacy
affinity
  of healthcare provider for patient,
    44–6, 47–8, 58
  medical gaze and, 44–6, 47–8
affirmative action, 4
Afghanistan, military spending in,
  32–3
Africa, compliance with AIDS
  therapy in, 33–4, 228n55
African Americans, see Black people;
  Black women facing breast
  cancer

Agency for Healthcare Research and
  Quality (AHRQ), 57–8, 158
aggressive treatment, racial-ethnic
  disparities in, 36
Aguirre-Molina, Marilyn, 60–1
alienation
  discrimination and, xvii
  healthcare disparities and,
    56, 58
Andre, Sophia, 72, 137–45
  advocacy and, 144–5
  bureaucracy\fee issues and, 143–4,
    164–5
  chemotherapy trial, 142–3
  on Christian theology and
    healthcare, 213–14
  continuity and choice of health
    care, 197–8
  described, 125–6
  gratitude of, 173, 176–7
  interplay of racial and
    socioeconomic assumptions,
    138–41, 147, 186–7
  opinions about healthcare system,
    199–200
  power dynamic between patient
    and healthcare providers,
    141–3, 151–2, 186–7
androcentrism, 78, 242n28
anti-Semitism
  in Holocaust, 72, 88–9, 103
  of Martin Luther, 72
Applied Research Center, 3

Asian people
    insured status of, 26, 26 (table)
    poverty rate of, 22–3, 24 (table)
    uninsured/underinsured status of,
        21 (table), 22, 24 (table)
    in U.S. population, 21
Association of American Medical
    Colleges, 42, 192–3
asthma
    as health status indicator, 13, 29
    relative availability of care and, 2

Balsa, A. I., 44, 50
bankruptcy filings, from illness or
    injury, 25
Beef Stew
    awareness of assumptions,
        189–90
    bottom-line focus and, 162–3,
        256n19
    healthcare providers of color
        and, 192
    interplay of socioeconomic status
        and race, 150, 205–6,
        251n27, 252n32, 256–7n26
Bettenhausen, Elizabeth, 84
bias
    of IRB members, 105
    patient and family, 58–9
    provider, see provider bias
    types of (Wacquant), 93–4
biomedical ethics, see medical ethics
Black people
    affiliative feelings of physicians
        toward patients, 44–6, 47–8
    "Black" as term and, 106, 108–9,
        220n9
    insured status of, 26 (table), 26–7
    lack of Black healthcare providers,
        42–3
    objectification of, xxi
    poverty rate of, 22–3, 24 (table)
    quality-of-life ratings for, 46–7
    relative availability of mental
        healthcare, 2–3

relative death rates from cancer
    and heart disease, 2
relative health status of, 12
relative levels of medical care
    for, 2
schizophrenia diagnoses among,
    2–3, 48
stereotypes concerning, 46–7
Tuskegee Syphilis Study, 59, 89,
    103, 233n95
uninsured/underinsured rate of,
    20, 21, 21 (table), 22,
    24 (table)
in U.S. population, 21, 98–101
Womanism, xvii, 64, 76, 79–84,
    204–5, 208–9, 219n2
    see also Black women facing
        breast cancer
Black women facing breast cancer
    Andre, Sophia, 72, 125–6,
        137–45, 147, 151–2, 164–5,
        173, 176–7, 186–7, 197–8,
        199–200, 213–14
    Gavin, Sandra, 125, 127, 128–35,
        154–5, 158–9, 164–5, 178,
        179–80, 196
    giving voice to, xix
    Hernandez, Luz, 116–20, 127,
        146, 148, 152, 157, 175–6,
        180–2
    Jacobs, Hannah, 112–15, 147,
        148–9, 157–8, 178, 183,
        184–5, 196
    Kelly, Wanda, 115–16, 156,
        174–5, 177, 181–2, 191, 206,
        254n9, 256n18
    languages and voices of, 86–7
    mortality rate versus white
        women, 12–13
    Slimfat Girl, 123–5, 127, 145–6,
        147, 151, 157, 173, 174,
        180, 183
    survival rate versus white
        women, 12
    themes concerning, 126–65

Bloche, Greg, 13–14
Bobo, Lawrence, 3–4
Boo, Katherine, 195
Botswana, compliance with AIDS
    therapy in, 33
Bourdieu, Pierre, 92–4, 247n71
Boyd, Donald J., 32
breast cancer study
    methodology of, 98–101, 103–4,
        217–18
    themes emerging from, 126–65
    see also Black women facing
        breast cancer; collaborators
        (healthcare providers);
        Institutional Review Board
        (IRB)
breast cancer support groups, 173–5
Bredsen, Phil, 31
Bristol, Lucy
    bureaucracy of healthcare and,
        160
    interplay of socioeconomic status
        and race, 146–9, 151, 205–6,
        251n26–7
    patient advocacy and, 155–6
bureaucracy of healthcare systems,
    50–7, 143–4
    bottom-line focus and, 162–5
    impact of, 193–4
    perceptions of, 156–62
Burke, Jane, 44–6, 49, 58
Bush, George W., 25, 30, 31,
    32, 193

Cahill, Lisa, 8
Canada
    healthcare spending in, 51
    prescription drugs from, 198
cancer
    relative death rates from, 2
    screenings for, relative availability
        of, 2
    screenings for, uninsured/
        underinsured status and,
        20–1

see also Black women facing
        breast cancer; breast cancer
        study; Latina women facing
        breast cancer
Cancer Care, 195–6
Carrillo, Emilio, 51, 53
Centers for Disease Control and
    Prevention (CDC)
    infant mortality rates and, 52
    Office of Minority Health and
        Health Disparities, 12
    reports on health status, 12–13
China, infant mortality rate of, 52
cholesterol levels, uninsured/
    underinsured status and, 20
Christian theology and ethics,
    171–209
    bloody legacy of, 65, 66
    as collaborative venture, 9,
        212–13
    death and, 171–2
    within healthcare ethics, 7–10
    healthcare in U.S. and, 65–7
    healthcare quality and, 15–16
    insights of women facing cancer,
        172–8
    methodological implications for
        doing of ethics, 200–9
    patient expectations of healthcare
        providers, 178–85
    social ethics for healthcare
        systems, 185–200
    see also theological anthropology
class, see socioeconomic status (SES)
Clemetson, Lynette, 30–1
Clifton, Lucille, 171–2
Clinton, Bill, 198
Closing the Gap, 198–9
COBRA (Consolidated Omnibus
    Budget Reconciliation Act), 33,
    128–9, 130, 143, 228n50,
    250n21
collaborators (general)
    accountability and, 96–8
    "human subjects" versus, 89–92

collaborators—*continued*
  "informant-expressed needs" and,
    96–8
  purpose of research and, 96–8
collaborators (healthcare providers)
  Beef Stew, 150, 162–3, 189–90,
    192, 205–6, 251n27,
    252n32, 256n19, 256–7n26
  Bristol, Lucy, 146–9, 151, 155–6,
    160, 205–6, 251n26–7
  Morales, Antonia, 149–50, 160–2,
    179, 187–9, 251–2n29
  O'Brian, Kathleen, 163, 169
  Orlando, Leonard, 163–4, 165,
    166–8, 194, 198, 236–7
  Williams, Rebecca, 163, 165,
    168–9, 198, 252n34
collaborators (women facing
    breast cancer)
  Andre, Sophia, 72, 125–6,
    137–45, 147, 151–2, 164–5,
    173, 176–7, 186–7, 197–8,
    199–200, 213–14
  described, 98–101
  Gavin, Sandra, 125, 127, 128–35,
    154–5, 158–9, 164–5, 178,
    179–80, 196, 254n3
  Hernandez, Luz, 116–20, 127, 146,
    148, 152, 157, 175–6, 180–2
  insurance coverage of, 112
  introductions to, 112–26
  Jacobs, Hannah, 112–15, 147,
    148–9, 157–8, 178, 183,
    184–5, 196
  Kelly, Wanda, 115–16, 156,
    174–5, 177, 181–2, 191, 206,
    254n9, 256n18
  listening by researcher and, 101
  Maldonado, María de Lourdes, 27,
    116, 135–7, 152, 156, 176, 181
  Rodriguez, Marcela, 120–3, 127,
    137, 152–4, 156, 159–60,
    173–5, 178, 182–4
  self-identification of racial-ethnic
    background, 112

Slimfat Girl, 123–5, 127, 145–6,
    147, 151, 157, 173, 174,
    180, 183
  themes concerning, 126–65
community networks, 173–5,
    194–6
compassion, importance of,
    181–2
confidentiality
  IRBs and, 103
  translators and, 41
Consolidated Omnibus Budget
    Reconciliation Act (COBRA),
    33, 128–9, 130, 143, 228n50,
    250n21
contract employees,
    uninsured/underinsured status
    of, 25
Copeland, M. Shawn, 64, 79–84,
    204–5, 208–9
critical theory, 78, 81, 244n45
cultural competency
  importance of, 187–91
  social medicine and, 56–7

death
  disparities around, xviii, 2
  as inevitable part of living, 16
  infant mortality, 2, 13, 52
  kinds of, 171–2
  mortality rates, 2, 12–13
deductive reasoning, in quantitative
    studies, 85–7
dehumanization
  discrimination as, xvii, xviii
  of healthcare bureaucracy, 138
diabetes
  as health status indicator, 13
  uninsured/underinsured status
    and, 20
Diallo, Amadou, 89
dignity, 175–6
  of women facing cancer, 176–7
discrimination
  alienation and, xvii

against communities of color, 44
as dehumanization, xvii, xviii
legal prohibition of, 3–4
methods of, xvii
negative racial stereotyping and, 4
see also racism
diversity
empowering of the other and,
    76–9
Fulkerson, Mary McClintock and,
    76–9
of general population versus
    healthcare providers, 192
solidarity and, 204–5
doctors, *see* healthcare providers
double consciousness
concept of, xxi–xxii
of people of color, xxi–xxii
of white people, xxii
Dovidio, J. F., 48

Emergency Medical Treatment and
    Labor Act (EMTALA), 30, 32
emergency rooms
Hispanic people and, 39
on-call coverage by physicians, 30
requirements to treat emergency
    cases, 30
uninsured/underinsured status
    and, 20
empathy
defining, 184
importance of, 54, 179–80
medical gaze and, 45–6
entitlement, attitude of, 205–6
environmental racism, 29, 227n37
ethics, *see* Christian theology and
    ethics; medical ethics
Ethnographic Interview, The
    (Spradley), 201–2
ethnography, 84–109
advantages of using, 100
ethic of white listening and, 87–98
fieldwork overview for study,
    98–101

IRB approval process in, 102–9
learning objectives of fieldwork, 6
methodology for study, 5–7,
    14–15, 98–101, 103–4,
    217–18
qualitative versus quantitative
    methodologies and, 85–7
themes of, 102–3
thick description in, 64, 108,
    249n90
value of acknowledged ignorance
    and, 201–3
see also listening; qualitative
    research
eugenics, 72, 88–9, 103
Evans, John, 7

Fadiman, Anne, 37
Farley, Margaret, 8, 208
Federal Employee's Group Health
    Insurance Program, 164
follow-up, racial-ethnic disparities
    in, 36
Fulkerson, Mary McClintock, 76–9
diversity and, 77
limitations of, 77–9
Fullilove, Mindy, 88, 91, 100,
    102, 185

Gavin, Sandra, 128–35
bottom-line focus and, 164–5
bureaucracy of healthcare and,
    158–9
continuity and choice of health
    care, 196
described, 125, 127, 254n3
expectations of healthcare
    providers, 178, 179–80
first doctor/hospital and, 128–30
patient advocacy and, 154–5
second doctor/hospital and, 130–3
third doctor/hospital and, 133–5
Gebara, Ivone, 67, 83–4, 215
Geiger, H. Jack, 57–8
Gilda's Club, 195–6

Good, Byron J., 55–7, 190, 193
Good, Mary-Jo DelVecchio, 55–7, 190, 193
Gore, Al, 198
gratitude, of women facing cancer, 172–8, 183

Harrison, Beverly, 73–4, 75
Harvard University, survey on quality of healthcare, 158
Hawaiian or Pacific Islander people, in U.S. population, 21
healthcare ethics, *see* medical ethics
healthcare in U.S.
    bureaucracy of, 50–7, 143–4, 156–62, 193–4
    as commodity, 59
    institutional context of, 99
    lack of universal coverage and, 59–60, 198
    as microcosm of society, 47–8
    objectification of human life and, xvii, xxi
    racial-ethnic disparities in, 4, 56–7
    reporting on, nature of, 17–18
    social ethics for, *see* medical ethics
    spending on, 50–2
    theological and ethical norms concerning, 66–7
    see also access to healthcare; healthcare providers; healthcare quality; health insurance; health status; hospitals
healthcare providers
    affiliative feelings toward patients, 44–6, 47–8, 58
    changing, by women in study, 128–37
    as collaborators in study, *see* collaborators (healthcare providers)
    compassion of, 181–2
    continuity and choice of, 196–200
    educating to see their own assumptions, 187–91
    empathy of, 45–6, 54, 179–80
    health testing by, 182–3
    honesty of, 180–1
    interplay of socioeconomic status and race, 146–51
    language issues and, 37–40, 41, 100–1
    listening by, 111–12, 178–81
    patient advocacy and, xviii, 54–5, 144–5, 154–6, 193–4
    patient expectations for, 43–4, 178–5, 195–6
    as people of color, 42–3, 54–5, 146–9, 191–3
    power dynamics between patients and, 3, 141–3, 151–4, 186–93
    stereotypes of, 48–9, 58, 150
    see also provider bias
healthcare quality
    access to healthcare and, 28–35
    barriers to, 27–8
    Christian theology and, 15–16
    disparities in U.S., 18, 57–62, 214
    health status versus, 11–14
    infant mortality rate and, 52
    language impact on, 37–40
    studies of, 1–2
    survey on perceptions of, 158
    variations across U.S., 52–3
health insurance
    appeal of denial of coverage, 54–5
    as basic healthcare commodity, 19–20
    bureaucracy\fee issues and, 143–4
    catastrophic coverage, 23
    Consolidated Omnibus Budget Reconciliation Act (COBRA), 33, 128–9, 130, 143, 228n50, 250n21
    crisis in, 19–20
    Federal Employee's Group Health Insurance Program, 164

private insurance as standard
for, 27
provider bias and, 44
see also Medicaid; Medicare;
uninsured/underinsured
status
health status
healthcare quality versus, 11–14
indicators of, 13
nature of, 11–12
racial-economic disparities in,
13–14, 223n27
research on disparities in,
11–13
socioeconomic status and, 13
of women of color, 12–13
Healthy People 2010, 60–1
heart disease
affiliative feelings of physicians
toward patients, 44–6,
47–8
discrimination against people of
color and, 44–6
as health status indicator, 13
relative death rates from, 2
relative quality of medical care
for, 2
Henry J. Kaiser Family Foundation,
2, 12, 158
Hernandez, Luz, 127
bureaucracy of healthcare
and, 157
described, 116–20
expectations of healthcare
providers, 180–2
individual agency and, 175–6
interplay of socioeconomic status
and race, 146, 148
power dynamic between patient
and healthcare providers, 152
Heyward, Carter, 74, 75, 80, 207
Hippocratic Oath, 43
Hispanic people, see Latina
women facing breast cancer;
Latinos/as

HIV-AIDS care
African compliance with AIDS
therapy, 33–4, 228n55
relative availability of, 2
Holocaust, 72, 88–9, 103
honesty, importance of, 180–1
hospitals
as diverse gatherings of people,
65–6
evolution of, 65–6
religious roots of, 66
requirements to treat emergency
cases, 20, 30, 39
respect for persons and, 191
see also emergency rooms
humility
ethnography and, 201–3
healthcare and, 67–8
importance of, xxiii
of women facing cancer, 176
hypertension, uninsured/
underinsured status and, 20

immigrants, expectations of
healthcare providers, 195–6
Indigenous people
objectification of, xxi
in U.S. population, 21
inductive reasoning
advantages of using, 88–9
listening in qualitative studies and,
87–9
in qualitative studies, 85–7
infant mortality
comparative rates of, 52
as health status indicator, 13
relative levels of, 2
informed consent, 91, 103, 143
Institute of Medicine (IOM), 1–2
research findings concerning
healthcare inequalities, 35–7,
44, 48, 53, 55, 58
Institutional Review Board (IRB), 11
accountability and, 94–5
approval process, 104–9

Institutional Review
    Board—*continued*
  autonomy of, 103
  bureaucracy and, 105
  informed consent and, 91, 103, 143
  membership demographics of,
      103–4
  origins of, 103
  qualitative versus quantitative
      approaches and, 103, 108–9
  review process, 100
  role of, 103
insurance, *see* health insurance
intellectualist bias, 93–4
interdependent relationship, 74, 80,
    207–9
interviews, *see* listening
Iraq, military spending in, 32–3
IRB, *see* Institutional Review
    Board (IRB)

Jacobs, Hannah
  bureaucracy of healthcare and,
      157–8
  continuity and choice of health
      care, 196
  described, 112–15
  expectations of healthcare
      providers, 178, 183, 184–5
  gratitude of, 183
  interplay of socioeconomic status
      and race, 147, 148–9
Jim Crow racism, 4
Johnson, Carol, 33
Jones, Serene, 244n45
justice
  love as expression of, 9
  minimalist notion of, 9

Kaiser Family Foundation, 2, 12, 158
Kaiser Women's Health Survey, 20
Kelly, Wanda
  cultural competency and, 191
  described, 115–16, 254n9
  dignity and, 177

expectations of healthcare
    providers, 181–2, 206,
    256n18
  gratitude of, 174–5
  patient advocacy and, 156
kidney transplants, affiliative
    feelings of physicians toward
    patients, 47–8
King, Martin Luther, Jr., 216
Kristof, Nicholas, 52

language issues, 37–3
  academic community and, 202
  challenges for non-English
      speakers, 53
  impact on quality of health care,
      37–40, 41, 100–1
  IRB perceptions of, 108–9
  lack of cultural understanding
      and, 41–3
  professional translators and, 38,
      39–40
  volunteer/ad hoc translators and,
      40–1
  women in study and, 86–7,
      136–7
Latina women facing breast cancer
  giving voice to, xix
  languages and voices of, 86–7, 136–7
  Maldonado, María de Lourdes,
      27, 116, 135–7, 152, 156,
      176, 181
  Rodriguez, Marcela, 120–3, 127,
      137, 152–4, 156, 159–60,
      173–5, 178, 182–4
  themes concerning, 126–65
Latinos/as
  barriers to health insurance,
      230n65
  insured status of, 26 (table),
      26–7
  lack of cultural understanding
      and, 41–3
  lack of Hispanic healthcare
      providers, 42–3

language barriers faced by, 37–43
Mujerista, 219n2
as non-homogenous population, 229n62
poverty rate of, 22–3, 24 (table)
relative availability of mental healthcare, 2–3
relative health status of, 12
relative levels of medical care for, 2
as term, 220n9
underrepresentation in policy research, 37–8
undocumented status and, 38
uninsured/underinsured rate of, 20, 21 (table), 21–2, 24 (table)
in U.S. population, 21, 37–8, 98–101
see also Latina women facing breast cancer
Lebacqz, Karen, 8
liberation theology, 79–84, 93
life expectancy
for Blacks versus whites, 12
as health status indicator, 13
listening, 87–98, 111–70
concerns of research collaborators and, 101
in ethnography, 100, 214
of healthcare providers, importance of, 111–12, 178–81
inductive learning through, 87–9
introductions to collaborators/women facing breast cancer, 112–26
language issues and, 100–1
to women facing breast cancer, 111–12
Lorde, Audre, 1, 63–4
Lourdes Maldonado, María de, 135–7
balance among humility, respect, and consideration for others, 176
described, 116

expectations of healthcare providers, 181
first doctor/hospital and, 135–6
gratitude and, 176
insurance coverage of, 27
patient advocacy and, 156
power dynamic between patient and healthcare providers, 152
second doctor/hospital and, 136–7
love
concrete expression of, 215–16
as expression of justice, 9
God and, 69–70, 174–5
neighbor-love, 83–4, 207
in white feminist anthropology, 83–4
Lu, Francis, 3
Luther, Martin, 64, 68–73
limitations of, 72–3, 78, 241–2n25
moral anthropology and, 68–9
Ten Commandments and, 70–2
views of God, 68–70

McGuire, T. G., 44, 50
McNeil, Donald, 33
Medicaid
costs of translator services and, 39–40
escalating costs of, 59
extent of health coverage under, 24–5, 197, 227n34
lack of universal coverage and, 59–60
limits of health coverage under, 24–5, 31–2
logistical and locational challenges for participants, 53–4
qualifying for, 31–2
recent changes in, 19, 31–2
reimbursement rates under, 28–9
shift to reliance on, 25–6
state role in designing, 25, 31–2

medical ethics, 185–200
    challenges to, 107, 211–12
    as collaborative venture with
        Christian theology, 9, 212–13
    healthcare quality disparities
        and, 18
    informed consent, 91, 103, 143
    Martin Luther and, 72–3
    methodological implications of,
        200–9
    nature of, 15
    norms for healthcare, 66–7
    task of social and medical
        ethicists, 61
    as term, 222n18
    theology in, 7–10, 72–3
medical gaze
    affiliative feelings of physician
        toward patient, 44–6, 47–8
    culture of medicine and, 55–7
    impact of, 193
    nature of, 43
    objectivity and, 5–6, 50
medical insurance, see health
    insurance
medical sociology, studies of relative
    quality of care, 1–2
medical students
    racial bias of, 46–8
    sexual bias of, 46–8
    see also healthcare providers
Medicare
    costs of translator services and,
        39–40
    decline in funding, 169
    escalating costs of, 59
    extent of health coverage under,
        24–5, 197
    limits of health coverage under,
        24–5
    logistical and locational challenges
        for participants, 53–4
    racial-ethnic disparities in,
        36, 54
    shift to reliance on, 25–6

mental healthcare
    affiliative feelings of physicians
        toward patients, 47–8
    relative availability of, 2–3
military spending, 32–3
Moe-Lobeda, Cynthia, 71–2,
    78, 204
Molina, Carlos, 60–1
Moraga, Cherrie, 63
Morales, Antonia
    awareness of assumptions, 187–9
    bureaucracy of healthcare and,
        160–2, 251–2n29
    interplay of socioeconomic status
        and race, 149–50
    patient expectations of healthcare
        providers, 179
moral principles, 7
mortality rates
    research on, 2
    of women facing breast cancer,
        12–13
Morton, Neil, xxii
Moses, Robert, 29, 227n37
Mujerista, defined, 219n2

National Center for Health
    Statistics, 12–13
Native American people, in U.S.
    population, 21
neutrality, in qualitative research,
    5–6
Northwest Federation of
    Community Organizations, 3
nurses, see healthcare providers

obesity, as health status indicator, 13
objectification, of human life,
    xvii, xxi
objectivity
    guise of, 50
    in qualitative research, 5–6
O'Brian, Kathleen
    bottom-line focus and, 163
    helping others and, 169

on-call coverage, 30
Organization for Economic
    Cooperating and Development
    (OECD), 51–2
Orlando, Leonard
    bottom-line focus and, 163–4,
        165, 194, 198
    ethnic identity of, 236–7n132
    listening and, 166–8

pain management
    language barriers and, 41–3
    relative availability of, 2
part-time employees,
    uninsured/underinsured status
    of, 25
paternalism, of white people, xxi
patient advocacy
    by community networks, 194–6
    by physicians, xviii, 54–5, 144–5,
        154–6, 193–4
Pear, Robert, 30, 31
people of color
    double consciousness and,
        xxi–xxii
    health status of, 12–13
    as healthcare providers, 42–3,
        54–5, 146–9, 191–3
    medical community discrimination
        against, 44
    studies of relative quality of
        medical care, 1–2
    uninsured/underinsured status of,
        19–22, 21 (table), 24 (table)
    see also Asian people; Black
        people; Black women facing
        breast cancer; Indigenous
        people; Latina women facing
        breast cancer; Latinos/as
physicians, see healthcare providers
poverty rate
    extent of, 30–1
    increase in, 22–3
    Medicaid coverage and, 24
    "officially poor" and, 23

racial differences in, 22–3, 24
    (table)
Powell, Annie Ruth, xviii–xx,
    xxii, 202
power dynamics
    in collaborator-researcher
        relationship, 90–1
    in healthcare, 3, 141–3, 151–4,
        186–93
    inductive reasoning and, 88–9
    IRB approval process and,
        108–9
    white feminist theology and, 80
praxis (concrete involvement),
    79–80
prenatal care, studies of relative
    quality of, 2
prescription drug coverage, 198
privacy
    IRBs and, 103
    translators and, 41
provider bias
    affiliative feelings of physicians
        toward patients, 44–6,
        47–8
    impact on lives of people, 33–4
    in medical diagnosis, 2–3
    insurance status and, 44
    medical enculturation and, 43–50
    of medical students, 46–8
    racial, 13–14
    socioeconomic status (SES) and,
        13–14, 44
psychiatric treatment
    affiliative feelings of physicians
        toward patients, 47–8
    relative availability of, 2–3
public clinics,
    uninsured/underinsured status
    and, 20

qualitative research
    accountability and, 92–8
    "collaborators" versus "human
        subjects" in, 89–92

qualitative research—*continued*
  comparison with challenges of
      women of color facing
      cancer, 109
  decentering of authority in, 90
  distinctiveness of methods of, 88
  as "feel-forward research"
      (Fullilove), 88
  inductive reasoning in, 85–7
  IRB and, 103–9
  methodology of ethnographic
      studies, 5–7, 14–15, 98–101,
      103–4, 217–18
  perception problems and, 211
  qualitative methods writing group
      and, 99–100
  quantitative research versus, 103–9
  reflexivity and, 92–4
  researcher role in, 86
  sample size and, 86
  themes of, 102–3, 126–65
  see also ethnography; listening
quality of healthcare, *see* healthcare
      quality
quantitative research
  deductive reasoning in, 85–7
  IRB and, 103–9
  qualitative research versus, 103–9

racial-ethnic inequalities, 3
  interplay of socioeconomic status
      and, 138–41, 145–51,
      186–93, 205–6, 251n26–7
  poverty and, 22–3, 24 (table)
racism
  contemporary manifestations of,
      88–9
  environmental, 29, 227n37
  eugenics and, 72, 88–9, 103
  Holocaust and, 72, 88–9, 103
  Jim Crow, 4
  stereotypes concerning healthcare,
      4, 33–4
  systemic, 98
  Tuskegee Syphilis Study, 59, 89,
      103, 233n95

white privilege and, xxii–xxiii,
      90–2, 169–70, 202–3,
      205–6
  see also discrimination;
      stereotypes
Rathore, Saif, 46
referrals
  for collaborators in study, 106
  by physicians of color, 55
  racial-ethnic disparities in, 36
reflexivity, 6–7, 79–80
  of Bourdieu, 92–4, 247n71
  self-critique and, 94, 205–6
  white entitlement syndrome and,
      205–6
respect for others, 54, 176
  concrete expression of, 215–16
  persons and difference, 208
  of women facing cancer, 176–8
Rodriguez, Marcela, 127, 137
  bureaucracy of healthcare and,
      156, 159–60
  described, 120–3
  dignity and, 175, 178
  expectations of healthcare
      providers, 182–4
  gratitude of, 173–5
  power dynamic between patient
      and healthcare providers,
      152–4

Satcher, David, 2
schizophrenia, differential diagnosis
      of, 2–3, 48
Schoen, Cathy, 23
school integration, 3–4
Senegal, compliance with AIDS
      therapy in, 33
Share, 195–6
Slimfat Girl, 127
  bureaucracy of healthcare
      and, 157
  described, 123–5
  expectations of healthcare
      providers, 180, 183
  gratitude of, 173, 174

interplay of socioeconomic status
    and race, 145–6, 147
power dynamic between patient
    and healthcare providers, 151
Smith, Michael, 3
social medicine, cultural competency
    and, 56–7
socioeconomic status (SES)
    access to healthcare and, 28–35
    affiliative feelings of physicians
        toward patients and, 44–6,
        47–8
    assumptions concerning, 186–93
    health status and, 13
    interplay of race and, 138–41,
        145–51, 186–93, 205–6,
        251n26–7
    poverty rate increase and, 22–3
    women facing breast cancer
        and, 126
solidarity, 203–6
    defined, 204
    recognition of others in, 204–6
South Africa, compliance with AIDS
    therapy in, 33, 228n55
Spradley, James, 87–8, 89, 96–7,
    201–2
stereotypes
    Black people and, 46–7
    clinical uncertainty and, 50
    cognitive shortcuts and, 49
    of emotional volatility, 138–9, 141
    of healthcare providers, 48–9,
        58, 150
    racism and, 4, 33–4
    as self-perpetuating, 48–9
Stoll, Kathleen, 19
storytelling, white feminist theology
    and, 77
Sullivan Commission on Diversity in
    the Workforce, 42, 192
systemic racism, 98

theological anthropology, 64–84
    of M. Shawn Copeland, 64,
        79–84

in healthcare forums, 65
of Martin Luther, 64, 68–73
as moral anthropology, 68–9, 75
nature of, 64–8
of twentieth-century white
    feminists, 73–9
see also Christian theology and
    ethics
theology, see Christian theology
    and ethics; theological
    anthropology
thick description, in ethnography,
    64, 108, 249n90
Thompson, Tommy G., 57
Tillich, Paul, 10
Townes, Emilie M., xvii, 8, 184,
    257n28
translation services
    professional translators and, 38,
        39–40
    quality of, 230n72
    volunteer/ad hoc translators and,
        40–1
trust, importance of, 184–5
Tuskegee Syphilis Study, 59, 89, 103,
    233n95

Uganda, compliance with AIDS
    therapy in, 33
uninsured/underinsured status
    defined, 18, 19
    delay in seeking healthcare and,
        20–1
    democratic principles and, 59–60
    escalating costs of, 59
    growth in population with, 18,
        25–6, 224n4, 225–6n12–13
    impact on healthcare, 195–7
    importance of human labor
        and, 59
    insurance crisis and, 19–20
    number of people with, 18–19,
        21 (table), 21–2,
        24 (table), 27
    "officially uninsured" and, 23
    underinsured and, 23

United States Agency for
    International Development
    (USAID), 33
U.S. Census
    composition of population, 21–3,
        21 (table)
    poverty rate, 31
    statistics on uninsured, 18–19
U.S. Department of Health and
    Human Services (DHHS)
    Agency for Healthcare Research
        and Quality (AHRQ) report
        and, 57–8
    Healthy People 2010, 60–1
    reports on health status, 12–13
Universal Declaration of Human
    Rights, 215
universal healthcare, 59–60, 198

van Ryn, Michelle, 44–6, 47–9, 58
Verhey, Allen, 7, 15
Veteran's Administration,
    differential diagnosis of
    schizophrenia, 2–3
vulnerable populations, defined,
    222n16

Wacquant, Loic, 93
white feminist theology, 73–9
    critical theory and, 78, 81,
        244n45
    differences in humanity and,
        80–1
    embodiment and, 74–6, 83
    feminists of color versus,
        239n8
    of Fulkerson, Mary McClintock,
        76–9
    interdependent relationship and,
        74, 75, 80, 207–9
    limitations of, 77–9, 80–1,
        83–4
    mutuality and, 74–7
    sensuality and, 74

white non-Hispanic people
    accountability of, xxii, 81
    attitudes toward affirmative
        action policies, 4
    attitudes toward school
        integration, 3–4
    comparative breast cancer
        mortality rates, 12
    comparative breast cancer survival
        rates, 12
    double consciousness of, xxii
    insured status of, 26, 26 (table)
    listening and, xx
    objectification of Black and
        Indigenous people, xxi
    paternalism and, xxi
    poverty rate of, 22–3, 24 (table)
    racism and white privilege of,
        xxii–xxiii, 90–2, 169–70,
        202–3, 205–6
    socialization into leadership roles,
        220n11
    uninsured/underinsured status of,
        21 (table), 22, 24 (table)
    in U.S. population, 21
    white consciousness and, xxii–xxiii
    see also white feminist theology
Williams, David, 2
Williams, Rebecca
    bottom-line focus and,
        163, 198
    racial-ethnic disparities and, 165,
        168–9, 252n34
Witness Project of Harlem, 195–6
Womanism, xvii, 76
    M. Shawn Copeland and, 64,
        79–84, 204–5, 208–9
    defined, 219n2
World Health Organization (WHO),
    51–2

Zambrana, Ruth Enid, 60–1
Zeber, John, 3
Zoloth, Laurie, 212